DISEASE AND ITS IMPACT
ON MODERN EUROPEAN HISTORY

Vincent J. Knapp

Studies in Health & Human Services
Volume 10

The Edwin Mellen Press
Lewiston/Queenston/Lampeter

Library of Congress Cataloging-in-Publication Data

Knapp, Vincent J., 1934-
  Disease and its impact on modern European history / Vincent J.
Knapp.
    p. cm. -- (Studies in health and human services ; v. 10)
  Includes index.
  ISBN 0-88946-135-X
  1. Communicable diseases--Europe--History. 2. Diseases and
history--Europe. 3. Social medicine--Europe--History. I. Title.
II. Series.
  RA643.7.E85K58 1989
  614.4' 24--dc19
                          88-13946
                        CIP

> This is volume 10 in the continuing series
> Studies in Health & Human Services
> Volume 10 ISBN 0-88946-135-X
> SHHS Series ISBN 0-88946-126-0

A CIP catalog record for this book
is available from the British Library.

The Edwin Mellen Press   The Edwin Mellen Press
Box 450   Box 67
Lewiston, NY   Queenston, Ontario
USA 14092   CANADA L0S 1L0

The Edwin Mellen Press, Ltd.
Lampeter, Dyfed, Wales,
UNITED KINGDOM SA48 7DY

Printed in the United States of America

To -- Janice, Derek, Colin and Kyle

TABLE OF CONTENTS

ACKNOWLEDGEMENTS

Years ago, when I first became intensely interested in doing a topic that meant combining both history and biology, I realized that I would have to engage in a great deal of both study and research. This project really began when a number of my colleagues in biology and chemistry allowed me into their courses and generously shared their knowledge with someone who was a trained historian, not only inside, but also outside of the classroom. To each of them, Professors Pei-Show Juo, Bruce Campbell, Charles Foster, Elizabeth Isenberg and William Peebles, all of the State University of New York, I owe a very special thank you.

I owe a similar debt to a number of other scientists who helped to enhance my knowledge of biology, chemistry and the way in which diseases attack human beings. In particular, I want to express my sincere gratitude here to Dr. Bruce Dracott of the Pathology Department at Cambridge University and to Dr. Leonard Poulter, formerly of the London College of Surgeons, and later associated with the Trudeau Institute for Immunobiological Research. It was truly a marvelous experience being able to test out some of my hypotheses about diseases on both of these extraordinarily helpful individuals.

My stay at the World Health Organization in Geneva was one of the highlights of this project. Once again, I was met with both warmth and generosity from the scientific community. Here I had an opportunity to work and talk with three men, each of whom measurably advanced my knowledge of the ways in which diseases operate. To each of them, Dr. Branko Cvjetanovic, Dr. Joel Breman and Dr. Andrew Arata, I can only express my thanks for the very magnanimous way in which they shared their knowledge of cholera, smallpox, and plague with me.

As it turned out, working with certain librarians, who found much of the material that I needed for this study, was just as great an experience as studying with the scientific community. My first debt of gratitude here goes to Mrs. Eleanor Vorse of the State University of New York, who never wavered in her efforts on my behalf and who was so instrumental in securing secondary sources for me. The primary sources that I have included in this study were gathered at three Bio-Medical Libraries in Europe. They were: the Wellcome Institute for the History of Medicine Library and the Royal Society of Medicine Library, both in London, along with the Library of the World Health Organization. In these three locations, I was aided by four librarians, Mr. Eric Freeman of the Wellcome Institute, Mr. David Stewart, of the Royal Society, and Mrs. Helen Rhee and Mrs. Erica Campanella-Sigerist of the WHO library. Each of them significantly helped to reduce the burden of searching out and finding some of the rare historical materials that I have included in this particular study.

I did the research for this book while I was on sabbatical leave at Cambridge University. There I was associated with the Cambridge Group for the History of Population and Social Structure, which was then directed by Professor Peter Laslett. Personally, it was a very rewarding experience to be associated with the Group and to be in an environment where novel approaches to history were constantly being explored.

I was also pleased to have my family with me in Europe while I was doing this project. The presence of my wife, Jan, and my three sons helped me to keep in touch with this world while I was simultaneously examining the rather unhappy world of those who had come before us.

INTRODUCTION

We still know far too little about the killing diseases . . . and their effect on the course of history. It is amazing how historians manage to ignore the subjects of hunger and disease altogether, yet they were the fundamental facts of life for most people until almost within living memory.

--W. G. Hoskins, "Epidemics in English History," The Listener, December, 1964, 1044.

The famous English historian Thomas B. Macauley called them the ministers of death. He was referring to the great deadly and disabling diseases that dominated everyday life in Europe from the 14th to the 20th centuries. Specifically, those diseases were plague, syphilis, smallpox, typhus, cholera, tuberculosis and influenza. All of these diseases were endemic to Europe at one time or another. Each was also an epidemic disorder, announcing its presence often either by disfiguring or destroying large numbers of Europeans in a short period of time. The first half of this essay will focus on those chronological moments when each of these diseases was at its height. Sometimes, as in the case of smallpox and tuberculosis these diseases gained sway slowly, growing more harmful over the course of either generations or centuries. In other instances, the diseases involved arrived in a truly spectacular manner. The Black Death which unceremoniously took the lives of nearly a quarter of the European population from 1347 to 1351 was just such a moment, so also was the disturbing arrival of malignant syphilis in the 1490s as well as the great cholera epidemics of the 19th century, particularly the first one.

Of all the diseases that would harass the European continent during these centuries none was more spectacular than plague. Plague, in its highly virulent pneumonic form, first penetrated Italy in 1347, spreading northward from there. No catastrophe down to the Second World War was as devastating to Europe as this one single experience. This disaster was followed by a series of other epidemics, in western Europe down to the 17th century and in eastern Europe until the 1770s. While obviously spectacular in its epidemic form, plague was just as distressing when it operated endemically. For long centuries, London barely knew a year when the disease was not present. Moreover, the bacteria responsible for plague was usually a rapid killer, apparently healthy individuals dying from this disorder in a matter of hours. In this sense, plague was very much like syphilis, another disease that produced a fairly high mortality but, in the case of syphilis, only during its early history.

The evidence that an extremely malignant form of syphilis entered Europe in the 1490s is really rather overwhelming. A milder form of the disease may have been known to an earlier period, but the kind of syphilis threatening Europe in this key decade was obviously quite severe. From the 1490s to the 1550s, this ugly disease spread steadily to the various corners of Europe before finally abating. By the end of that period, the disease had grown considerably tamer. After this, right into the 20th century, syphilis operated more subterraneously. Its actual presence was often difficult to detect, largely because its symptoms tended to fade and ostensibly, at least, it took very few lives. It was still present, however, passed on innocently to infants or picked up promiscuously by young adults. By the 19th century, hospital records, just beginning to be meticulously kept, would finally prove just how ubiquitous this disease actually was.

Yet another disease that disabled far more people than it managed to kill was smallpox. All told, some 60 million Europeans probably died from this disease, while in all likelihood hundreds of millions had it at one time or another. Smallpox has been justly regarded as the most universal of all the European diseases. This had not always been the case. For smallpox did not come to the continent all that suddenly. It developed slowly within European society, in a very evolutionary fashion. True, smallpox was known to the Middle Ages, but the full peak of its impact did not come until the 18th century. Characteristically, smallpox struck every country in Europe and, as far as can be reasonably estimated, all classes. But unlike plague, smallpox was not stopped by a loss of infectivity, but intriguingly by human effort. Vaccination, first developed by Edward Jenner, definitely overpowered this disease during the 19th century, bringing to an end its previously escalating affect upon the European population.

From a purely biological point of view there is little reason for linking typhus and cholera. The first is caused by a rickettsia, the second by a bacteria. Still, historically, the two diseases were quite commonly the result of the same social circumstances. Almost inevitably, dirty and squalid conditions were principally responsible for proliferating cases of both diseases. Typhus existed in Europe long before cholera came crashing into the continent in the early 1830s. Typhus was first recognized as a separate disorder when it broke out among Spanish troops besieging the Arab stronghold of Granada in 1489 and 1490. Ever after this, the development of this particular disease seemed to be tied to the existence of military squalor. Meanwhile, unsanitary living conditions, prevalent in the cities of Europe, kept encouraging the further spread of both typhus and cholera. Finally, improved sanitation along with the perfection of vaccines would by the early 20th century help to reduce these two notorious diseases to insignificance.

At the every moment in European history when typhus and cholera were on the decline, tuberculosis was beginning to rage out of control.

This subtle killer was by the latter decades of the 19th century reaching truly epidemic proportions, although it was rarely listed as an epidemic disorder. By the early 1900s, three million Europeans were annually dying from tuberculosis. Robert Koch, the man who ultimately discovered the microorganism responsible for tuberculosis, sadly recorded in the 1880s that one out of every three adults was now succumbing to one or another of the various forms of this disease. The history of this lingering disease goes back to ancient times, but it was not a widespread disorder in Europe until the early part of the 18th century. Beginning in that century, tuberculosis was clearly taking on menacing proportions, soon to become the most prevalent cause of death for the next two hundred years. For an extended period of time, tuberculosis was thought by the medical profession to be incurable, but then that is how most Europeans fatalistically regarded most of the diseases that they had to confront in the period before the coming of Industrial Revolution.

Influenza, the last of the seven deadly diseases that will be analyzed in the first part of this essay, is best remembered by 20th-century audiences as "the Spanish lady" of 1918-1919, a disease that came trailing into Europe right at the end of the First World War. The Spanish flu of those two years ultimately claimed two million lives, adding to the already heavy tolls incurred during four years of fighting. Apart from typhus, which was exceedingly difficult to identify medically over the course of time, influenza was perhaps the least perceived of all the diseases under discussion here. Often disguised, influenza was known to different countries and various ages by such highly distinctive names as "the English sweat" and "the Trousse-Galants." In spite of the fact that this disease was recognized only regionally, its symptoms were remarkably similar from one time to another. Primarily a disabling disease, influenza like all the other infectious disorders locked into European history could produce truly murderous epidemics.

Morbidity and mortality will, of necessity, be discussed at some length in this study. This essay will likewise take a look at the chronological history of these diseases, their etiology, their major focal points and their geographic range. This work will also try to trace, at least in outline, the natural history of these diseases, suggesting those historic moments when certain diseases mutated, sometimes surprisingly, in the direction of either greater mildness or, as it happened, greater virulence. The second half of this essay will go on to assess both the social and the psychological impact of these diseases. In the centuries-long struggle between the parasites, causing these diseases, and their human hosts, man was too often the loser. True, both government authorities and the medical profession desperately tried to fight back, but they largely failed. In the centuries before the 1850s, the microbes involved here really had the advantage, progressively determining the fate of armies, monarchies, cities, family-life and, as it turned out, even life-expectancy itself.

The long history of constantly recurring diseases from the Black Death of the 1340s to the Spanish flu of the late 1910s obviously affected popular attitudes. As far as can be determined from relatively sparse pieces of information, the mass of Europeans grew fatalistic in the face of so much suffering and adversity. Throughout this era, most intellectual observers simply explained away the presence of disease as the result of either divine, astrological or miasmatic influences. Either way, the actual cause of disease remained an ongoing mystery, quite beyond human understanding. In this era dominated by customary beliefs, the medical profession was one of the few agencies dedicated to the containment of disease. Part of their effort included a rather heavy dependence, at certain critical moments, on the use of drugs. Unfortunately, physicians in the past rarely used the right ones. In spite of its toxicity, mercury, for example, was repeatedly used as an unfailing cure for syphilis. Moreover, it took the medical profession nearly two hundred years to learn the appropriate way to use digitalis. Only during the 20th century were drugs and chemotherapy finally used in an effective way to help bring about the conquest of infectious disease.

Medical opinion in Europe's historic past, whether it involved the administration of drugs or the search for etiology was, from the point of view of a modern audience, often ridiculously faulty. The problem to a large extent was distinctly conceptual. Prevailing medical thought from the time of Hippocrates and Galen until far into the 19th century kept overconcentrating medical perceptions on the air. Throughout this era, it was unfailingly assumed that corrupt, or foul, air was the devastating cause of all sorts of diseases. It was only when this miasmatic view on the origins of disease came falling apart in the 19th century that the more realistic microscopic explanation for the presence of disease finally had a chance to emerge. The two names most closely associated with this new and more daring way of thinking were, of course, Louis Pasteur and Robert Koch. They are usually identified as the pioneers of this new age, now so dependent upon microbiological thinking. What can not be forgotten, however, is that microbiological thinking was not the exclusive monopoly of Pasteur and Koch. In a rudimentary form from the Italian Fracastoro to the German von Asch, certain doctors, with tremendous intellectual efforts and going against the dominant intellectual views of their own age, had, indeed, perceived the key to all modern medical thinking.

If doctors were continually struggling to separate mystery from truth, they were not the only ones seeking to combat disease. Governments were also actively involved. The classic techniques that they used were first isolation and then quarantine. A few decades after the Black Death subsided, both Venice and Dubrovnik established quarantine stations at the head of the Adriatic. These institutions were only partially effective. Later on, the Italian city-states went even further creating public health boards as part of their never-ending battle to limit the impact of one or another of these infectious diseases. Even the army, the strongest expression of the growing political absolutism of the day, was regularly involved. Austrian troops were constantly patrolling the Turkish border, seeking to prevent spreading epidemics from reaching the empire's population centers. Their quarantine stations were a marvel of efficiency, but they were only momentarily effective when it came to stopping the advance of disease. Governments helped much more in the 19th and 20th centuries when they began advocating vaccination and other public health measures that significantly reduced the incidences of smallpox, typhus and tuberculosis.

The ultimate decline of infectious diseases in the 19th century, the combined result of medical and governmental action, gave an immediate impetus to population growth. Between 1800 and 1900, the population of Europe leaped from 189 million to over 400 million. By this time, Europe was obviously no longer paying the demographic price it had been for infectious diseases. For nearly five hundred years prior to this pivotal century, harmful pathogens had been dampening down Europe's population growth. Each disease had taken its own toll. Smallpox, by way of illustration, was primarily a disease of childhood that in its milder form only scarred. But in its malignant form it could easily take the lives of up to 20 percent of the young in a given geographic area. Tuberculosis and typhus were, by contrast, conspicuously diseases of young adults. When these two disorders killed, they, of course, had an immediate effect on fertility, taking many who had been recently married. Inevitably, disease had other dire demographic consequences, either tearing families apart, or in the case of truly intense epidemics, causing whole families to disappear.

The historian of disease knows that millions of Europeans died from one or another of the great deadly and disabling diseases. It has been manifestly much more difficult to dig deeper and determine exactly what social classes and groups suffered the most. However, a vague pattern is beginning to emerge from a host of rather imprecise information. The poor do seem to have died more frequently and at an earlier age from the great bacterial killers, plague, syphilis, tuberculosis and cholera. Typhus, which is not a bacterial but a rickettsial disease, was likewise definitely rife among the downtrodden. What can be said with some assurance about bacterial disease is probably not true of smallpox and influenza, Europe's two outstanding viral disorders. Their sociological impact is difficult to determine, but then much less is known about viruses, evidently the very last category of microscopic agents that medical science has yet to vanquish.

While some of the major viral diseases ranging perhaps from cancer to the common cold are still prevalent in modern European society, the great historic diseases are, for the most part, gone. Names like plague, cholera and typhus provoke, at best, only distant memories of what had been in the past truly terrifying diseases. The vast majority of Europeans now alive probably have never seen even a mild case of plague, smallpox or tuberculosis. Yet it has been reasonably estimated that more than 600 million Europeans, over the centuries, died directly from one of these three diseases. Even influenza, which in 1889-1891 and 1918-1919 caused widespread mortality, is now viewed more as an inconvenience than a mortal threat. The diseases of the past have largely passed into our collective memory. Yet, in former decades, they were constantly on people's minds, shaping their lives in a way that a modern audience can only understand with a great deal of determined effort. The purpose of this study is to tell the story of how Europe's great historic diseases came and went.

PART ONE

THE DISEASES

> **It is hardly too much to say that infectious disease has now ceased to have any serious social significance in the advanced countries of the world.**
>
> **--MacFarlane Burnet, <u>Natural History of Infectious Disease</u>, 2nd edition (Cambridge, 1953), p. ix.**

A number of themes will course their way through the first half of this book. By way of illustration, it is now generally agreed that individual diseases have their own history. This insight, far from being exclusively modern, can easily be traced back to the 17th century and the time of the great English physician Thomas Sydenham. Obviously impressed by the evidence that entirely new diseases were coming forward and replacing older ones, Sydenham described the whole process metaphorically. He insisted that diseases were historically similar to empires in that they both rose and fell. Sydenham's description, it would seem, was only partially correct. The study of epidemiological trends strongly suggests that diseases do have their own natural history, but it is highly doubtful that they rise and decline in the same rhythmic pattern that Sydenham originally ascribed to them.[1] The way that diseases have acted over long periods of time, as this study will attempt to show, is far more uneven than that, for the actual history of most diseases strongly suggests that the great pathogenic agents that have most affected Europe were, if anything, somewhat unpredictable in their impact. The microorganisms that dominated Europe for long centuries exercised their power, it now appears, in a much more random than systematic way.[2]

The constantly changing nature of the microorganisms affecting man, along with their uncanny ability to grow virulent and then, after either a long or short period of time, quite innocuous was first pointed out by a number of scientists around the turn of the 20th century. The process that regulates both the limited as well as the gigantic changes that can take place within a microorganism is known, of course, as mutation.[3] The exact biochemical changes that govern this process are still relatively mysterious. Even though the basic mechanism by which mutation takes place is still somewhat unknown, few can doubt the capacity of most microorganisms to perform this rather intricate biochemical manuever.[4] Knowledge of this fact has led to a great deal of speculation about the overall performance of diseases, including interpretations which claim that formerly virulent strains, like the bacilli that were once responsible for plague, have actually undergone a metamorphosis so complete they now exist in a entirely different state.[5] Speculation in this area has also encouraged the belief that certain pathogens, during a relatively dynamic state in their history, have progressively changed one previously identifiable disease into another.[6] The capacity of microorganisms to change their pathogenic character over generations and even centuries will be one of the central concerns of this study, which will not only seek to identify the biological consequences of Europe's great deadly and disabling diseases but to explain their social impact as well.

The notion that diseases follow their own internal pattern of development can be traced back to ancient times. The basic assumption that diseases have both an endemic and epidemic stage can, for example, be found in the writings of the noted Greek medical thinker, Hippocrates.[7] The two terms, used for long centuries to describe the presence of disease, are, by themselves, really quite limiting.[8] All of the diseases included in this particular study have had readily identifiable endemic and epidemic stages. Still, these two references are extremely restrictive terms primarily because when they are used they do not tell the student of historical epidemiology just how devastating one or another disease actually was. As an example, malignant syphilis certainly exploded onto the European scene epidemiologically in the decade of the 1490s. Yet, by comparison, tuberculosis, which around 1900 was taking up to three million lives a year in Europe has repeatedly been referred to as an endemic disorder. It has been described as endemic in spite of the fact that its death-dealing impact was much greater than syphilis had ever been, all of which suggests that medical history needs to use these two terms much more carefully than it has. Unfortunately from the point of view of the historian who is interested in diseases, the specific pathogenic agents that kept unsettling European society in the past have not left any artifacts.[9] Essentially deprived of archaeological evidence, historians working in this area have instead become almost totally dependent upon literary works, tracts that focus almost exclusively on symptomatic evidence.[10] Admittedly, this is only secondary evidence, but it is, nonetheless, crucial. It is also a highly authentic way of studying disease patterns. It is legitimate because most diseases in the past produced their own unique symptoms. It is true that diagnostically bubonic plague is sometimes difficult to separate from malignant syphilis, but this kind of overlapping of symptoms is, historically-speaking, the exception. Most of the physical disorders that will be analyzed here are so individual that they do permit the historian to approximate, with at least a fair degree of accuracy, the actual historic path that each one of these diseases has taken through the course of European history.

This study will not only attempt to assess just how diseases have acted in the past, it will also examine their influence upon the larger society in which they took place. One of the most important considerations here is the long-standing connection between disease and urban life. It is clear from the historical evidence that has accumulated up to now that most of the highly infectious diseases of the past favored the cities. Because they did, many interpreters have come to see them as essentially crowd disorders. Why they were so prevalent in the urban environment is very easy to understand. After all, the pathogenic agents that were involved here were parasites that obviously needed human hosts in order to survive.[11] That need for numbers was demonstrated in the case of cholera, which came shooting through the cities of Europe in the early 1830s.[12] It was just as characteristic of the history of other diseases such as plague and tuberculosis, both of which seemed to seek out the larger population areas. This inevitability meant, of course, that urban growth was often stifled by the recurrent tendency of disease to attack urban elements, most partially those lower down in the social order.

Beyond these biological and sociological considerations, the presence of so many diseases was psychologically such an overpowering experience that it undoubtedly deprived most Europeans of their optimism. Pain, suffering, deformity and death from one or more of the more common infections of the past must have created a totally unyielding type of fatalism in the popular mind.[13] Men in the European past simply bowed submissively to what Phillippe Ariès has called their "familiarity with death."[14] The close acquaintanceship which previous generations had with death tended to produce in them a kind of passiveness. That sense of resignation in the face of the inevitable was reinforced over the course of many centuries either by some new "plague" or by the sudden resurgence of a disease in epidemic form that was once thought to be tame.[15] Either way, for more than a millennium, most Europeans must have felt like the commentator for the Economist who opposed the first Public Health Act of 1848, insisting as he did that "suffering and evil are Nature's abominations, they cannot be got rid of."[16] That comment so characteristic of the way in which Europeans thought in the past would not be heard again in the decades after the 1840s. For the universal pessimism that underscored popular attitudes before this was just about to end. That older way of thinking would soon be driven out by the new age of microbiological thinking. Within half a century, the etiology of most of Europe's great deadly and disabling diseases would be uncovered and some of them would soon be on the way to extinction. In time, most of them would be conquered, so much so that by the middle of the 20th century the majority of them would begin to fade from the collective memory of contemporary Europeans.

CHAPTER 1

PLAGUE

> The plague is an acute, contagious, epidemical and poisonous Fever. . . . That it is Acute, is seen by the effects; for it killeth within foure or five days . . . ; it is contagious because its poison is easily imparted . . . ; it is Epidemical because it seazeth upon all kinds of people . . . ; it is Poisonous because it flighteth all remedies.
>
> --Theophilus Garencieres, <u>A Mite Cast into the Treasury of the Famous City of London</u>, (London, 1665), p. 1.

Plague was known to Europe more or less constantly, from the middle of the 14th to the end of the 18th century, when it finally and mysteriously disappeared. It first arrived in the form of the Black Death in 1347. Its last serious outburst took place in Moscow in 1772. In between those two key dates up to 50 million Europeans died, the majority of them agonizingly, as a direct result of this disease. Though it began as a Medieval disorder, plague lived on for centuries significantly influencing the course of European history right into early Modern times. For the most part powerless during an attack of plague, the medical profession could do little either to stem its advance or relieve the suffering of those who came down with it. During its long stay in Europe, plague inevitably had its social consequences either stifling economic growth, affecting the rise of empires, dislocating family life, or, most particularly, checking the overall expansion of population.

Within Europe's pre-industrial society, the coming of plague was often regarded as a curse. In the words of one contemporary moralist, plague was a form of divine punishment visited upon God's erring followers, for as he pointed out "when God speaks by ordinary diseases and is not heard, then sometimes he sends a Plague."[1] The appearance of plague was usually a terrifying experience. It was made all the more frightening because the disease killed so suddenly. As late as 1820, one Maltese physician, who was still familiar with the disease, could write: "The suddenness with which the Plague makes its attack is very remarkable, many being apparently in the full enjoyment of health but a few hours before death."[2] Striking in an instant and killing off sometimes thousands, sometimes millions, plague must have been one of Europe's most unnerving and disquieting experiences. When it penetrated Europe in the form of the Black Death between 1347 and 1351, it literally shocked European society. Some elements were so badly dislocated that they took their wrath out on outsiders, in this case Jews and gypsies.[3] For nearly all concerned then, the coming of plague both in the 1340s and in the period thereafter was, to say the least, a rather disillusioning and maddening time.

Plague is one of the world's oldest diseases, more than likely dating back some 2,000 years.[4] The ancestral home of plague, according to Wu Lien-teh, one of this century's leading epidemiologists, was Central Asia.[5] Sometime before the birth of Christ, plague became migratory, spreading out to other parts of the globe and establishing itself in certain well-defined focal points. Today, according to the World Health Organization, plague is still present in Central Asia, its geographic range now concentrated from the Caspian Sea to the Mongolian desert.[6] Like most other infectious diseases, plague periodically seems to abandon its normal habitat and to burst forward into other areas. One of those moments took place between 1347 and 1351, when plague virtually overran the whole of the European continent. That invasion was probably not the first time that plague had troubled Europe. There is ample literary evidence available that in the first centuries after Christ plague kept attacking the Mediterranean littoral, occasionally spilling over into Europe. The great pandemic of the 6th century A.D., known to history as the plague of Justinian, definitely penetrated Europe.[7] A milder outbreak of the disease also touched Europe in the 660s, infecting Scotland and parts of Scandinavia and Germany.[8] Medieval Europe knew a variety of diseases from scabies to leprosy, but by the middle of the 14th century, it had long since forgotten its earlier experiences with plague. Lacking a common memory of this disease, European society was all the more startled by the arrival of plague, and in particular by its capacity to kill so quickly and so unsparingly.

The pneumonic form of plague that first struck the Sicilian port of Messina in October of 1347 was extraordinarily virulent. The original infection that started here had been carried to Messina by twelve Genoese galleys, which had just been trading along the Crimean coast.[9] From the very inception of plague, then, sea-borne trade became one of the classic means by which this disease was to be spread. From Sicily, this very deadly form of plague was transferred to the Italian mainland, again by ship. Three of the Genoese galleys that had originally been responsible for depositing the disease in the south moved northward, docking in Genoa in January, 1348. From there, the disease spread rapidly through much of northern and central Italy. In the early part of 1348, pneumonic plague entered the central Italian city of Perugia.[10] A few weeks later, it attacked the neighboring town of Florence, where the well-known Italian writer Boccaccio, caught in its midst, has left us with a moving account of what life was actually like in those first few frightening days after the disease had invaded a city. Plague was evidently a ghastly disease to watch taking hold, for normally it spotted its victims, producing ugly black sores up and down the length of the body. Those marks were, as Boccaccio testified in the Decameron, a rather sure sign that death was on its way. Writing in 1348, Boccaccio reported:

. . . after a while the fashion of the contagion began to change into black or livid blotches which showed themselves in many first on the arms and about the thighs, and afterwards spread to every other part of the person, in some large and sparse, and in others small and thick sown; and like as the plague-boils had been first (and yet were) a very certain token of coming death. . . . Not only did a few recover thereof but well-nigh all died within the third day after the appearance of the aforesaid signs.[11]

Town officials, faced with the desperate demands of their own populations for protection, tried to contain plague as best they could. But no amount of cleanliness, quarantine or medical advice was adequate enough to stop the disease's unrelenting advance. Most health officials were quick to assume that the disease was contagious, for it was, apparently at least, being passed from one victim to another. Again, Boccaccio has left us with a very vivid account, this time of plague's supposed lightening-like capacity to infect. Recording his observations once more in the Decameron, he commented:

. . . this pestilence was all the more violent, because, by communication from the sick to the sound, it spread no less rapidly than a fire will spread to dry or oily things that lie close at hand. And, worse still, not only did the speaking or association with sick folk bring disease to the sound, or involve both in a common death, but even to touch their clothes, or anything else which the sick had touched or handled, seemed in itself to convey the same sickness to him who had touched.[12]

From Florence, the disease moved on to several other major Italian populations centers, including Venice and Siena. When it did, one anonymous 14-century Sienese chronicler reported somewhat laconically that: "In 1348 there was a great pestilence in Siena and through the world, and it lasted three months, June, July, and August, and out of [every] four, three died."[13] The endlessly tragic character of this period, brought on by the death of so many, has been aptly described by Agnoli di Tura, who wrote of these times that:

> Father abandoned child, wife, husband; one brother another, for this illness seemed to strike through the breath and the sight. And so they died. And no one could be found to bury the dead for money or for friendship. . . . And in many places in Siena great pits were dug and piled deep with huge heaps of the dead. . . . And there were also many dead throughout the city who were so sparsely covered with earth that the dogs dragged them forth and devoured their bodies.[14]

Scenes like those which di Tura portrayed were soon being repeated in Venice, where at its height the Black Death was claiming up to 600 lives a day. City fathers in Venice were all but helpless against the disease. They could do little else beyond providing for sanitary burial, usually by carrying the bodies away in barges to be buried at some distant spot.[15]

At the very same moment that this disease was punishing most of Italy, it was rapidly spreading through the Greek portions of the Byzantine Empire. The Emperor of Byzantium Ioannes Cantacuzenos soon became aware of the terrible human toll that the disease was taking in his empire. Here, as in Italy, plague took hundreds of thousands of lives. Describing that ferocity, Cantacuzenos reported:

> So incurable was the evil, that neither any regularity of life, nor any bodily strength could resist it. Strong and weak bodies were all similarly carried away, and those best cared for died in the same manner as the poor. If some had a previous illness he always succumbed to this disease and no physician's art was sufficient, neither did the disease take the

same course in all persons, but the others, [those] unable to resist, died the same day, a few within an hour. Those who could resist for two or three days had a very violent fever at first, the disease in such cases attacking the head.[16]

If the continuously expanding epidemic of 1347 and 1348 had stopped at this juncture, its geographic spread would not have been any greater than the outbreak that had occurred during the 6th century A.D. That particular epidemic had, after all, touched Europe marginally. And as of 1348, plague, as devastating as it had been, was still essentially confined to the Mediterranean littoral. However, beginning in 1349, plague began slicing into northern Europe. Within a matter of months, it was ominously ranging into Germany, spreading so far afield that historians would later be forced to identify it by the broader geographic term pandemic.

After it had invaded Italy and Greece, the Black Death moved directly northward, following the traditional commercial path through the Alps provided by the Brenner Pass.[17] The pace of the disease, while it was generally fast, was now somewhat slower than it had been largely because plague was now travelling overland rather than by sea.[18] Throughout the early part of 1349, it ranged far beyond the Alps, spreading panic and promoting despair whenever and wherever it struck. North of the Alps, the disease pushed out in four directions, penetrating, in turn, Germany and southern Norway, the Hungarian plain, southern France and England and Scotland. Rather appropriately the Germans kept referring to this period as "the Great Dying."[19] As in 1347 and 1348, the disease seemed to single out the major commercial centers, always producing a significant loss of life. In the future German University town of Erfurt, the so-called Sampetrium Chronicle of 1349 reported, somewhat graphically, that: "The people are dying most of the time by the glands."[20] Evidence from this and other chronicles strongly suggests that bubonic plague had now broken out and was actually accompanying the pneumonic form of the disease that had been so prevalent during the first two years of the pandemic. Everywhere the loss of life was great. Hungarian royal officials quickly estimated that the disease had carried off nearly a quarter of the kingdom's population.[21]

Plague continued to wend its way across the continent, soon spreading into France and England. By now the Black Death was taking on the proportions of a universal catastrophe. No one really knew just how extensive the death-toll actually was. It was rumored in Marseilles, either rightly or wrongly, that four-fifths of the population had been killed. Further to the north at Avignon, along the Rhone, death-tolls were extremely high. At that moment when about half of Avignon's population had already perished, Guy de Chauliac wrote the following description of the disease's impact upon the city; he said:

> The mortality commenced in the month of January, 1348, and lasted for the space of seven months: the first type lasted two months with constant fever and blood spitting, and with this people died within two days. The second lasted the rest of the time. In this, together with constant fever, there were external carbuncles or buboes under the arm or in the groin, and the disease ran its course in five days.[22]

From the symptomatic evidence presented here by de Chauliac it is abundantly clear the the two major forms of plague, the pneumonic and bubonic forms, were both operating within Avignon. At the very same time, both types of the disease were also invading England.[23] In London, the session of Parliament scheduled for January, 1349, was abruptly cancelled due to the "sudden visitation of deadly pestilence [which] had broken out at Westminster and the neighborhood."[24] By the following year, plague, completing its deadly sweep of the continent, had entered Scotland with the usual devastating results.[25]

By the beginning of 1351, the pandemic was starting to abate. During the years when it reigned, it produced an extraordinary amount of public distress. Popular reaction to plague during this period of upheaval was both panicky and excessive. The public had frequent recourse to prayer, with millions of Europeans hoping for divine intercession. In 1349, the Pope, Clement VI, responding to the popular outcry, called for a European-wide pilgrimage against the plague. All together, nearly a million Christians from all over the continent converged on Rome, each praying for deliverance from what was one of Europe's greatest tragedies ever.[26] The sight that frightened most men and woman was the horrifying spectacle of so many suffering and dying without any apparent cause. Countless Europeans saw scores of people writhing, in the rather classic description of one French observer, from:

> an internal Heat, an extream Anxiety and Depression of the Spirits, a restless Agitation of the Body, accompanied with a Fever, Pains of the Head and Stomach, Phrensy and Delirium; a conclusive Motion of the Tendons, and small Contraction of the Limbs, . . . a fetid Scent proceeded from the Mouth and Skin. . . . The Bowels were likewise affected the following Symptoms: A malignant Diarrhea . . . with . . . a Propensity to Vomit.[27]

In its terminal stage, the pneumonic form of the disease added the equally disquieting sight of mass hemorrhaging. In the words of the noted German chronicler, Adam Lonicerus: "the nose of the victim was very bloody, with blood bubbling up through the various parts of the head."[28] These maddening sights provoked some into violence. A few blamed themselves and their own sinfullness. These types, described at the time as Flagellants, could be seen parading their way through certain cities of the Netherlands and western Germany. Usually, they whipped and lacerated one another, in this way hoping to atone for the sins that they thought had bought on the pestilence. On several other occasions, half-crazed mobs turned against the Jewish population in certain cities, accusing them of having poisoned wells thus bringing on the misery that all had to endure. In one urban area after another, completely innocent Jews were barbarously tortured and in a number of instances burned alive.[29]

Although up to 25 million people died during the Great Pandemic of 1347-1351, medical men in Europe viewed the appearance of plague as a deep-seated mystery.[30] As circumstances would have it, the actual cause of plague was not discovered until 1894, more than a century after the disease had virtually disappeared from the European scene. For almost five centuries before this, the various forms of plague had been harassing the European continent, with few ever suspecting its true etiology. The microorganism that caused the disease, Pasteurella pestis, or as it is sometimes called, Yersinia pestis, was finally brought to light in 1894 during an outbreak of plague which was then raging in the British Crown Colony of Hong Kong. The co-discoverers of this still highly toxic microorganism were the French pathologist, A. Yersin, and the Japanese bacteriologist, S. Kitsato, both of whom were investigating the disease in one of its principal focal points in the Far East.[31] Whether the pathogenic agent that they first saw under their microscopes was the same poisonous substance that had been engulfing Europe since the middle of the 14th century is still not analytically clear. No microfossils of the original pathogen obviously exist. But, if one takes into account the rather compelling symptomatic evidence from the past, it is fair to say that the two germs were probably the same. Descriptions of the symptoms produced by the plague are remarkably similar from the 14th century on down. Making use of this kind of evidence, it is relatively safe to assume that the microorganism that Yersin and Kitsato first isolated in the 1890s was anatomically similar to the pathogen that had been attacking the European population over time. Still, a potential killer in both Africa and Asia, the bacterium responsible for plague continues to live on in a variety of forms.[32] Over the past few decades, modern research in the area of bacteriology has systematically stripped this microorganism of much of its previous mystery. It has firmly been established, for example, that plague exists in a number of different strains, each biologically capable of producing an almost endless combination of symptoms in its victims.[33]

Modern medical science has established that plague has an unusual capacity to vary its symptoms, both from one day to another and from one patient to another. This current perception about the plague was not lost to previous generations of medical men in Europe. While the medical profession never successfully defined the etiology of plague, it did progressively identify the disease's numerous symptoms. The 17th-century English physician Nathaniel Hodges noticed the fluctuating character of plague's symptoms during the London epidemic of 1665.[34] So did the Frenchman Jean Astruc, who kept commentating on this peculiar aspect of the disease during the rather unexpected attack of plague on Marseilles in 1720 and 1721. Later on in the 18th century, one of Europe's more acute medical officers, the German Georg von Asch stated it more succinctly than most when he declared that since there were varying symptoms, "there were different kinds of pestes."[35] The various strains of Pasteurella Pestis have evidently then always had the capacity to alter symptoms from one plague victim to another. It is true that during some epidemics of plague in Europe the sequence of identifiable symptoms from one patient to another was only slightly altered, but they did change. Fevers, for example, came and went in most patients in a very irregular fashion, occurring early in some cases and later in others, with the severity of the fever varying quite individually.[36] Once again, the English physician Hodges pointed to the capacity of plague to run a rather erratic course. Commenting in 1665, Hodges declared: "Many patients were lost when they were thought in a safe Recovery; and when we thought the Conquest quite obtained, Death ran away with the Victory; . . . whereas other[s] got over it who were quite given over for lost, much to the Disreputation of the Art."[37] These conspicuous turn-abouts were not, of course, the fault of the medical profession. They were instead the direct result of the antigens at work here, progressively changing the body chemistry of those that they were attacking. This last consideration was, needless to say, unknown to Hodges and other observers, who simply viewed the disease as an arbitrary one.

Diagnostically, it took generations for physicians in Europe to come up with all the symptoms that plague was capable of producing. The much more sophisticated microscopic evidence building up after 1894 was, of course, not theirs. But, even though, the medical profession was almost exclusively dependent upon external evidence for its insights, the three forms of Pasteurella pestis were over time progressively identified by previous medical observers. The pneumonic form of plague has historically been the most devastating. The bacteria involved here have a strong propensity for lung tissue. Eating away at the lungs and breaking down both capillaries and veins, this extremely lethal form of plague soon produces a characteristic bleeding from both the nose and mouth, a symptom often reported upon in the past. The second form of the disease that appeared in Europe was bubonic. Its name derives from the fact that it always attacks the lymphatic system, causing pronounced swelling around the groin, under the arm-pits and in the neck. These carbuncles, or buboes as they were called, soon ulcerated, producing, in turn, a seeping pus. After 1351, the bubonic form of plague became the predominant type in Europe. The last form of plague, septicaemic, was less well known to the past primarily because it did not produce truly outstanding symptoms such as bleeding and ulceration. Instead, it usually just raced through the body, in a matter of hours, moving past organs but soon saturating the blood with huge quantities of plague bacillus. In this instance, death was almost immediate as over and opposed to the pneumonic and bubonic forms of the disease which usually took several days to run their course.[38]

Most historians are agreed that the Black Death of 1347-1351 was initially a severe outbreak of pneumonic plague.[39] That form of the disease is easily passed from one victim to another by means of air-droplets, making it highly contagious. At the very same time, bubonic plague also began to break out in Europe.[40] While bubonic plague is antigenetically similar to the pneumonic form of the disease, its appearance during these years must be regarded as a chance occurrence, for the bubonic form of this disease is only incidentally a disease of human beings. Bubonic plague is primarily a disease of burrowing rodents, principally rats, squirrels and gerbils.[41]   The animal that was most responsible for moving this form of plague around Europe was the black rat (Rattus rattus). The actual transfer of bubonic plague from rat to man, however, is the work of two vectors. The primary carriers are two rat fleas, Xenopsylla Cheopsis and Nosopsyllus fasciatus. Usually gorged with the blood of septicaemic rats, these fleas often bit humans producing in them a quickly proliferating type of plague that is only slightly less deadly than the pneumonic form.[42]   The surprising appearance of bubonic plague, probably in the year 1349, as a companion to the pneumonic type, obviously compounded the misery that was then being experienced. Just how and why these two forms of plague, one involving man and the other rats, broke out almost simultaneously in Europe, both after such a long absence, has never been adequately explained. What is clear, however, is that the pneumonic form of the disease became relatively rare, while bubonic plague, helped along by Rattus rattus quickly became commonplace.[43]

Modern medical science along with 20th-century means of detection have gone a long way toward subduing plague, even though ground animals are still carrying the disease in certain parts of the globe. There has been a workable vaccine against the disease in existence since 1902. The vaccine, originally made from dead bacteria, while not providing truly long-lasting immunity was and is momentarily effective for at least a few months.[44]   A more promising possibility in the search for a more potent vaccine has emerged since World War II. This work involves a specific bacteria known as Pasteurella pseudo-tuberculosis. This particular bacillus has an antigenic structure that is amazingly similar to Pasteurella pestis.[45] It is the belief of some that this kind of bacteria will eventually guarantee the type of immunity which cowpox vaccine has continually provided against smallpox. Beyond this hope, epidemiologists, working today for the World Health Organization, have been able to stymie the growth of plague by monitoring and policing the traditional habitats of rodents who often carry this disease. The big breakthrough in the field of detection actually came in the 1920s when an international team of epidemiologists discovered the

Eurasian homeland of most infected rodents.[46] Since then, scientists from first the League of Nations and then the World Health Organization have systematically combed these infected areas, eliminating whenever possible potentially dangerous rodent colonies.[47]

The terrifying sweep of the Black Death was never to be repeated again in the period after 1351. The bubonic form of plague operated more casually in succeeding generations, attacking here and there but never with the intensity or scope of plague's first coming. A medical cartographer, mapping the advance of the Black Death in the 1340s could easily have finished up his study by representing its movement in flood-like proportions. Penetrating both urban and rural areas, the Black Death spared only a few fortunate pockets on the entire continent.[48] As plague settled in during the decades after 1351, it seemed to confine itself to certain well-defined focal points, its geographic pattern now apparently fragmenting. The Great Pandemic of 1347-1351 had advanced so relentlessly that it missed neither town nor countryside, although the cities do seem to have been the avenue for the disease's entry into entirely new areas. In the generations and centuries that followed, plague increasingly became an urban phenomena, periodically draining off tens of thousands of people from a number of key European cities. The major commercial ports in Europe were the hardest hit, with London, Vienna and Venice suffering the disease almost regularly.[49]

The pathogenic agents involved in this new spread of plague were evidently less numerous than during the Great Pandemic, but they were only slightly less infectious,[50] for the fatality rates from both the pneumonic and bubonic forms of plague were extraordinarily high. The number of Europeans who perished during the ongoing epidemic of 1347-1351 was probably close to one-quarter of the whole population. Some estimates go higher than that, but even erring conservatively the figure was probably about 25 million people.[51] The disease, of course, kept reoccurring during succeeding centuries, often sapping cities and sometimes villages of a fair proportion of their population. During the majority of the epidemics that occurred between the 14th and 18th centuries, mortality rates among those struck down during the early weeks of an epidemic normally hovered around 90 percent. Contrastingly, as plague spent itself in a certain locale, death rates among clinical cases began to ease, on occasion dropping as low as 30 percent. Before the discovery of modern antibiotics, capable of controlling this disease, mortality rates in Asia and Africa, where plague was still common in the early 20th century, remained in and around 65 percent of all those contracting the disorder.[52]   No other disease in European history permitted so few of its victims to escape. Throughout the era then, when bubonic plague was still mostly endemic, but also periodically epidemic, death-rates remained exorbitantly high. This killing disease wiped out a third of Warsaw's population in 1567-1568.[53] It took an additional 40,000 lives in Paris in 1580.[54] Routinely, whole families just disappeared from parish roles, as they did in Carlisle after the plague of 1597-1598 had passed through that city in northern England.[55]   Villages frequently escaped the reach of plague at this time, but in 1645-1646 one-fifth of the population of Colyton, in Devonshire, was wiped out in the wake of a single attack from plague.[56]

The era that knew plague intimately could think of little else except panicky flight as soon as the news spread of its arrival. The Italian physician Pietro de Tossignano was, at this time, among those who were totally convinced that plague was spread by means of human contact. Writing in 1398, he advised the healthy to flee from infected areas and to seek safer places that had not recently known the disease.[57] Shunning others became a common bit of medical advice. In the middle of the 15th century, Bengt Knutsson from Vastoras, in the neighborhood of Stockholm, warned of plague's contagiousness saying, "Beware of any multitude of people leste that be the brethe of summe of them may be enffecte." He also counselled against the frequenting of public baths declaring: "Let them beware of allytyl ferment do corrupte halle the body."[58] The social pathology and fear that plague repeatedly instilled in the European population has been acutely described by the Italian writer

Benvenuto Cellini. Taken ill with plague during the Roman epidemic of 1523, Cellini recorded what he thought were his last anguished moments in his Autobiography. He commented:

> I rose upon the hour of breaking fast, and felt tired, for I had travelled many miles that night, and was wanting to take food, when a crushing headache seized me: several boils appeared upon my left arm, together with a carbuncle which showed itself just beyond the palm of the left hand, where it joins the wrist. Everybody in the house was in a panic: my friend, the cow [a prostitute] and the calf [the serving girl] all fled. Left alone there with my poor little [ap]prentice, who refused to abandon me, I felt stifled at the heart and made up my mind for certain I was a dead man.[59]

As it turned out, Cellini somehow recovered, one of the minority that did.

As Pietro de Tossignano knew, there were areas on the European continent where bubonic plague was not present. For the disease was arbitrary, attacking some locales with a chilling regularity, wholly ignoring others, while penetrating yet others only now and then. Its very arbitrariness, made bubonic plague a disillusioning experience. London was, by many accounts, one of the disease's major focal points. Directing attention to its endemic presence there, the Venetian ambassador to the Court of London declared in 1554: "They have some plague in England well nigh every year, for which they are not accustomed to make sanitary provisions, as it usually does not make great progress."[60] Plague never really left the English capital, one historian estimating that between 1500 and 1665 the disease was absent from London for only 12 years.[61] Vienna had a similar experience. The Klosterneuburg Chronicle related that no area in Austria suffered a greater loss of life in 1349 than the Austrian capital did. Records dutifully kept by the University of Vienna over subsequent periods prove that the disease was constantly reoccurring here. In the 15th century, it attacked, epidemically, four times and in the

16th century, a total of eight. In the epidemic of 1521, approximately 10,000 people perished, while in 1541, some 40,000 died.[62] Venice, meanwhile, probably suffered more intensely from plague than any other European city. Over the course of four centuries, it was wracked by no less than 70 different documented epidemics.[63] Whether bubonic plague was continuously present in Vienna and Venice, the way it was in London, is not clear from the historical record.

The large commercial centers, located either on the coastline or along the great rivers, were not the only ones that experienced plague. Small inland cities also knew the disease, with sporadic outbursts of the disease attesting to its presence here as well. By way of example, the Papal center of Avignon was hit by plague at six different intervals between 1348 and 1390. Yet, somewhat mysteriously, the city of Carpentras, located just 14 miles to the north and east of Avignon, completely escaped the disease.[64] Singularly unlucky in comparison with Carpentras, was the river town of Chalons, on the Marne in eastern France. That small port-city was virtually paralyzed by 15 separate outbreaks of bubonic plague between 1455 and 1522. The pattern of attack in Chalons was completely unpredictable. Sometimes the disease broke out yearly and other times after an absence of a decade or more.[65] The cities of Mecklenburg in northern Germany also experienced the seemingly quixotic comings and goings of the bubonic form of plague. In this area of Germany, the disease was almost exclusively confined to urban centers, the villages of Mecklenburg being continually spared. Again, the cities were struck randomly. The city of Wismar was rather unfortunate being engulfed by every single outbreak in the province between 1348 and 1639. Meanwhile, neighboring Schwerin was curiously attacked only 50 percent of the time, while Plau and Parchin, in close geographical proximity to the other two towns, were spared the disease almost entirely.[66] Like Wismar, the small Tuscan town of Azeppo, in north central Italy, was one of those well-known urban centers where the presence of plague became legendary. Between 1389 and 1531, the disease desolated Azeppo 11 different times, claiming an average of 1,150 lives during each catastrophe.[67]

DEATH TOLL IN SELECTED EUROPEAN CITIES
FROM PNEUMONIC AND BUBONIC PLAGUE, 1349-1771.[68]

City	Date	Number Killed
London	1349	20,000
Lübeck	1371	80,000
Florence	1418	16,000
Paris	1418	50,000
Venice	1477-78	30,000
Vienna	1542	18,000
London	1593	23,000
London	1603	34,000
Amsterdam	1655 + 1664	41,000
London	1665	100,000
Vienna	1679	141,000
Prague	1681	81,000
Marseilles	1720-21	40,000
Moscow	1771	57,000

By the 16th century, the medical profession was becoming progressively more sophisticated in its diagnosis, especially of bubonic plague. For one thing, the disease was prevalent enough in certain key places to allow physicians the opportunity to investigate its more pronounced symptoms. During this period, the medical profession was seriously divided as to just what symptom, out of the many associated with plague, was the most significant. The German medical observer Thomas Jordanus kept pointing to the rather grotesque boils erupting on the skin as the disease's most abiding feature. He described them as scabies, using a Medieval term, insisting that these carbuncles were the physiological source of the disease's contagiousness.[69] Quite apart from these unsightly sores, the Italian physician Nicholas Massa was personally convinced that the fever which inevitably went along with this disease was its most distinguishing trait. Massa repeatedly referred to plague in his writings as pestilential fever, arguing that it was the high fever caused by plague which was the principal cause of death.[70] The Scottish doctor Albert Skeyne, writing in the same time period, broadened his diagnosis of plague, arguing that the disease had a whole variety of symptoms that one could characteristically identify with it. Somewhat more analytically, he declared: "The prinicipall signs . . . in pestilentiall personis, ar frequent swoning, cauld Sweiting, Vomitting . . . dieuris . . . , principallie inclining to blak, . . . crampe . . . in exterior membranes . . . , with imperfectioun of speche and stink and breathe, . . . with red spottes on the bodie."[71]

By the 17th century, most physicians would have agreed with the overall assessment of plague given by the well-known Russian doctor Athanasius Shafonski. Shafonski tersely described plague as " . . . more dangerous than all other diseases, highly contagious and producing external signs upon the body . . . buboes, carbuncles, and large and small black spots; for the most part ending in death."[72] Although the symptoms of plague varied endlessly from one clinical case to another, the onset of the disease was remarkably similar in each instance. Describing in the 1660s, the initial stages of bubonic plague, the London diagnostician Thomas Sydenham could only report what other physicians had observed for long centuries. He stated: "The plague usually begins with chillness and shivering, like the fit of an intermittent [fever]; soon after, a violent vomiting, a painful oppression at the breast, and a burning fever."[73] Not in a position to fathom plague's etiology, the medical profession became increasingly fascinated by its symptoms. This highly externalized approach to the disease was encouraged, at this time, by the rather excruciating pain that was brought on by the seething carbuncles that regularly covered the body. One doctor, obviously trying to describe these boils with as much clinical detachment as possible, simply recorded that: "The Carbuncle is a malignant pustule proceeding from blood very hote and grosse in substance, which causeth . . . an ulcer with an Eschare or crust in the skin, swelling and red, raising the inflammation thereof . . . and procuring exceeding pain in him that is possessed therewith."[74] The very severity of the pain that had to be endured seemed to make the boils clinically important. The Englishman Thomas Culpepper argued, credibly in his own age, that these carbuncles were the actual key to the disease's cure. For the putrid matter causing the plague, he explained, needed to be liberated by means of bloodletting. The specific location of the carbuncles on the neck and groin was highly significant to Culpepper because it actually revealed where the offending matter was lurking and, in turn, told the physician where the cutting should take place.[75]

During the course of the 17th century, plague ominously began to take on the proportions of yet another pandemic. But, unlike the Great Pandemic of 1347-1351, Europe's last great pandemic was not confined to an extremely short and wholly intense period of time. Instead, the disease lasted a good deal longer, extending itself over two easily recognizable time periods. The first was the rather wide-ranging explosion of bubonic plague that occurred in the 1620s and 1630s. As disastrous as it was, this outbreak was only the prelude to a much more extensive epidemic, one that literally riddled whole areas of the European continent in the years from 1664 to 1681. Taken as a whole, these two renewals of the disease represent the widest geographic extension of plague since the sorrowful days of the Black Death. Ever since the early 1350s, plague had been operating as a purely regional affliction striking here and there, sometimes often, sometimes on occasion, but never really spilling over a truly wide geographic area. But, disturbingly, in the 1620s, the disease, evidently being carried further afield by the fighting associated with the Thirty Years War, seemed to be pushing out of its former enclaves entering entirely new territory. The kind of plague that was now running rampant was the bubonic variety, meaning that its spread was very much dependent on the movement of infected rats and fleas. Rat migrations, aided and abetted presumably by the invasions of armies, must had been taking place at this time. While they were, Europe was once more subjected to all of the terrifying scenes that had so disrupted normal life during the 14th century, only this time the suffering was to be spread over several decades not just a few years.[76]

The epidemic of plague that struck London in 1625 was the first indication that a new pandemic was about to occur. John Graunt, often regarded as Europe's first historical epidemiologist traced, with rather intricate statistics, the disease's path through the city. Under normal circumstances, according to Graunt, the principal causes of death in the English capital were tuberculosis, various kinds of fevers and smallpox. But in 1625, plague deaths suddenly took precedence. In the historic inner part of the city, a section that was still walled, out of a recorded 14,340 deaths that year, 9,197 perished from plague. This deadly pathogen also took the lives of a full 75 percent of those dying in the 25 London parishes that lay outside of the walls, all told, some 22,000 people.[77] The disease next jumped the Channel, making an appearance in northern Germany. From here, plague was evidently carried by German troops into the south of Germany and the northern parts of Italy. The Thirty Years War was now at its height and troop movements were dramatically accelerating the spread of this dangerous disease. In 1629, bubonic plague broke out in the southern German commercial center of Augsburg. From there, invading German military units most likely passed it on to centers in northern Italy. Here, one Italian health official mournfully reported that: "Most of these Germans are infected with plague because of their wantonness and their dirtiness. Unbearable odors surround them," he went on, "due to the rotting straw whereon they sleep and die."[78] The disease was soon passing on to Venice, a city that was to have its last great epidemic of plague ever in the year 1630.[79] After attacking Venice, the disease next moved on to Bologna where it hit with characteristic fury, carrying off a half of that city's population.[80]

During the next few decades, plague seemed to subside in virulence, becoming as before a purely local disorder. In this interim period, the disease continued to strike at urban centers, but now only occasionally. In 1648, it broke out unexpectedly in the Spanish city of Oriheula in Valencia. One tract after another, written at the time, definitely identified the outbreak as yet another case of bubonic plague. Beyond this, most observers noticed all over again the classic tendency of this disorder to vary its symptoms from one victim to another. One symptom, in particular, however, did not change, for all those falling ill had a "large number of carbuncles covering different parts of the body."[81] In another isolated incident, the Jewish ghetto in Rome felt the harsh consequences of this disease in 1656. The officials in charge of the Roman ghetto organized both swift medical attention and quick burials in an attempt to stem the impact of plague. But, in spite of these efforts, the disease just seemed to carry away all of the potential susceptibles in the community.[82] A few years after these widely-separated events, a pronounced upswing in the disease's virulence was becoming increasingly noticeable. Then starting in 1664 and continuing for the next 17 years, plague began cutting a wide geographic swath across the length of the European continent. During this terrifying period, plague, acting almost as it had in the 1340's, engulfed one population center after another, killing some 100,000 people in London in 1665, with 140,000 dying in Vienna in 1679 and 83,000 in Prague in 1681 before it was all over.[83] What this age did not know was that plague was making its last murderous attack on western Europe. For after long centuries, this one ubiquitous disease was curiously about to disappear.

The accelerating expansion of bubonic plague, beginning in the 1660s, most likely originated in Amsterdam, probably starting in the year 1663. Highly disturbing reports that: "The plague it seems to grow more and more at Amsterdam," were heard on numerous occasions in London.[84] After this initial outbreak, the disease spread precipitously into southern England, northern France and western Germany.[85] Plague ravaged London, for the last time historically, in 1665. It is unlikely that any epidemic in the history of plague was so thoroughly described by contemporaries as this one particular event. Moreover, it is clear from the abundance of symptomatic descriptions piling up at the time that it was bubonic plague that was racing so relentlessly through the English capital. One chronicler, Dr. Thomas Vincent, focusing on the disease's symptoms commented on how the popular mind had come to identify the appearance of boils and carbuncles as a sure sign of impending death. Writing two years after the event, he pointed out that:

When the disease had invaded . . . and first began with a pain and dizziness in their head, then trembling in their other members; when they had felt boils to arise under their arms, and in their groines, and seen blains [carbuncles] to come forth in other parts; when the Disease hath wrought to them at that height, as to send spots which (most think) are the certain Tokens of neer approaching death; and now they have received the sentence of death within themselves. . . .[86]

The true source of plague remained a mystery in 1665 to most Londoners. But, interestingly, one London commentator Theophilus Garencieres came extraordinarily close to the actual origins of the disease when he described plague as: "an acute, contagious, epidemical and poisonous Fever, accompanied by either a Blotch, a Carbuncle, or Red-spotts, like Flea-bites, vulgarly called the Tokens."[87] While he came close, Garencieres, like most physicians during plague's long presence in European society never even consciously suspected that either rats or fleas were implicated in the spread of the disease.

The all too obvious fact that in London plague did "killeth within foure or five days,"[88] was not only well known to the city's masses, it was also the cause of considerable panic. Among others, Nathaniel Hodges derided the masses for being so frightened at the mere appearance of plague. Sarcastically, he wrote:

As soon as it was rumoured amongst the common People, who are always astonished at any Thing new, that the Plague was in the City, it was impossible to relate what Accounts were spread of its Fatality, . . . every one predicted its future Devastations, and they terrified each other with Remembrances of a former Pestilence; for it was a received Notion amongst the common people, that the Plague visited England once in Twenty years, as if after a certain Interval by some inevitable necessity, it must return again.[89]

Actually, mass elements in the city had good reason to be fearful. The average death rate in London for the weeks preceding the outbreak of 1665 was 352. By the middle of July in 1665, plague was taking a thousand lives a week, and by early August the figure was up to two thousand. By the height of the epidemic, which came in September, the death-toll had escalated to nearly six thousand a week.[90] Almost desperately, Dr. Vincent described some of the scenes taking place during these weeks when the disease was killing so uncompromisingly. He noted:

> Now the Grave doth open its mouth without measure. Multitudes, multitudes, in the valley of the shadow of death thronging daily in Eternity; the Churchyards now are stuft so full with dead corpses, that they are in many places swell'd two or three foot higher than they were before, and new ground is broken up to bury the dead.[91]

The desperation that was common to those living through a plague was recorded by yet another Englishman, the diarist Samuel Pepys. Describing what London was like in September when the epidemic was at full force, Pepys wrote rather soulfully: "Thence I walked to the tower, but Lord! how empty the streets are and melancholy, so many poor sick people in the streets full of sores, and so many sad stories overheard as I walk, everybody talking of this dead and that man sick."[92] Almost as compelling as Pepys' description was the partially fictional account of the great London plague written decades later by Daniel Defoe. Even though he composed his story a half century after the event, Defoe, nevertheless, succeeded in capturing the pathos of those harrowing days. Poignantly, he told of how:

> The misery of that time lay upon the poor, who, being infected, had neither food nor physic; neither physician nor apothecary to assist them, nor nurse to attend them. Many

of them died calling for help, and even for sustenance, out at
their windows, in a most miserable and deplorable
manner.[93]

Defoe's sociological analysis of the plague was amazingly accurate. The
rich tended to flee the city, leaving the less fortunate to a rather predictable
fate.[94]

From southern England, the disease moved back across the
Channel, its pandemic sweep carrying it through northern France, the Low
Centuries and western Germany. Throughout 1666, plague steadily
advanced, saturating, in turn, Normandy, Picardy and the Paris Basin. At
Rouen, in the heart of Normandy, the disease again displayed its long-
standing characteristic of killing off the overwhelming majority of those who
came down with it. Death-rates in Rouen over a three-year period kept
hovering at around 80 percent of all clincial cases, with most patients dying
shortly after they had been infected.[95] Bubonic plague subsequently
made it to Paris in 1668, where the Minister of Finance, Colbert, demanded
that immediate steps be taken to arrest the disease's advance. A
quarantine was established in the French capital and the disease's path
was closely mapped so that communities could have ample forewarning of
its approach. Yet, in spite of these precautions, plague kept intensifying its
attack on the population centers in the whole Paris region.[96] At about the
same moment in time, plague was also attacking in the Rhineland. By
August of 1666, Cologne, like other urban areas along the river, had lost
up to one-third of its overall population. Right after these electrifying
visitations, plague all but vanished from western Europe. The explanation
that is generally given for plague's sudden disappearance centers
specifically on the fate of the black rat. According to this argument, the
black rat, which historically had been so susceptible to infection from
plague, dies off as a species. The black rat, it is again assumed, is soon
replaced by the grey rat, a mammalian species known to be resistant to
plague.[97] This zootic explanation is the one that has been most frequently
given to explain Europe's sudden and almost miraculous emancipation

from plague.   Much of what has been said is, however, somewhat speculative, since solid archeological evidence for this contention is as of yet not all that plentiful.

Nevertheless, as of the early 1670s, plague was definitely gone from western Europe. The same could not be said in that decade for central Europe. For in 1679, a revival of plague in Vienna, quickly left, according to one of the most reliable accounts, some 140,000 people dead. The worst part of Vienna's last experience with plague ever was that the city had been anticipating its arrival. The Austrian imperial government had already posted descriptions of the disease, warning the city's population that the disease acted mercilessly. Posters nailed up in Vienna ahead of time described plague rather accurately as "a poisonous illness . . . which in the majority of cases is untreatable and deadly. . . . For the most part it is characterized by seizures, intense heat and either carbuncles or brown spots . . . death normally ensuing within a few hours or a few days."[98] After decimating Vienna, this epidemic moved on to Prague, taking in 1681 some 83,000 lives, before it finally spent itself.[99] After 1681, the large geographic area from Ireland in the west to the Carpathians in the east, which for centuries had known one plague visitation after another, was now totally free of the disease. There were, it is true, three notable exceptions. There was a minor outbreak of plague in the Baltic in 1710 and another in the eastern part of Austria in 1718,[100] along with one truly devastating attack of bubonic plague in the port of Marseilles in 1720. That epidemic was western Europe's last deadly reminder of what had been regularly happening to her over the course of the last four hundred years.

Plague was brought to Marseilles in the summer of 1720 by a trading ship which had most recently docked in Sidon in Syria. By July, deaths from the disease were beginning to occur randomly. As before, the news panicked thousands into fleeing the city. Before long, the city itself was completely encircled by French troops drawn up in a desperate attempt to build a sanitary cordon against the spread of the disease. Marseilles was soon turned into a living hell, half of its remaining population of 80,000 dying excruciating deaths within a very short period of time.[101] The scenes that this particular epidemic of plague engendered were among the most gruesome that have ever been recorded. Pichatty de Croissante, trapped in the city during the outbreak, later told of some of them. Reporting in his history, he wrote:

> There lie extended about a thousand Bodies close to each other, the freshest of which have lain there about three Weeks, so that had they not been infected, the lying so long in a Place exposed to the hot Sun all the Day, might have sufficed to render them contagious: All one's Senses are arrested at approaching a Place, whence one smells afar the contagious Vapours which Exhale from it: Nature shrinks, and the firmest Eyes cannot bear so hideous a Sight; those Bodies have no longer any human Form, they are Monsters that give Horror, and one would think all their Limbs stir, the Worms are in such Motion about them[102]

De Croissante also listed the symptoms of the disease that he saw, pointing out that the most prominent were: "the Carbuncles, Buboes and other bad Tumors [that] appeared in sundry parts of the Body."[103]

Except for the surprise epidemic of 1720, western and central Europe were from here on in free from the plague. The disease was also fading into insignificance in eastern Europe during the 18th century. There were only two short-lived exceptions to this general trend. The disease was unquestionably present in epidemic form in the Ukraine in 1738 and 1739.[104] Beyond this, it made one last devastating attack on the Balkans and southern Russia in the late 1760s and early 1770s. Originating in present-day Bulgaria and Rumania, plague penetrated Russia, being carried along by Russian troops involved in the fighting against the Turks. By the latter part of 1770, the first cases of plague were being reported in Moscow. The disease began among impoverished textile workers and from there quickly spread to all corners of the city. As so often in the past, the culprit was again the bubonic form of the disease, with carbuncles and ugly black spots regularly appearing on those who came down with the illness. Before the epidemic exhausted itself in 1771, one-third of Moscow's population had perished.[105] Among the handful of physicians working with the sick was the Russian medical officer, Danilo Samoilowitz. Samoilowitz's observations on the onset of plague represent in themselves the most advanced medical thinking that there was in his day. That thinking still rested, for the most part, on the importance of symptoms. Rather typically, Samoilowitz dismissed the whole notion that plague might conceivably be caused by microscopic objects that he described as "insects," a phrase that obviously meant germs.[106] The germ theory did have its exponents in the 18th century, but their approach was almost always denigrated in favor of the more commonly held belief that disease was caused by stale, putrid air.

Even at the moment when plague was disappearing from European society, the medical profession was still stymied when it came to explaining the disease's etiology. Moreover, without the advantage of microscopic evidence, the medical profession was left with a series of often perplexing observations. Medical men since the Middle Ages were philosophically committed to the miasmatic view that disease was caused by unclean air. Few, historically, ever really challenged this assumption largely because it had behind it the full force of custom. The attention of the entire medical profession for centuries then had been traditionally focused upon investigating the air, a point of view that was distinctly macroscopic rather than microscopic in its orientation. Holding to the views that they did about the danger involved in inhaling air that had been corrupted by putrid smells, doctors could prescribe all sorts of seemingly logical remedies such as "the burning of Goats Horn, as good Fume against pestilence and infected air."[107] The major problem with this time-honored interpretation was that physicians kept observing that some could operate right in the midst of what was assumed to be corrupt air with little or no bad effect. To his own amazement, Samoilowitz saw this happen over and over again during the epidemic in Moscow in 1771. Numbers of priests and physicians escaped infection even though they were continuously exposed to the "bad air" which most believed surrounded the victims of plague.[108] If plague was the consequence of foul and putrid air, how was it that so many breathing it managed to escape its ill effects? The well-known English publicist, John Howard, was so puzzled by this that at one point he asked: "How is it possible if the plague be communicated by infected air, that a whole body of men in a town where it rages should be capable of being preserved from it?"[109]

The answer that was increasingly being given for this rather perplexing development was almost mathematical in its formulation. Howard attempted to explain this dilemma, but in doing so he also sought to preserve as much of the prevailing view on the origin of disease as was possible. He did this in one instance by declaring that:

> it may be observed that the infection in the air does not extend far from the infected object, but lurks chiefly (like that near carrion) to the leeward of it. I am so assured of this, that I have no scruples going, in the open air, to the windward of a person ill of the plague and feeling his pulse.[110]

Almost equally as ingenious was the explanation put forward by Theophilus Lobb. Like Howard, he was convinced that infection was possible only if one actually breathed in a sufficient quantity of infected air. Expanding on this point, Lobb wrote:

> the Danger of being infected with Plague very much depended on the Quantity of infected matter emitted into the Air, and the Nearness of Persons to receive it, before it is so much diluted with the Air, as to have lost its Power of producing the Distemper.[111]

Beyond these speculations, medical thought on plague during the 18th century added little that was really new. After this, plague disappeared from Europe, and as it did, the medical profession, preoccupied with the coming of other disorders, began to lose all interest in what once had been the deadliest of all diseases. Further, as far as the etiology of plague was concerned, it may be said, with some justification, that medical men were just as confused about this disease at the end of its long tenure in Europe as they had been at its beginning.

Historically, plague was a disease that always seemed to act erratically. From the very start, contemporaries regarded it as unpredictable. It entered European society suddenly in the 1340s, disappearing centuries later just as precipitously. Not only did plague come and go rather quickly, it also fluctuated in its impact while it was actively present. This was obvious by 1349 when both forms of the disease, pneumonic and bubonic, even though they are acquired in very different ways, broke out in some of the same localities. Almost arbitrarily, the pneumonic form of plague just faded away in the 1350s. After this, it was difficult to find. The same was not, however, true of bubonic plague. It lived on permanently residing in some places like London, which may very well have been the focal point for the disease in Europe. Every year at least a few people died of it in London, a fact that attests to its endemic presence there. In other cities, such as Basle, plague struck only on widely separated occasions, but usually with much greater force as an epidemic.[112] While sometimes operating endemically, plague could and did at certain crucial times turn extremely virulent as it did in the 1340s and later on in the 17th century.[113] Taking into account the overall history of this disease, it would appear then that plague often acted in an uneven fashion. And what was apparently true of the disease as a whole was also seemingly the case when it came to individual instances of plague. For the overwhelming bulk of symptomatic evidence concerning plague suggests that the disease operated then, as it often does now, in a highly individualistic way.[114] It is true that plague killed in the great majority of cases, but before it did it produced rather vacillating symptoms from one patient to another.

Like all other diseases, plague has a history that is all its own.[115] What determined that particular course of events was not only the environment in which plague operated, but also its own natural history. The great pathogenic agents that have caused so much misery in the European past fall into three possible categories, bacteria, rickettsia and viruses. Plague was, of course, a bacterial disorder. And like most bacterial diseases it proved susceptible to climatic influences, especially temperature. Most physicians in the past knew that plague was a warm-weather disease. This knowledge was substantiated on numerous occasions. The epidemic that struck Bologna in 1630 was most prominent during the months of July and August.[116] The disastrous London plague of 1665 likewise reached its peak during August and continued on into September.[117] In this regard, at least, plague was consistent. For the full fury of the disease did not normally abate until the coming of colder temperatures.[118] Vienna, for instance, was spared in 1679 only with coming of colder weather in November.[119] All three of these outbreaks were the result of bubonic plague, meaning that its spread was simultaneously dependent upon the movement of rats and fleas. Their actions were likewise influenced by temperature and so also was the activity of the pathogen involved here, Pastueurella pestis. Bacteria tend to respond to temperature changes and undoubtedly warmer-type weather likewise effected the metabolism of these highly dangerous microorganisms. Beyond this vital consideration, plague itself may have arisen, gained force and then ultimately declined not only because of environmental factors, but also because some kind of biological imperative had been at work. Men evidently did help to transfer this disease from place to place. But, the life-cycle of the bacteria that caused the plague may just as well explain the recurrent outbreaks of this disease historically as other more commonly held environmental factors.

Like all other bacteria, Pasteurella pestis is subject to mutation at least three percent of the time. Being itself a somewhat arbitrary process, mutation can sometimes weaken a strain, and at other moments make it much more virulent.[120] The periodic decline and then resurgence of plague may perhaps best be explained by the way that bacteria act over extremely long periods of time. The microorganisms that operated in the past may not be the same pathogenic agents that cause plague in Africa and Asia, but more than likely they are probably similar. The question as to why plague came on suddenly and then ultimately disappeared may presumably be explained by examining the life-cycle of the black rat and its final extinction. But, as things now stand, there is very little evidence in existence either about its original susceptibility or its rather astonishing disappearance as a species.[121] Rats may have conveyed fleas to man, but the mystery of plague's coming and going may just as well be tied to the existential history of the bacteria responsible for the disease. The changing nature of the pathogen due to mutation also satisfactorily explains its extraordinary behavior in the past. The arbitrary impact of plague, both socially and individually, so often commented upon in the past, was more than likely caused by the relatively powerful propensity of this microorganism to alter its own biochemical make-up. Its arbitrary impact over time; its tendency to grow first virulent and then harmless, may logically have been due to its own genetic variability.

CHAPTER 2

SYPHILIS

> Whoremongers, Adulterers and
> lascivious Persons must in my
> opinion have been most liable
> to the Diseases of the private
> Parts, as from their proneness
> to Lust they have conversed
> with Strumpets who were
> always very unclean.
>
> --John Astruc, <u>A Treatise of
> the Venereal Disease</u> (Lon-
> don, 1737), Vol. I, p. 41.

During the decade of the 1490s, a highly malignant form of syphilis settled into Europe, disfiguring the faces and bodies of its victims in a way that had never been seen before. Unlike plague, syphilis killed in an outright fashion only occasionally.[1] But far more startling to those unlucky enough to catch it were the unsightly sores that it produced. The rather terrifying psychological toll that this disease exacted from a man's pride was graphically described by one of its more articulate victims, the German man-of-letters, Ulrich von Hütten. Speaking of his ordeal, he declared:

> There were boils, sharp and outstanding, having the
> consistency and quantity of acorns, from which came such
> foul humours, and so great a stench, that whoever smelled it,
> thought himself infected. The colour of these pustules was
> dark green and the sight of them was more grievous to the

patient than the pain itself; and yet their pains were as though one had laid in fire.[2]

The sight of so much ugliness led almost immediately to the banning of syphilitics, many of whom were driven from the cities of Europe because it was thought that they might contaminate others. The Renaissance writer, Desiderius Erasmus, believed that syphilis was a totally unique disease, one that was astonishingly different from anything that Europeans had ever before known. Referring to syphilis, he commented: "Its a most presumptuous pox . . . In a showdown, it wouldn't yield to leprosy, elephantiasis, ringworm, gout or sycosis."[3]

It has never been fully established whether or not syphilis was an ancient disease. For the early history of syphilis is still surrounded by a great deal of controversy. The actual origins of syphilis have always been hidden, so much so that in 1772 N. D. Flack, commenting on the disputes that were raging in his own day, insisted that: "There is perhaps no ailment incident to the human specie, which has caused so much altercation amongst modern physicians, as the Origin of the Venereal Disease."[4] The arguments heard then are still going on right into the second half of the 20th century. In spite of the various interpretations that are still being given, the most commonly accepted explanation for the sudden appearance of malignant syphilis is that it was brought, unknowingly, from the New World to Europe by crewmen sailing with Columbus on his voyages of discovery. This notion, often referred to as the Columbian theory, holds that Columbus' crew became infected with the disease in Haiti and, in turn, passed it on to the population of Spain most probably either in 1493 or 1494.[5] The belief that malignant syphilis actually penetrated Europe at this time was backed by later propagandists like Hütten, who, several decades after these key events, declared: "In the year of Christ 1493 or thereabouts the evil began among the People, not only of France, but originally at Naples in the French camp."[6] Hutten's contention here skips over the more widely accepted belief that the disease was first present in Spain, from where it was quickly passed on to

French troops fighting the Spanish for control of the southern Italian city of Naples.[7] Cases of malignant syphilis were reliably reported in Barcelona months before syphilis actually broke out among French troops in Italy. Moreover, the Spanish physician Francesco Lopez de Villalobos had evidently treated the disease there. Writing about its presence, he described syphilis as a widespread disorder in Spain. He also insisted that its symptoms were entirely novel, saying unhesitantly that: "This was a pestilence, which prior to that time [1493 or 1494] was unknown to poet, man-of-letters, philosopher or historian. None had ever spoke of it before. Malicious, filthy, cruel to the excess and very contagious, it was a terrible disease, impossible to conquer."[8]

From Spain, the disease was evidently carried to southern Italy. There, the spread of the disease became entwined with the political history of the Italian peninsula. In the early part of 1494, Ferdinand, king of Naples, died without leaving an heir. The throne was immediately claimed by Charles VIII, king of France. In the latter part of 1494, Charles invaded Italy to insure his claim, marching south with a combined force of French nationals and foreign mercenaries. His army of 30,000 men included not only French troops, but Dutch, Swiss, Spanish, Italian, English, Hungarian and Slavic soldiers, most of them free-booters.[9] During the military campaign for Naples, syphilis was apparently transferred from the Spanish to the French, initially by a group of high-priced Courtesans.[10] The disease quickly spread through Charles' army, decimating it even as it started to retreat back up the peninsula.[11] As was common at this time, Charles' army was trailed by a group of hangers-on, including according to one source, some 500 prostitutes, most of whom presumably helped to spread the disease to the civilian population. The symptoms of syphilis were so grotesque and so dreadfully easy to identify that the progress of the disease was astonishingly simple for observers to follow.[12] Few other diseases historically were capable of producing such grizzly sights, with intense pain, ulceration and the actual eating away of flesh being quite common. The 16th-century English physician William Clowes has left a truly memorable description of one of his syphilitic patients, a description that must have been repeated thousands of times during the heyday of malignant syphilis. Clowes wrote:

> He had upon his head a mightie great node, which dyd corrupt the bones through both the tables [skull]: his throte and the roof of his mouth was deeply infected with evil ulcers of hard curation. . . . He had painful hard swellings upon his legges commonly called the shinne bones, were with the mallis of this sickness, corrupted and perforated very deeply in certain places, so that they were for the most part, taken away.[13]

The disturbing advance of syphilis up the Italian peninsula rather reminds one of plague's conquering movement along a similar route some 150 years earlier. Most contemporary accounts insist that the epidemic did indeed begin in Naples. The Spanish observer, Juan de Vigo, for example, was certainly shocked by the number of cases of disease left behind in Naples right after the departure of Charles' army. Since the disease, or so it seemed to him, started among French troops, de Vigo kept referring to syphilis as the French disease, thereby blaming them rather than the Spanish both for its origin and its spread. That condemnation lived on for centuries. For from here on in, syphilis would be popularly known as the French pox. As it moved its way up the Italian peninsula, the presence of syphilis was noted by one chronicler after another, first in Rome and then Perugia, Bologna, Verona and finally Venice. All of them reported the exact same symptoms. Typically, according to Natale Montesauro, victims of the disease fell ill with excruciating pain throughout the body, followed by the classic appearance of sores that soon began to ulcerate.[14] The precise number of those contracting the disease has been historically impossible to determine. However, the growing volume of commentaries at this time readily attested to its unrelenting spread. Throughout the 1490s, syphilis remained a perplexing disease for those who had been trying to treat it. Like many others, de Vigo was able to describe its symptoms, but its origin remained undefined. At first most did not even observe that the disease was primarily venereal. Still, when it struck it produced an all-pervading sense of disillusionment, a feeling suggested by de Vigo when he wrote:

> In the year of our Lord 1494 in the month of December there appeared a certain disease throughout all Italy of an unknown nature which sundry nations have called by sundry names. This disease is contagious with little pustules which could not be healed by medicine applied within or without. Furthermore, a month after the said pustules the patient was vexed with great pain in the head, the shoulders, the arms and the legs, after which . . . hard things like bones were engendered in the patient with exceeding pain in the night which ceased during the daytime. [15]

De Vigo's symptomatic findings were confirmed by a number of other equally well-known accounts, including the famous Chronicle of Perugia written a short while before this. From this evidence, it is abundantly clear that syphilis acted very differently than plague. For it produced symptoms that were ruthlessly similar from one patient to another.[16]

In a matter of months, Charles VIII's army had pushed its way out of Italy leaving behind a mounting human toll. His army had already begun to disintegrate long before he ever reached his intended destination of Lyons. Moreover, his army was still evidently carrying the disease, for cases of syphilis were now breaking out in France, Germany and Switzerland. By 1496, syphilis, with all of its ugly and frightening consequences, was now commonplace in Holland. In the following year, it entered both England and Scotland. By the late 1490s syphilis had also veered eastward, with both Hungary and Russia having reported its sudden awesome appearance.[17] A few decades after the introduction of malignant syphilis, Girolamo Fracastoro, the Veronese physician and historian, confirmed what everybody already knew that the disease was by then universal in Europe. Writing in 1530, he referred to syphilis as "a contagion which small in the beginning, but soon gaining strength and matter on by degree spread itself throughout all lands."[18] A little before this, around 1500, most town councils, like most doctors at the time, were still unaware that the disease was a venereal disorder. On the other hand, they did regard it as extraordinarily contagious. They, therefore, took drastic steps to isolate the unsightly victims of this disease from those who were still healthy. In the past, local officials had handled the victims of leprosy and then plague by ostracizing them both physically and morally. Not too surprisingly, syphilitics were recipients of similar treatment. In 1496, for example, anyone found to have syphilitic pustules on the body was summarily driven from the city limits of Paris.[19] Other town councils were soon acting in an equally draconian way. In a number of German cities, public baths were promptly suspected as the centers for the transfer of this disease. Motivated by this suspicion, both Nuremberg and Würzberg banned all known syphilitics from using them.[20] Yet another German city, Augsburg, went much further, establishing in 1497, a <u>Blaterhaus</u>, a virtual prison, to house all of its syphilitic cases.[21]

After penetrating the major urban areas of France and Germany in a very punishing way, syphilis next moved on to England and Scotland. It arrived in those two countries in epidemic form in the late 1490s, claiming untold victims. Even before this, however, there were some scattered references to the disease's presence in England. The East Anglican Chronicler Wyllam Amfflays, writing about events occurring in 1494 asserted that: "In this year beganne the ffrence pockes."[22] Scotland, like England, in commercial touch with the Continent, seems to have known the disease on a wide scale by the late 1490s. And once again the military was implicated in the spread of this malignant disease. Theory has it that syphilis was brought to Edinburgh by a disorganized band of mercenaries, some 1,400 followers of the military adventurer Perkin Warbeck. In any event, shortly after their arrival in the Scottish capital, the disease was running rampant. The king, James IV, immediately issued a decree ordering all "incurables," as they were known, to be seized and taken forcibly to the island of Inchkeith so as to protect the King's "lieges fra this seikness."[23] As syphilis made its way from one country to another, impressions about it naturally began to build up. The number of people killed by malignant syphilis does not appear to have been great, although there were fears that it would act in the same way as plague. Albrecht Dürer, the German portrait and landscape painter, was one of the many who anticipated this happening.[24] Much more hideous than it was murderous, syphilis turned out to be no respecter whatsoever of either person or place. It attacked both rich and poor at the same time.[25] Virulent on its own, human folly significantly contributed to the further spread of this disease. Those who were afflicted with syphilis, covered as they were by grotesque boils and ulcerated flesh, were evidently so hideous to others that they were often driven from sight. As a consequence, country roads were packed with syphilitics, wandering from one locale to another and in the process helping to spread the disease ever further.

By the early 1500s, the suspicion began to grow that syphilis was radically different from leprosy and plague and that it was actually being spread by sexual intercourse. Prior to this, it had always been assumed that syphilis was dangerously contagious, but not necessarily venereal. There was at the start no reason to suspect this possible cause. After all, plague had also produced ugly and disfiguring sores on the body, but no one had ever assumed that it was venereal in origin. Medical opinion about syphilis, initially at least, fell back on tradition believing as always that "the source and seat of the evil must exist in the air."[26] This customary, but unproductive view, soon gave way to more exacting evidence that kept pointing out that the disease was unquestionably sexual. De Vigo, among the first to treat the disease, was increasingly convinced, along with other physicians, that syphilis was being passed on through its pustules and that the genitalia were directly involved in producing the infection.[27] Von Hütten put it more bluntly, saying: "In Women the Disease resteth in their secret Places, wherein are little pretty sores, full of venomous Poison, being very dangerous for such as unknowingly meddle with them."[28] Women were now being singled out for condemnation as the potential carriers of this extremely disgusting disease. By the 1510s, syphilis had become fully identified with women, especially those who were now being classified as bad and evil. The age quickly assumed, thereafter, that it was immoral women who were passing on this fearsome disorder and, what was even worse, they were doing it surreptitiously, for "the most commonly held opinion about the cause of venereal chancre is that . . . it is debauched women who manage to hide it in their vaginas."[29] It was not a matter of coincidence that the Puritan ethic was born at this time. For the fear of syphilis among Europeans had grown to such proportions that chastity was increasingly being seen as the only acceptable way of preventing syphilis from entering a family-line.

Popular attitudes toward immoral women, if the literature of the day is a test, turned vicious and cruel. In one of his more famous colloquies, Erasmus rather neatly expressed a generations growing animosity toward promiscuous women who, it was held, kept inflicting this degenerate disease both upon themselves and others. In a then well-known dialogue between a repentant blade and his former mistress, now a harlot, Erasmus poignantly warned the young lady that:

Thou makest thyself a common sewer, into which all the base, nasty, pocky Fellows resort, and empty their Filthiness and if not [the] leprous infection they called the French pox hasn't seized thee, thou will not escape it long. And if once thou gettist it how miserable wilt thou be, though all things go favourably on thy Side, I mean thy Substance and Reputation. Thou wouldst be nothing but a living Carcase.[30]

According to one of the leading medical thinkers of the 16th century, Ambroise Paré, syphilis was definitely a sexual disorder.[31] By the 1520s, this belief about the disease was firmly established in the popular mind. It was also subsequently surrounded by myths and tales. The most popular myth of the day, as related by Joannes Manardus and others, told of how a noble prostitute from Valencia had originally sold herself to a leprous cavalier, who in turn, somewhat ingraciously, had infected her with "the

French disease." Within a matter of months, the story had it, she had successfully passed the disease on to hundreds of youths, many of whom were members of the army of Charles VIII.[32]

   While it is true that syphilis was increasingly identified in the popular mind with sexual promiscuity, the disease may not have been a purely venereal one. Circumstantial evidence, accumulated during the epidemic of the 1490s and early 1500s, strongly suggests that the bacteria involved here, Treponema pallidum, may have been so extraordinarily virulent that it could easily have been transferred to others merely by touch. The highly respected English physician, William Clowes, was personally convinced from what he saw that the disease could be passed on by eating with infected persons, by lying with them or by touching their bedding.[33] Lending further evidence to this possibility was von Hütten's own demoralizing experience with syphilis, for he contracted the disease at the age of eight, long before the normal age for sexual intercourse.[34] Beyond these two examples, there were other bits and pieces of information suggesting that syphilis could, indeed, be acquired by extragenital means. The most likely way in which it was transferred, other than sexually, was as a result of bleeding. Bleeding was, in the 16th century, a common medical practice. It was not only performed by physicians, but also by barber-surgeons in the numerous bath houses dotting the cities of Europe, usually in the form of cupping. The term cupping simply referred to the well-established practice of lancing sores, something that was commonly done in these bath houses. The scalpels that were used over and over again for lancing were evidently not kept very clean. Even worse, the microorganisms involved here were proving so powerful that they were also being transmitted from one bather to another simply by means of touch. While most of these assumptions here are admittedly speculative, bathhouses in Frankfurt, Nuremberg and Brünn were, at the time, all directly linked to the spread of syphilis. Along with many others, Thomas Jordanus observed that the punishing outbreak of malignant syphilis in the city of Brünn in 1578 was directly traceable to the city's bathhouse.[35] So much evidence, attesting to these occurrences, was piling up in this period, that the extragenital transmission of syphilis may have been taking place.

If the etiological origins of syphilis were continually baffling to those living during the first half of the 16th century, its geographical origins were not. For most Europeans were by the 1520s and 1530s overwhelmingly convinced that the disease had come to Europe from America. It is true, that many of the early chroniclers like Joseph Grünpeck had initially referred to syphilis as the French disease.[36] But the very novelty of the disease along with its surprising impact kept troubling others, like the Spaniard de Villalobos, who was personally convinced that the disease had originated outside of Europe.[37] By the 1520s and 1530s, a rather influential group of Spanish historians had come to the conclusion that it had been imported from the New World and that Columbus' crew had been responsible for planting it in Spain. The evidence that they were able to put together in favor of this thesis was, to say the least, massive.[38] It was, and had been for centuries, so convincing that one of the leading 20th-century historians of the disease, the German Iwan Bloch, could not resist summing it all up dogmatically, insisting, as he did, that: "Syphilis was unknown in Europe before the year 1493. Its home is America, or, as far as Europe is concerned, the island of Espænola or Haiti, whence the crew of Columbus brought it after the latter's voyage."[39] Syphilis may actually have existed in Europe before 1493 in a much more disguised form, but this possibility was almost never taken into account. For, as far as this age was concerned, syphilis was indisputably American, and Columbian, in origin.

The three Spanish historians of the early 16th century who contributed the most to the development of the Columbian theory were Ruy Dias de Isla, Gonzalo Fernandez de Oviedo and Batholome de la Casas. Dias de Isla had been a practicing physician in both Barcelona and Lisbon in the 1490s, where he acquired a great deal of first-hand experience treating cases of malignant syphilis. Moreover, de Isla was in Barcelona in 1493 at the time of Columbus' triumphant return from the New

World.[40]   There, he saw the disease for the first time, stating in his historical memoirs that: "Of the disease I had much experience, for I had the care of persons from the first expedition to America, and I treated them for the disease at Barcelona."[41]   Yet another Spanish writer, de Oviedo, came up with formidable evidence, drawn from his own experience, supporting the Columbian theory.   De Oviedo was by training a diplomat, who made any number of trips to the West Indies.   During his travels, he became convinced that syphilis had indeed originated in the Caribbean for he saw innumerable cases of the disease there although usually in a much milder form.[42]   Visiting Italy when the disease was rampaging out of control, de Oviedo commented, somewhat knowingly: "Many times in Italy I laughed, hearing the Italians speak of the French disease and the French called it the disease of Naples; and in truth both would have had the name better, if they called it the disease of the Indies."[43]   De Oviedo went on to establish the Columbian connection even more firmly, not only in his own mind but also for future generations.   Writing years later in his Natural History of the Indies, he declared:

> The first time that this malady was seen in Spain was after the Admiral, Don Christobel Colon [Columbus] had discovered the Indies and returned.   Then in the year 1495, when the grand Captain Gonzales Hernandes de Cordoba took an army to Naples to the aid of Don Fernando, by the order of Ferdinand and Isabella of immortal memory, they carried the malady with them.[44]

The Spanish cleric and historian de la Casas proceeded, after this, to confirm the findings of de Isla and de Oviedo even more convincingly. Like de Oviedo, de la Casas had extensive knowledge of the West Indies. Intensely curious about the true origin of syphilis, de la Casas periodically questioned the local Indians concerning the disease's presence among them. Telling of his experience, de la Casas commented:

I took the trouble on several occasions to interrogate the
Indians of the Island (Haiti) as to whether this disease was of
great antiquity, and they answered "Yes," that it dated from a
period long before the advent of the Christians, the origin of it
beyond the memory of any men, and nobody can disbelieve
this.[45]

For hundreds of years after this, educated Europeans automatically
assumed that syphilis had been brought to Europe as a result of the
voyages of discovery. One writer summed up that conclusion poetically.
Seeking to explain all of the consequences of Columbus' monumental
accomplishment, he declared: "Columbus discovered a continent of many
isles, with treasures of gold and silver. But amongst the precious metals
was a thorn . . . For the trireme [three ships] of Columbus carried the Mal
Français to Europe."[46] Between the 1490s and the 1550s, European
society was supremely conscious of the presence of syphilis. Having been
made aware of the unsightly and horrifying effects of malignant syphilis,
Europeans were understandably eager to explain to themselves the
sudden appearance of this truly frightening disease. They accepted the
Columbian explanation largely because all the circumstantial evidence at
their disposal kept pointing to the Caribbean as the source of this disease.

It took the medical profession in Europe literally centuries to identify
all of the symptoms that are now classically associated with syphilis.
During the era when it was still malignant, it was initially thought to be
primarily a painful skin disorder. The characteristic boils and festering
sores that the disease produced certainly fooled de Villalobos into
believing that it was exclusively a disease of the skin.[47] De Villalobos'
contemporary, de Vigo, likewise focused on these skin eruptions, instantly
classifying syphilis in the same category as such other Medieval skin
infections as scabies and leprosy.[48] Both men actually looked right past
the characteristic first stage of the disease, normally a chancre sore
erupting on or in the genitalia. This diagnosis was admittedly difficult to
make in this day and age, especially when one considers that skin

disorders of almost every imaginable type were exceedingly common. Syphilis itself is caused by a bacteria, <u>Treponema</u> <u>pallidum</u>. This particular bacteria has a strange, indeed, somewhat schizophrenic character, for its survival largely depends upon the environment in which it finds itself. Outside of the human body it is a delicate organism, so fragile that it easily dies. By contrast, inside of the body it is extraordinarily powerful, innately capable of preying on its host for long periods of time. Both the malignant syphilis of the 16th century and the congenital or chronic form that succeeded it historically were individually capable of passing through three distinct stages of development. Two of those stages were overt and obvious, the third subcutaneous and, for several centuries, virtually impossible to discern. The first stage of syphilis, usually appearing one or two weeks after the original infection, was then and is now characterized by a hard chancre emerging on the genitalia, a sore that quickly begins to ulcerate.[49] The German Alexander Grünpeck noticed this initial stage of the disease in the late 1490s, but it took several decades before his insight into the actual course of the disease became universally accepted.[50] By the 1550s, however, what the then famous French physician Ambroise Paré described as "the pustule of the testes" was being progressively recognized as the true beginning of syphilis in most patients.[51]

The second and third stages of syphilis, it is now known, are radically different from one another. These two stages are so unique that it took nearly three hundred and fifty years before the medical profession perceived that they were part of the same syphilitic syndrome. The second stage of malignant syphilis was and is much more sensational than the first. For in its second stage, malignant syphilis is characterized by extremely painful constitutional symptoms.[52] These symptoms, which include intense headaches, pains in the bones and ugly swellings all over the body, were by 1500 in Europe being unmistakably identified as characteristic of syphilitic attack. Although, the chancre was at this time being steadily identified as the true start of this disease, syphilis was thought to have taken full hold only with the eruption of sores and lesions. In the words of one physician diagnosing cases of syphilis in the early 16th century, only with "nodes and bumps like young claves' horns, sprouting out about the skull, may you safely pronounc him poxed."[53] These lesions soon began to ulcerate creating a sight so frightening that some physicians actually refused to treat syphilitics. In the year 1578, an outbreak of malignant syphilis occurred, without warning, in the Moravian city of Brünn. During that localized epidemic, Jordanus described the symptoms that he saw, in particular those that are now known to be a feature of the second stage of malignant syphilis. Pointing to the abcesses that he saw most often, he remarked:

> the discharge was corrosive. The flesh surrounding the boils . . . became foul and corroded and gave forth a stench. . . .In many the entire body was covered with pustules, the countenance was horrifying to look at. The back, chest, abdomen, feet, indeed the whole body from head to toes was defiled by scabs and itchiness, with crusted ulcers. . . . From these oozes a thick sluggish mucous. When the scabs fall away and the lesions heal, there are left dark spots, of a greyish or brownish color.[54]

As Jordanus reported so graphically, the ugly and painful ulceration eventually healed. Once these sores were gone, it was commonly believed for centuries, both in and out of the medical profession, that the disease was cured and that the patient had recovered. All that it really meant, medical science in the last part of the 19th century finally realized, was that the pathogen had gone deeper into the body and had become insidiously latent. The bacteria at work here, Treponema pallidum, was perfectly capable of long periods of dormancy. But, periodically, it was equally capable of reviving, irritating and inflaming, in turn, certain body organs, along with the arterial system and the nerves covering the spinal chord and brain.[55] This mysterious tertiary stage of syphilis was never actually discovered until late in the 19th century. It was only then that modern-day autopsies were able to prove that the bacterium that caused syphilis lived on long past the disease's first two easily recognizable stages. Taking into account the symptomatic evidence that appeared over and over again in the chronicles, there is little reason to doubt that the epidemic that first broke out in 1490s was, in fact, malignant syphilis. After a stay of nearly 60 years, however, this highly virulent form of syphilis began to disappear among Europeans. After this, it became extraordinarily rare. In the 19th century, one Munich doctor, specializing in venereal cases, recorded that of the 12,000 syphilitics that he had treated, he had seen only four cases of malignant syphilis.[56] Today, malignant syphilis, while still infrequent, does occur often enough to be able to check its symptoms against those of the past. Much more is, of course, now known about this extreme form of the disease. Sometimes referred to as galloping syphilis from the way it spreads through the body, malignant syphilis still leads to headaches, ulceration and pains in the bones. All of these symptoms were described innumerable times by 16th-century chroniclers interested in mapping the disease's growing dominance in Europe.[57]

The cause of syphilis, an unsolved mystery in Europe for long centuries, was finally uncovered in 1905. In that year, the microorganism responsible for the disease was discovered by the German bacteriologist Fritz Schaudinn. Working in close conjunction with Erich Hofman at the world-renowned Imperial Health Institute in Berlin, Schaudinn was the first to identify the spiral-shaped bacterium responsible for syphilis, a microorganism known more precisely as a spirochaete. Shortly after this, Schaudinn and others began to describe the bacteria that he had discovered by its more common scientific name, Treponema pallidum.[58] The discovery of this microorganism ended long decades of baffling speculation about the cause of syphilis. One observer, taking note of the ever expanding number of explanations that had been piling up, caustically remarked that no less than: "One hundred and twenty-five causes had been established during the last 25 years."[59] For nearly 400 years prior to Schaudinn's breakthrough, the more modern form of chronic syphilis had been steadily spreading through European society. Throughout that era, medical men had precious little at their disposal with which to fight the disease. It is true that for several hundred years, the medical profession thought that it had a cure in mercury, a product which it had been using externally as a salve and internally as a compound. Like many physicians, the noted English medical pioneer, John Hunter had unhesitantly praised mercury for its curative powers, saying at one point that: "Mercury in the lues venera [syphilis], as in the chancre, is the great specific and hardly any thing else is to be depended upon."[60] In spite of its reputation, mercury was not a dependable drug. Too often it was used in the wrong way, and when it was, it proved to be astonishingly toxic.[61]

Schuadinn's and Hofman's widely acclaimed discovery of the syphilitic pathogen led almost immediately to several other major breakthroughs. In the following year, 1906, August von Wasserman, a noted Berlin toxicologist, significantly advanced the cause of medical detection by devising a blood test, which in numerous instances, was capable of determining the disease's presence in previously undiagnosed cases.[62] The introduction of this unique laboratory technique was followed a few years later by the development of modern chemotherapy in the hands of Schaudinn's fellow national, Paul Ehrlich. In 1912, Ehrlich succeeding in producing a compound based on arsenic that was apparently capable of limiting, and even sometimes arresting, the advance of syphilis within the body.[63] The medical war against syphilis was at least partially being won in the years prior to World War I. The final victory, however, did not come until the 1940s when antibiotics were successfully used for the first time to subdue the disease.[64] These modern means of identification, detection and cure came, of course, too late for millions of Europeans who had already succumbed to syphilis. Just exactly how many Europeans had experienced this progressively debilitating disease over the centuries is a figure that will never be known. Not even the number of those who came down with syphilis during its first great epidemic sweep in the 1490s has been accurately estimated. One thing, however, is clear: during its congenital or chronic stage, which came after the 1550s, it was probably far more widespread than most commentators have previously reported. Precisely how extensive the disease actually was in European society was finally revealed in the 19th century in the growing number of hospital records, detailing the disease's presence, that were then being published.

In the decade of the 1550s in Europe, the malignant form of syphilis underwent a gigantic metamorphosis, one that turned it into a much milder disorder.[65] The terrifying symptoms of an earlier period that had disfigured so many were from here on in seen only rarely. For malignant syphilis was now being replaced by what came to be known as congenital syphilis, but which would be described more properly as chronic or latent syphilis. Chronic syphilis was a much more subtle disease than its malignant predecessor. It still produced a chancre, but its follow-up symptoms were mild, usually not much more than isolated spotting or swelling of the lymph nodes. Once these symptoms, so characteristic of the first and second stages of the disease, vanished, the disorder was still exceedingly dangerous. Few physicians in the past, however, saw it that way. They believed that the disease was cured once the symptoms faded.[66] Because the tertiary form of syphilis was for them impossible to detect, the widespread presence of this lingering disease in European society was not even suspected by medical men. Doctors, on the other hand, did see enough of syphilis to know that it was communicable. Fearing its potential spread, government agencies and charitable institutions did try to take decisive action. In the 17th century, for example, syphilitics were legally banned from all Parisian hospitals. But later, investigations proved that they were nearly always there, usually infecting others.[67] In the 18th century, some Russian doctors, perhaps more observant than others, began to suspect that syphilis was making substantial headway among that country's peasant population.[68] Meanwhile, epidemics of the disease were also taking place, although sporadically. The two Norwegian cities of Bergen and Christiana were both struck by an epidemic of malignant syphilis in the 1750s. Victims of the disease were covered with sores and ulcers in a way that reminded some of the disease's original onslaught in the 1490s.[69] At the very same time, some rural areas in France seemed inundated with the disease. Peasant girls were particularly susceptible, they, in turn, often infecting local military garrisons.[70]   Meanwhile, syphilis was a growing social problem in a number of French cities, including Bayeux in Normandy and Lyons much further to the south.[71]   None of this, of course, adds up to a coherent picture, but bits and pieces of evidence recently brought to light do suggest that syphilis was over the course of generations silently making its way through European society.

Just how extensive syphilis actually was did not become apparent until the 19th century, when government and hospital records began to reveal its presence more accurately than ever before. These reports, taken together, suggest that syphilis had been functioning in the past in a very subterranean way, more than likely growing more dominant from the 1550s on with each passing century. This last point, admittedly, cannot be finally proven until more studies investigating its presence in pre-industrial times are completed. But, what can be established, to some degree, through the more thorough record-keeping of the 19th century is that syphilis had by then grown to such a point that it constituted an extremely serious social problem. Before this, the diagnosis of syphilis in the 18th and early 19th centuries had always been hampered by the prevailing medical belief that syphilis was a curable disorder. Even the occasional case of malignant syphilis was deemed to be readily curable.[72] The third, and potentially deadly stage of syphilis, was never even recognized, much less taken into account. Even as late as 1886, Vienna's main General Hospital was able to boast that 93 percent of all the syphilitic cases it admitted were eventually discharged as completely cured.[73] This conclusion was possible because the focus of the medical profession, as it had been since the Middle Ages, was still on observable symptoms, and once these outward signs disappeared patients were thought to be free of the disease. In this age, medical men, given the limited scientific knowledge of the time, had no way of even guessing that syphilis was in actuality a deep-seated and not a short-lived disorder. Given these conditions, misdiagnosis was virtually inevitable and the case of one Michael Whelan admitted to the Lock Hospital in Dublin in 1813 was just one example of the inability of medicine to see this disease in all of its ramifications. His particular report ran:

Michael Whelan was admitted April 19th, 1813. His complaints were superficial ulcers on the corona and glans; a large ulcerated bubo in the right groin, of a projecting fungoes appearance, and a papular eruption on his breast, back and face. . . . He complained also of pains in his shoulders, elbows and ankles. . . . The lotion of muriate of mercury and lime-water, [along with] antimonial solution were directed for him. (May 3rd). The ulcers of the penis were healed, and the pains lessened . . . he was discharged the hospital cured on the 23rd of the same month [May].[74]

Even though the medical profession as a whole was not conscious of the disease's tertiary stage, enough cases of symptomatic syphilis were encountered by health officials to approximate its somewhat subtle presence in 19th and 20th-century society. Some medical men were, in fact, beginning to note its spread very early on. In the late 1840s, the Bulletin of the French Medical Society issued a major report warning all physicians that syphilis was definitely on the rise in French society.[75] That report could have just as easily been published by any one of the leading urban hospitals in Europe, for they were all being made acutely aware of the presence of syphilis. In 1861, for instance, syphilis was the leading cause of admission to the Steeven Hospital in Dublin, followed thereafter by bronchitis, a disease most believed to be far more prevalent than syphilis.[76] This trend continued; two decades after this, a thorough examination of the records of the Rudolphean General Hospital in Vienna proved that syphilis was the second leading cause of confinement, trailing only tuberculosis, the great killer of the age.[77] In comparison with other diseases like cholera and tuberculosis, syphilis did not through its long history appear to kill in an outright fashion. St. Bartholomew's Hospital, one of the best known in all of London, annually took in about 100 syphilitics. But the death-rate among them was really quite low, an average of only one percent a year.[78] Yet, even past the turn of the 20th century, syphilis continued to be a serious medical problem, with the hospitals of the day compelled to treat hundreds of thousands of cases each year. Beyond this, the amount of symptomatic syphilis, the only kind that could be identified diagnostically, among pregnant women in certain hospitals had apparently reached truly staggering proportions. For example, of the 1,460 pregnant women admitted to Glascow's Royal Maternity and Women's Hospital in 1926, 48 of them were found to be syphilitics. By comparison, only two in this group were discovered to have tuberculosis, supposedly the most widespread disease of the times.[79] These figures were all the more ominous when one considers that advanced research into syphilis had by the 1920s already proven that up to one-half of all cases of latent syphilis were still not being diagnosed short of surgery.

Probably, the most pitiful victims of syphilis were the young. The disease was thought to run in certain families, but exactly how the disease was being passed on from one generation to another was not clear to the medical profession during most of the 19th century. However, its disintegrating consequences were being recognized more and more. Demented children were, in some instances, the result of congenital syphilis being passed from mother to child, a process which was not then even remotely suspected. A prime example of the impact that this disease could have on the young was reported by the General Hospital for Sick Children in Manchester. This one child's overall medical report ran:

Congenital Syphilis Dementia. John Ed. W., aged 3 3/4 years. No history of Syphilis in mother; this is only child. Father weak in mind and body, addicted to drink, has had Syphilis 6 months ago, and probably previously also. Patient had rash and snuffles [noisy breathing] when 2 months old; rash led to sores on the buttocks; he had attacks similar to present one at intervals; present attack has lasted for 8 months, never seems to be himself and does not understand what is said to him, . . . no rigidity of limbs, but arms are liable to sudden spasm when moved; constantly crying and howling, makes no intelligible sound; appears to be almost devoid of understanding, gait unsteady, often walks backwards and now and then jumps about and clasps his hands.[80]

The bacteria at work here was now obviously attacking the boy's nervous system, one of the sure signs, by the way, of tertiary syphilis.

Medical perceptions about syphilis did steadily improve as the 19th century moved along. One of the most commonly held beliefs about this disease in the early 1800s was that syphilis ran in certain families and that more than likely it was inherited. This notion was eventually discarded once it was finally perceived that the disease was being picked up congenitally, sometimes in the womb and sometimes in the birth-tract at the time of delivery. Physicians were also becoming more conscious of the ways in which the disease acted in adults. A number of new discoveries were made by the French surgeon, Philippe Ricord, who had the unique advantage of being able to work at the highly specialized Venereal Hospital in Paris, where he was able to observe the victims of syphilis over long periods. Ricord noticed, among other things, that syphilis usually attacked young adults for the first time between the ages of 17 and 28, only to reoccur in some years later. Supposedly cured patients were reporting back to the hospital with relapsed cases of the disease.[81] This characteristic of syphilis, which was, of course, the tertiary stage of the disease asserting itself all over again was noticed more and more by others as the century went on. But, even up to the early 1900s, it was not clear to the medical profession whether this was the result of reinfection from the outside or the revitalization of bacteria already housed in the body. Syphilis was now, however, definitely known to reoccur, and progressively more instances like the one reported by the Manchester doctor S. Messenger Bradley were, in fact, coming to the conscious attention of the medical profession. Still a little surprised by the disease's return, Bradley reported on one of the these cases saying:

He was a spare man, forty years old, who ten years before had contracted syphilis, for which he had been treated non-mercurially. The secondary symptoms which ensued were of an ordinary and not very grave nature, but after an interval of apparent cure, which lasted over four years, he began, about the middle of 1873, to notice a gradual and painless enlargement of the cartilaginous part, which very slowly increased up to the time when I first saw him.[82]

Even if all of the symptoms of syphilis were not in the 1870s and 1880s totally known, its actual presence in European society was being increasingly mapped and pointed out largely as a result of improved record keeping. For not only was its advancing presence in the civilian population being detected more accurately by hospital records, its rather extensive presence was also being discovered through investigations being conducted by the military. The long-standing connection between the military and syphilis, previously often suspected, was finally confirmed in the 19th century by military records. British troops, fighting the French in Spain, were generally known to be carrying the disease, although the true extent of the disease in their ranks has never been absolutely established.[83] Far more exact information was, however, compiled later on especially in regard to the incidences of syphilis among German forces on occupation duty in 1871 after the Franco-Prussian War. A rather thorough-going medical investigation of German soldiers in France in July of 1871 showed that of 97,333 men, 1,478 had external signs of syphilis. Moreover, in August and September of the same year, the Department of the Army discovered a total of 1,307 and 996 fresh cases respectively.[84] Considering just how long the disease tended to reside in the body and that the tertiary stage still could not be distinguished, these figures were a shock. The wide-scale presence of syphilis in the German army was paralleled, both before and after this, by records published by the British navy. A study done in 1859 of 61 British warships, with crews totalling 19,300 men, revealed that 1,442 of them were overtly suffering from syphilis.[85] Beyond this, the problem, first revealed in 1859, hardly subsided. For in 1905, yet another inquiry showed that of 108,190 men in the British navy, 6,480 were known to have gonorrhea and another 5,041 were suffering from either the primary or secondary stage of syphilis.[86] Even in the face of growing medical knowledge about this disease, syphilis was the only major infection that actually flourished among troops during World War I.[87] Any kind of analysis of the amount of syphilis in the pre-war German army and British navy would have made this development seem quite likely.

From the literary evidence that has accumulated in the past, it would seem that syphilis, both in its older malignant form and its more modern congenital or chronic form, was never really an unrelenting killer. The commentaries from bygone eras suggest that it was disabling, but not particularly deadly. Even in 19th-century London, Europe's largest city, the number of those reportedly dying from syphilis was extremely low, between 1858 and 1870 on average only about 350 a year.[88] Ostensively then, death from syphilis was not all that common historically - or was it? By the 1920s, the medical profession had, at long last, learned to look past the disease's external symptoms. Investigating the deep-seated physiological consequences of syphilis, coroners and researchers were now looking for both organic and neurological damage as a tell-tale sign of the disease's presence. As methods for detecting the tertiary stage of syphilis improved, so, somewhat interestingly, did the actual number of deaths attributed to the disease. By 1925, in Germany alone, 5.7 percent of all autopsies being done revealed the unmistakable presence of organic syphilis.[89] If this particular figure was speculatively extended to the whole of the European population in the 1920s, it would have meant that there were 25 million syphilitics in the society. Given this highly revealing statistic from Germany, one can only imagine how many millions of Europeans may have died in previous centuries from equally undiagnosed cases of deep-seated syphilis.

Few diseases have been more difficult to trace both medically and historically than syphilis. This inability was, in part, the result of a long-standing pattern of medical thinking that kept associating disease with readily observable symptoms. If those external symptoms were not there, the disease was automatically assumed to have gone away. During the very last part of the 19th century, syphilis was discovered to be an asymptomatic disease, meaning essentially that its symptoms were more internal than external. Once this aspect of syphilis was uncovered, the medical profession was much more willing to admit that numerous cases of the disease were still, practically-speaking, eluding them. As late as 1944, just prior to the discovery of antibiotics capable of reaching syphilis in the deepest recesses of the body, conscientious medical opinion was still obviously aware how difficult it actually was to search out this particular disease. Writing at the end of World War II and addressing himself specifically to the neurological form of the disease, Dr. Bernhard Dattner cautioned that:

> Neurosyphilis represents many problems in diagnosis and treatment. There are patients whose chancres date back twenty or thirty years and even more, but who nevertheless do not manifest the slightest signs of the disease even when the most thorough examination is performed. However, when one realizes that syphilis of the central nervous system is eminently a chronic disease, the later effects of which sometimes become apparent in old age, one will understand how important it is for the physician to make certain whether the chronic inflammatry process is still going on, smouldering beneath the surface, or whether it is already arrested.[90]

If modern medical science was still perplexed in the 1940s by this disease, then the highly imaginative explanations of syphilis commonly put forward in the past, and obviously born of ignorance, become a little more understandable. The 18th century, for example, was very much removed from any real answers about syphilis. As a consequence many of the explanations that they gave for the presence of syphilis really fall into the category of speculation. As an illustration, the well-known Italian doctor

Georgi Baglivi assumed, along with numerous others, that both gonorrhea and syphilis were glandular diseases. He came to this particular conclusion by examining the disease's characteristic inflammations and eruptions, most of which, he observed, were relatively close to the body's glandular system.[91] The Englishman John Hunter came somewhat closer to the truth when he insisted that the disease was a constitutional disorder. But, instead of seeing that the disease was capable of retreating further into the body, he believed that "the venereal pus" surfaced again, after the disappearance of the chancre to do more localized damage on the surface of the skin. According to his assessment:

> The venereal poison is capable of affecting the body in two different ways; locally, that is, in those parts only to which it is first applied [the genitalia]; and constitutionally, that is in consequence of the absorption of the venereal pus. . . . When the matter has got into the constitution, and is circulating with the blood, it there irritates to action. There are produced from that irritation many local diseases, as blotches on the skin, ulcers in the tonsils, thickening of the . . . bones.[92]

In actuality, even the physical method by which syphilis was acquired still remained a mystery to some physicians in the 18th century. One of them, N. D. Flack, for instance, argued that it originated with women who acquired "an ulceration in the vagina," resulting from "excessive friction" and "promiscuous venery." It was passed on by such a woman, according to Flack, to a "man who copulates with her, particularly if he is young and fiery, and especially if he ejaculates; though she herself may not strictly be said to have the disorder, which she communicates."[93] The widely-held notion that syphilis was the direct consequence of promiscuity led the Frenchman, Jean Astruc, in the 1730s to denounce those who kept the disease going. Arguing this point, he said: "Whoremongers, Adulterers, and lascivious Persons must in my opinion have been most liable to the Diseases of the private Parts, as from their proneness to Lust they conversed generally with Strumpets, who are always very unclean."[94]   This age knew then that syphilis was communicated venereally and that it had a variety of recognizable symptoms. Those symptoms, as described by Astruc, were spotting, scaling, itching, ulcers, loss of hair and inflammation.[95] But beyond these obvious characteristics, medical thinking on syphilis did not really advance for long generations.

Gradually as the 19th century unfolded, more precise information about syphilis did begin to accumulate. Ricord made an important breakthrough when, as a result of his research, he insisted that gonorrhea and syphilis were entirely different diseases. Prior to this, it was generally believed that they were just two different initial expressions of the same disorder.[96] Even more vital, in this regard, were the monumental discoveries that emerged out of modern autopsy. By the 1860s, autopsies performed on those who had died of syphilis were finally proving that chronic inflammation of the arteries, certain organs and some nerves were, indeed, a definite feature of this disease.[97] Moreover, by the second half of the 19th century, the medical profession was finally beginning to see the true consequences of the tertiary stage of syphilis. This new knowledge, however, did not necessarily aid detection. The Wasserman test was an advance, but it was able to uncover only about one-half of the suspected cases of syphilis.[98] Deep-seated syphilis, now definitely known to exist, was still extremely difficult to find in many. Beyond this particular dilemma, doctors, in the 1910s, knew for a fact that the disease was reoccurring in some patients, but they were uncertain whether this was the result of reinfection or relapse. Puzzling over these two possibilities, two British doctors around the time of World War I, described their own confusion on this point by saying:

Unfortunately, however, nearly every case which may be reviewed from the point of view of reinfection is also necessarily open to the criticism that it is not a reinfection but a relapse. The sore on the penis may not be due to an introduction of a new sprionemes but to a renewed outbreak of old.[99]

As it was, this last remaining mystery about syphilis, and how its tertiary stage actually worked, was just about to be cleared up. Within a few short years, this extremely complicated disease, which over the centuries had confused some of Europe's best medical minds, would, at long last, be brought within the range of human understanding.

Syphilis entered Europe, but unlike plague it never left. Historically, it passed through two distinct stages. The epidemic of syphilis that broke out in the 1490s and came to everyone's notice was demonstrably an extremely virulent form of this particular disease. Its symptoms, from several accounts, were even more hideous and frightening than those previously associated with plague. The sheer ugliness of this disease coupled with its sudden and startling appearance obviously confused many. But just as perplexing to this age was the equally dramatic moderation in syphilis that occurred in the middle of the 16th century. That transformation was so great that malignant syphilis and the congenital or chronic form which followed it seemed like two entirely different diseases. In fact, the symptoms were often similar to one another, but in congenital or chronic syphilis they were often barely perceptible. The striking way in which syphilis flared up and then all of a sudden moderated seems to lead naturally to the conclusion put forward by the 17th-century epidemiologist J. B. van Helmont. Speaking of diseases in general, van Helmont remarked: "Truly, diseases are changed, are masked, are increased and do degenerate."[100] His insight was, of course, apparently correct, especially if one considers the overall history of bacterial disorders like plague and syphilis. Even under laboratory conditions bacteria act this way, for not only can highly infectious bacteria be deprived of their virulence, they can also be restored back to their initial pathogenic state.[101] Rising virulence, in such instances, can be caused by either a grand mutation of some sort or a process now known as bacterial proliferation. Either way, relatively tame strains can become extraordinarily virulent. And what happens in the lab can evidently also occur in nature.

These two biological considerations can cast some light on the still-disputed question of where syphilis came from. It may possibly have been present in Europe prior to the 1490s. There is some partial evidence that there were cases of the disease during the Medieval period.[102] They were not identified as such, some believe, because in its milder form syphilis could have been easily confused with leprosy, a much more prevalent disorder at that time.[103] One thing is, however, true: malignant syphilis was not known to Europe before the time of Columbus. Anthropological studies of more than 16,000 skeletons in Europe, all dating back to the period before the 1490s, have failed to reveal a trace of the disease's presence.[104] This evidence is critical because malignant syphilis classically ulcerates to the bone leaving a tell-tale scar. If malignant syphilis was unknown then before the great epidemic of the late 15th century, where did it come from? Two very reasonable possibilities have emerged from the rather extensive literature that has examined this question. Both explanations combine history and biology. The first has been put forward by the American historian Alfred W. Crosby, Jr. Crosby readily admits the possibility that syphilis may have been present in Europe prior to the age of exploration. But he personally favors the contention that Treponema pallidum first developed into syphilis in America and that it was then exported to Europe, where it grew more virulent in what was for it a new and more hospitable environment.[105] Just as intriguing are the ideas advanced by the late English historian, J. F. D. Shrewsbury. Just prior to his death in the early 1970s, Shrewsbury had become convinced that the disease was already present in European society before the time of Columbus' first voyage. But, he went on, in the 1490s, the pathogen involved here mutated radically producing an epidemic that was only coincidental with Columbus' return from the new world.[106]

Shrewsbury's basic assumption here could be expanded to provide an even further explanation of the way in which both plague and syphilis have acted in the past. For his entire conclusion rests on the belief that the process of mutation has not been sufficiently taken into account in the study of past diseases. It is true that the sudden appearance of plague can be readily explained by the fact that in its pneumonic form it is easily transferred by man and in its bubonic form by vectors. But, the all too rapid disappearance of bubonic plague, the surprising onset of malignant syphilis and the almost miraculous modification of the syphilitic pathogen in the 1550s are historic events that are manifestly much more difficult to explain by conventional arguments. What strikes the observer of disease patterns here, as it did Shrewsbury, is the idea that radical mutations have taken place. The pathogens that were involved here obviously changed their level of toxicity in an exceedingly short period of time. Those changes came so fast that they immediately suggest a process of mutation that must have affected nearly all the bacteria alive at the time. It is well known that this process can take place artificially. For, sometimes in the laboratory, bacteria can multiply at an incredible rate of speed. Studying disease patterns in the past, one is sorely tempted to argue that this is exactly what has happened historically, only in what obviously was a much larger environment. In the final analysis then, bacterial proliferation, occurring over a wide geographic area and within a relatively short period of time, is just as plausible an explanation for the sudden emergence of syphilis in the 1490s as any other that has so far been advanced.

CHAPTER 3

SMALLPOX

> The smallpox has spread so widely over the world, and has, for so many ages, been allowed to destroy a very large proportion of mankind, that it is, and long has been regarded as one of the necessary evils of humanity.
>
> --John Haygarth, A Sketch of a Plan to Exterminate the Casual Smallpox from Great Britain (London, 1793), Vol. I, pp. 59-60.

Unlike plague and syphilis, smallpox did not strike Europe either suddenly or dramatically. Instead, it evolved over the course of several generations and centuries. For an extended period, it was only a secondary disease, one that affected people's lives marginally. By the early part of the 17th century, however, smallpox was beginning to emerge as a much more common disease.[1] As the decades of the 17th century unfolded, smallpox progressively became universal, steadily spreading across both western and central Europe. By the turn of the 18th century, it had become so commonplace that those who escaped it were looked upon as an oddity. By then, few areas on the European continent had been spared. Less murderous than plague and less disabling than syphilis, smallpox was still seen as a very dangerous disorder. For it did hit hardest at the young, taking the lives of up to 10 percent of its youthful victims. By the late 1700s smallpox had come to replace plague as the most spectacular cause of death in the whole of European society. Everywhere, it was taking a heavy toll of population, attacking in the cities evidently a little more than it did in the countryside. Smallpox was a significant check on population growth in the 18th century and would have continued to take life on a truly gigantic scale had it not been for Edward Jenner and the discovery of vaccination. After the development of his vaccine, smallpox lived on for several decades as a serious endemic and epidemic disease. But, in time, with the gradual acceptance of vaccination by all levels of European society, the disease was progressively conquered. When it was, it marked the very first time that any of Europe's great deadly and disabling diseases had ever been vanquished by means of human ingenuity.

Because of its outstanding symptoms, which last on average for up to two weeks, the presence of smallpox inside of European society during certain centuries has been relatively easy for historical epidemiologists to trace. Those symptoms were, by the end of the 17th and beginning of the 18th centuries, well known to both physicians and laymen alike. Even though smallpox normally lasted for only a short period of time, its impact could be both physically and psychologically devastating. For not only did it kill off a significant portion of the young, it left many of those who survived it pock-marked for life. In a rather memorable passage, the English historian Thomas B. Macauley recalled the truly depressing effect that this disease often had on previous generations. Writing in the 19th century, he commented:

> The smallpox was always present, filling the churchyards with corpses, tormenting with constant fears all whom it had not yet stricken, leaving on those who lives it spared the hideous traces of its power, turning the babe into a changeling at which the mother shuddered, and making the eyes and cheeks of the bethrothed maiden objects of horror to her lover.[2]

For nearly two hundred years, the medical profession had nothing at hand with which to fight this disease. That sense of helplessness came to an end with the introduction of vaccination, a novel medical procedure that quickly won the support of a large number of practicing physicians. Once the medical profession was successful in encouraging its use, millions of Europeans were spared the grief and agony of a disease which had previously saturated the general European population.

The historical origins of smallpox are still somewhat obscure. Many believe that its original habitat was either Central Africa, India or China.[3] No matter where it developed, smallpox first came to public notice during the decades immediately following the death of Christ. By the third century A.D., it was rampaging its way through China. Here, the disease evidently took on greater virulence, for the description of smallpox given at this time by the Chinese alchemist Ko Hung is remarkably similar to those that would be recorded later on in 18th-century Europe. Reporting on what was obviously a very malignant form of the disease, Ko Hung wrote:

> Recently there have been persons suffering from epidemic sores which have attacked, face and trunk. In a short time the sores spread all over the body. They have the appearance of hot boils containing some white matter. While some of the pustules are drying up, a fresh crop appears. If it is not treated early the patients usually die. Those who recovered are disfigured by purplish scars which do not fade until after a year.[4]

This description, with only minor variations, matches very closely the type of smallpox which the World Health Organization currently refers to as variola major. Smallpox first penetrated the European continent sometime during the Middle Ages. It was more than likely introduced to the continent by merchants who had recently been trading in Byzantium and the Middle East.[5]

Some historical epidemiologists believe that smallpox existed in Greece and Rome, from where it was passed on to Europe. However, evidence for this particular conclusion is really quite inconclusive.[6] More probably, the disease first began to creep into European society sometime during the 6th century A.D. Gregory of Tours mentions the presence of smallpox in France in the 560s, arguing that it was a highly contagious disease.[7] It was also during this particular period, when the disease was momentarily passing through parts of France and Italy, that it was repeatedly referred to as variola. It would keep that name for many centuries to come. Smallpox in the early Middle Ages was a purely local disease, operating quietly and striking here and there only after a very prolonged interval. Nevertheless, by the 10th century, both England and Ireland were evidently fairly familiar with the symptoms of this disease. Still, by all accounts, the disease was not spreading all that rapidly, for smallpox did not even reach northern Europe until the 1400s, places like Denmark having never experienced the disease up to that time. By contrast, for some as yet unexplained reason, Iceland was singled out for attack by smallpox. At certain periods, it seems to have been the major cause of death on that rather remote island. Even though the presence of smallpox was reported by a few Medieval chroniclers, it was at best little more than a tertiary phenomenon, drawing little or no public notice. The medical profession virtually ignored its sometimes subtle presence. Normally, medical literature tends to concentrate on the most important ailments of the period. The profession's silence on this disease further attests to its rather inconsequential influence during the Middle Ages. Even more interesting here is the fact that the Crusaders undoubtedly came into contact with smallpox in the Holy Land. But, not even this potential avenue of infection proved sufficient to bring the disease back to Europe.[8] Still, on occasion, the Middle Ages did come to know an isolated case or two of the extreme form of smallpox, one that would today be classified under the title of malignant smallpox. When it did strike, it caused excruciating pain, one Medieval chronicler declaring: "It is shocking to hear the groans of the sufferers, to see parts of their bodies as if burnt, dissolving away and to smell the intolerable foetor of their putrid flesh"[9] Both the pustules which caused the pain and the burning sensation mentioned here are symptoms of variola major, a form of smallpox that would be all too common in Europe by the 1700s.

After centuries of apparent quiescence, smallpox began to spread across the European continent in the 16th and 17th centuries, infecting a larger and larger percentage of the population. It came on at about the same time that malignant syphilis, typhus and influenza were also invading European society, a society that was now becoming, or so it seemed, more disease-ridden than ever before. Gaining momentum with each passing decade, smallpox was fast becoming an endemic disease. By the 1650s, it was familiar to physicians and the general public alike, "the marks of smallpox being everywhere."[10] One hundred years after this, smallpox would be the most widespread and prevalent disease in all of Europe.[11] Even though the more extreme form of smallpox was known, a much milder form of the disease dominated 17th-century Europe. In 1689, the very first English text ever published on the acute illnesses of childhood stressed this fact, the authors telling their public that: "Smallpox and measles in infants, being for the most part a mild and tranquil effervescence of the blood, are wont to have often no bad character, where neither the helping hand of the physicians are called, nor the unbounding skill of the complacent nurse is put to requisition."[12] Shortly after this, however, smallpox turned considerably more virulent. Right away, Europeans from all levels became alarmed. They were disturbed not only because the disease was spreading, but more importantly because the disease was enigmatically becoming more murderous. The noted French philosopher Helvetius watched this transformation take place. Reporting on the growing apprehension that this change was causing in the 1730s, he pointed out:

Mankind for a long time thought there was little Danger in the Smallpox. They were grown as it were familiar with them, by being accustomed to see the recovery of most children who had them, effected by a very easy plain Method of Cure. Twas with some Amazement they beheld their fatal Effects even upon Persons more advanced in years.[13]

By the 18th century, smallpox had become a universal scourge, saturating both urban and rural areas on the continent. Mostly endemic, the disease would also periodically break out in epidemic form, claiming thousands of lives in a single stroke. In some urban areas like Geneva, Lyons and London, the disease was positively ubiquitous, taking lives each and every year. In other locales, it returned with depressing regularity, occurring often enough, here, to convince the French observer Pierre de Baux that endemic smallpox came and went in predictable cycles," reoccurring naturally every four, five or six years."[14] Whether it was constantly there in some places or only reoccurring periodically, smallpox was a continuous drain on population. In Geneva, to give just one example, smallpox was an unrelenting killer throughout the period from 1580 to 1760. During those long decades, a total of 21,149 Genevans died from this disease. The average number of deaths annually was around 120, meaning, of course, that the antigens responsible for this disease must have been continually present in the city.[15] Municipal records for the French city of Lyons for the period stretching from 1581 to 1800 show a decidedly similar pattern. Throughout this period smallpox never relaxed its grip on this city, killing off an average of 38 persons a year.[16] As far as can be estimated at the time, the ratio of morbidity to mortality for smallpox was very close to one in 10. According to these standards, then, about 1,200 Genevans had the disease each year and about 380 in Lyons, at a moment when the population of both cities was relatively small. These statistics imply, in turn, that only a fortunate few ever escaped coming down with this type of infection. This fact of life in 18th-century Europe was made obvious by a survey that was conducted in the northern English city of Chester in 1775. Here, it was discovered that 85 percent of the city's population had already had the disease at one time or another in their lives.[17]

By the 1770s, smallpox had become so common that its comings and goings were viewed rather fatalistically by nearly all levels of European society. Those who took it upon themselves to try and fight the influence of this disease were constantly frustrated by the public apathy that inevitably surrounded the disease. The English physician John Haygarth recorded in 1793 just how disillusioned he had become in trying to break down this attitude. Speaking of his experience, he wrote:

> The smallpox has spread so widely over the world, and has for so many ages, been allowed to destroy a very large proportion of mankind, that it is, and long has been regarded as one of the necessary evils of humanity. This opinion so universally prevails among all, even the wisest men, that every attempt to exterminate, or even to regulate, and control the progress of this fatal distemper, may be thought too visionary and chimerical to deserve any serious attention. [18]

As in an earlier age and with other diseases, the constant presence of smallpox was frequently seen as a form of divine punishment. Referring specifically to smallpox, the Reverend Edmund Massey declared during this time that: "Diseases . . . are sent unto us for the Trial of our Faith, or the Punishment of our Sins; He alone to whom our Faith must approve it self, and our Sins are manifest, has properly the Power of inflicting them. [19] This explanation seemed just as logical as any other to an age that was helpless to prevent smallpox's almost endless return.

Not only was smallpox endemic to 18th-century Europe, it was perfectly capable of producing periodic epidemics as well. Like most other European cities, London experienced the merciless staccato influence of this disease. Throughout the 16th century, smallpox was steadily gaining prominence in the English capital. By the 1660s, it was the third leading cause of death, right behind tuberculosis and the all-too-frequent fevers of the day. [20] For nearly 100 years after this, death-rates from smallpox in proportion to London's overall population kept moving upwards. [21] As a consequence, smallpox was continually depleting the city's population, taking the lives of a full nine percent of all those who died within the city's limits.[22] Eventually, the disease peaked and death-rates from smallpox in relation to London's total population did begin to fall by the latter part of the 18th century. However, this does not mean that London lost this disease, for deep into the 19th century, the number of those dying from smallpox in the world's largest city remained set at between 1,000 and 3,000 a year. Beyond this, London was still experiencing anywhere between 10,000 and 30,000 cases of the disease annually, the variation being dependent on whether an epidemic had taken place or not.[23] A century before this in the 1700s, London had been shocked by especially virulent outbreaks of the disease in 1710, 1752 and 1772.[24] If anything, London was far more fortunate during the 19th century because epidemics of this deadly and disfiguring disease were occurring much less frequently.

During the 18th century, smallpox seemed to be growing in force all over Europe. Even areas on the fringe of Europe, such as Malta, were reporting ever-escalating incidences of the disease.[25] By the 1770s, the Hungarian physician J. J. Plenck, who once regarded smallpox in his country as a rather tame disorder, was by then listing it as an ever-increasing threat to public health.[26] For a while it was believed that Russia, with its extremely cold climate, might be spared the disease.[27] That myth was dramatically exploded in 1779-1780 when an unexpected epidemic sickened hundreds of thousands, according to government records, and took more than 20,000 lives.[28] Everywhere the story was the same. The Irish physician Timoteo O'Scanlan, who at this time was working in Spain, reported that the number of victims of smallpox in that country ranged up into the many millions.[29] By the end of the 18th century, governments all over Europe were becoming increasingly alarmed over the loss of population that was taking place. That worry and concern led to a more accurate system of record-keeping which revealed, among other things, that Prussia in the 1790s was losing 75,000 a year to the surging influence of this disease.[30] Moreover, the impression was definitely growing among health officials that smallpox itself was increasing in virulence. Since adequate records to support such a belief have not yet surfaced, this particular point can not be easily proven. But the popular impression of the time was that the disease was becoming more and more infectious. Summing up that widely-held belief, the Italian physician M. Gatti commented: "There seemed to be a larger and larger pool of victims for smallpox."[31]

Additional evidence that smallpox had, indeed, taken a disturbing new turn in the direction of greater and greater virulence came out of Belgium. Scarring, which had apparently occurred only rarely in the 17th century when the disease was first gaining ground, was by 1800 becoming quite frequent. An inquiry carried out in Belgium in the early part of the 19th century showed that a full 25 percent of the Belgian population was permanently pock-marked as a result of this disease.[32] Being pock-marked, it turned out, was one of the characteristic features of the criminal element inside of Belgium. This popular belief gained acceptance most likely because the poor were especially vulnerable to smallpox and because a substantial number of them evidently drifted into crime later on in their lives. In any event, one very revealing study done of the jails in Liège during the 1780s discovered that 47 percent of the city's inmates had serious facial scarring.[33] With death, disfigurement and illness from smallpox constantly present for all to see, it is little wonder that the conservative minded tended to view this disease as a natural part of their existence. When the idea of vaccination was first put forward in the early part of the 19th century, it very often produced a nearly hysterical response. It was as though some commentators believed that the natural and inevitable order of things had somehow been interrupted. Almost quizzically one William Rowley asked how this disease, then so universal and commonplace, could possibly be eliminated. Obviously attacking Jenner and the whole idea of vaccination, Rowley asked:

> But the most glaring and striking assertion is, that if the innoculation of the Cow Pox should become universal, it would totally exterminate the Small Pox. How is it possible?

When the Almighty God permits this epidemic disease to rage at certain seasons in the air, and some years more than others, which ages of experience confirm? Can presumptious vain man alter the decree of Providence . . . ? Is it not an impious supposition, unthinking, irrational, profane?[34]

The constantly spiralling effect that smallpox was obviously having around 1800 must have been the direct result of changes in the antigenic structure of the virus that causes this disease. Smallpox is, to start with, an extremely contagious disease. It is easily transferred from one person to another either by touch or by air-droplets. The viral agent specifically responsible for smallpox is now known by the name of Variola virus.[35] As it was, vaccination succeeded in overcoming this disease more than 125 years before medical men actually saw the tiny microorganism that was directly responsible for its toxicity. While the etiology of smallpox was never even suspected in the past, the medical profession knew from the start that it was a highly contagious disease. Physicians may never have known how plague was actually acquired, but they did come intriguingly close to judging the exact way in which smallpox was transmitted from one individual to another. Haygarth hit on it exactly when he insisted that: "the natural small-pox appears to be communicated thro' the air. Hence it proved incontestibly that the pestilential effluvia, or miasma, exist in the air near to the small pox patient, or to variolous matter."[36] Even the best of appraisals, however, in this era could be marred by a lack of information. For Haygarth went on from here to declare: "That the breath . . . and perspiration of a patient are infectious nobody disputes."[37] For the most part, Haygarth was correct, but his analysis of smallpox probably owed more to his deep-seated belief in the miasmatic origins of disease than it did to any real empirical observations on his part.

The beginnings of smallpox in a patient were not then and they are not now all that easy to pick out. During its initial stage, which normally follows about two weeks after incubation, smallpox characteristically appears to be just another febrile disorder, with accompanying backaches. Today, such indistinct symptoms would barely differentiate it from one of several different types of influenza.[38] The medical profession of the 18th century, usually quite good at seeing symptoms close up, readily understood that smallpox was all but impossible to diagnose during its early stages. This would not, of course, be a feature of the disease later on. For after a rather slow start, the symptoms of smallpox would come bursting forth. The English physician Thomas Dimsdale, who in the 1760s worked rather extensively with the victims of smallpox in Russia, suggested to other doctors that there were, however, some early signs of the disease that they might conceivably look for. Describing them more exactly, he pointed out that:

> The first attack of the small pox is so much like the beginnings of some other fevers as not easily to be distinguished; though a diligent attention to the symptoms will generally . . . enable us to form a pretty certain prognostic. For if the attack of the cold fit be severe and the subsequent fever unusually high; if a nausea and vomiting succeed, together with great pains in the head, back and loins . . . if a delirium, great restlessness, disagreeable taste in the mouth, and a peculiar foetid smell in the breath, or even if several of these symptoms are observed, the smallpox may with great reason be expected.[39]

These rather ill-defined symptoms were inevitably followed in the 18th century by the onset of a rash. The spotting that now began to occur usually passed through four escalating stages: the first was characterized by small spots, the second by reddish sores, the third by watery blisters and the last by pus-filled blisters.[40] Describing these eruptions, one Englishman, Theophilus Lobb, chose not only to list them, but to classify them with a kind of mathematical exactness. Writing in an obviously clinical tone, he said of them:

1.   ... the sooner the Eruption begins, the more numerous the Pustules are likely to be.
2.   ... The Pustules commonly appear first in the Face, then the Neck, Arms, Hands, Body and Legs.
3.   ... the Pustules suppurate in the same Order in which they come forth; so that they, which come out first, do first come to Ripeness.
4.   ... the Pustules tho' exceedingly small at their first appearance, do grow, and daily increase in Bulk dilating and become more red and inflammed. [41]

Extreme cases of smallpox, commonly featured by pustules that entirely covered the body, were just as ordinary a sight as the disease itself. Those who were compelled to suffer through this kind of ordeal were almost absolutely certain that they would come out of it scarred for life. The diary of one physician included just such a case. The unfortunate woman involved here was of aristocratic origins. Describing her tragic situation, he noted that: "the pustules came out in great Numbers . . . so thick, indeed, that as the Distemper encreased they adherred almost every where together."[42]

Smallpox, during its extended stay in Europe, existed essentially in two forms. During a significant portion of the 17th century, smallpox functioned in its milder form, one that is often referred to medically as variola minor. This kind of smallpox regularly produced symptoms that were extraordinarily similar to the extreme form of the disease, but they were much less conspicuous. Moreover, the death-rate from variola minor was historically quite low, usually not more than one percent of those who came down with the disease. Today, this relatively weak form of smallpox has become well known to medical teams working for the World Health Organization in such places as Africa and South America. There was, at the same moment, a much more virulent form of smallpox generally known as variola major. It was this type, with symptoms grossly exaggerated over variola minor, that was gaining momentum in Europe in the 18th and early

19th centuries. Much more contagious than variola minor and capable of being communicated by touch, variola major was also much more deadly. In the extreme form of this disease, the fever was much more pronounced and the rash and pustules significantly more plentiful. The extreme form is also physically much more taxing with the result that when it strikes, death-rates usually go shooting up.[43] There is, of course, ample literary and statistical evidence available to prove that it was variola major which ravaged Europe from the late 17th to the 19th centuries. In that time period, deaths from the disease consistently reached nine percent of those taken ill. Beyond this, they could occasionally soar to 20 percent or more during an especially virulent attack of the disease.[44]

Unlike syphilis, which was overtreated medically, smallpox was normally permitted to run its natural course. The orthodox remedy for this disease in the 17th century simply consisted of isolating the patient, in a hot, unventilated room, plenty of bed rest and, if need be, bloodletting. Drugs were almost never prescribed for this particular disorder.[45] The reason why smallpox was originally treated so lightly was because the disease was so mild to begin with that it hardly called for sophisticated treatment. According to Sydenham and many other experts, smallpox was, in the 17th century, not even a serious disorder. Commenting on its mildness, Sydenham declared: "This disease in its self is very salutary and when not mishandled kills few or none, nature haveing annexed thereunto both a full and convenient discharge of the morbifick matter."[46] The only real dispute among medical men in regard to this disease was exactly how the fever accompanying it should be handled. Some thought that it should be brought down by hot applications, others favored cold.[47] The rather relaxed attitude of the medical profession towards smallpox came to an abrupt end around the year 1700. By then, this disease was undergoing a gigantic metamorphosis, one that was about to turn smallpox into one of the most dangerous diseases of the age. Trying to cope with what was rapidly becoming a "new" disease was an extremely frustrating experience for most physicians. As the disease gained in fury, an ever-increasing number of doctors began to look first upon inoculation and then vaccination as the best means that they had for checking smallpox's spiralling impact upon the European population. While some latched onto newer methods of treatment, others simply fell back on older remedies, including bloodletting, purging and vomiting, hoping thereby to drive out of the body "the morbifick matter" that was making it ill.[48]

During the century and a half between the rise of variola major and the final acceptance by most of vaccination, death-rates from smallpox kept soaring. During the extended period in which he practiced in Spain, O'Scanlan, a strong advocate of inoculation, found that the Iberian Peninsula was rife with the disease. He concluded that the disease had literally taken over Spanish society and was killing off, on a yearly basis, a full 10 percent of all those that it infected.[49] Other statistics gathered together at the time invariably produced similar findings. Haygarth, for example, reporting back to his English colleagues in the 1790s on the impact of smallpox elsewhere, noted that: "The celebrated M. de la Condamine computes that in France one in ten of all who are born, dies of smallpox. Dr. Rosenstein . . . shews that every tenth boy and ninth girl, dies of it in Sweden."[50] These percentages assembled over the course of decades largely represent deaths from endemic attacks of smallpox. Epidemics inevitably produced higher tolls. Typically, when an epidemic of variola major struck the German city of Halle and the area surrounding it in 1806, the mortality rate jumped immediately to some 17 percent of those affected.[51] In a day and age when average life expectancy normally hovered at around 28 or 30, smallpox was obviously a major factor contributing to the extremely short rate of life expectancy in 18th century Europe.[52] Europe was in these trying decades a disease-ridden society, with the bulk of the population dying at one or another stage of life from a variety of highly infectious diseases. The impact of some of those diseases was not all that easy to uncover. For a number of them including syphilis, tuberculosis and the countless fevers of the time, often took lives almost secretly. The same could not be said for smallpox. Its death-dealing effects, usually after just a few short weeks, were there for all to see. In fact, smallpox, which killed openly, and tuberculosis, which was now coming on as a major disease, were effectively holding down population growth during much of the period up to the beginning of the Industrial Revolution.[53]

The highly virulent form of smallpox that was, as of the 1700s, rampaging its way through European society was principally taking the lives of children. Children, and in particular infants, were especially susceptible to smallpox largely because they had never had the disease and, therefore, had no real immunity against it. Even then, it was well-known that a single case of this disease normally conferred immunity on those fortunate enough to survive smallpox the first time around. However, given the growing potency of the antigens involved here and the poorly developed immune systems of the young, it was almost inevitable that smallpox would during these decades take an uncompromisingly heavy toll among infants. Physicians and laymen alike tended to look upon this disease as one of the hazards of childhood. In the villages that surrounded Lyons, for example, every official report on the incidences of smallpox regularly listed large numbers of children among the dead.[54] Within that group, the very young were the ones who were normally victimized the most. This eventuality showed up in the records of one English provincial town, where some 589 children died from smallpox between the years 1769 and 1774. Of that total, the overwhelming majority, 466, were below the age of three and only one was older than 10.[55] Haygarth certainly regarded smallpox as the greatest killer of the young that there was. Speaking in 1785 to a meeting of the Chester Society for Promoting General Inoculation, he stated categorically that: "Before the society commenced, half as many children under ten years old died of the Small-pox, in Chester, as all other diseases."[56] A very similar pattern existed in Geneva. Here, municipal records, dutifully kept for the years 1580 to 1760, revealed an exceedingly high rate of infant mortality. In this period, half of those dying in the city from smallpox infections were under the age of two, while a full four-fifths of those who passed away were six or less.

SMALLPOX DEATHS AT VARIOUS AGES UP
TO SEVEN YEARS, GENEVA, 1580-1760.[57]

Number Dying	Ages	Percentage of Smallpox Deaths
6,792	0-1	26.8
5,416	1-2	21.4
4,116	2-3	16.2
2,826	3-4	11.1
1,928	4-5	7.6
1,325	5-6	5.2
944	6-7	3.7

Over this entire span, 96 percent of those killed by the disease in Geneva were under the age of ten. National figures published a short while after this for France in the early 1800s also proved that smallpox was primarily an infantile disorder.[58]

Smallpox continued to pose a serious health problem to European society right into the latter part of the 19th century. Living on as both an endemic and an epidemic disease, smallpox, if anything, seemed to be growing in virulence with each passing decade, all of which means that the vaccine that Jenner developed around the year 1800 was most probably intercepting a form of smallpox that was steadily becoming much more toxic. Notwithstanding the partial acceptance of vaccination, smallpox was still a disease that was intrinsically capable of causing epidemics. This became obvious when major outbreaks occurred covering the periods 1824-1829, 1837-1840 and 1870-1874.[59] Early in the 19th century, moreover, many individual countries were still being mercilessly attacked by this disease. In 1822, for instance, an epidemic of smallpox struck Hungary and Transylvania, immediately killing some 42,000 in an area which already experienced some 350,000 cases of the disease each and every year.[60] One despondent Hungarian physician, commenting on the perpetual presence of smallpox in his country, pointed out that many "did not know any other drug except the bitter tears of men who groaned under the yoke of variola."[61] Recurrent epidemics, each in turn taking so much young life, were becoming such fearful experiences that they were driving many into an acceptance of vaccination. This is exactly what happened in Turin in the wake of the deadly epidemic of 1824-1830 that hit that city in northern Italy.[62] Large numbers volunteered to be vaccinated in spite of their own loudly-expressed apprehension about this new medical technique. Public suspicion of vaccination in Italy and elsewhere was actually very high through the first half of the 19th century, with the vast majority really not knowing what to think of it. Nevertheless, vaccination programs did gain favor among mass elements largely because there was no perceptible let-up in the virulence of smallpox attacks during most of the 19th century. In this situation, many were driven to accept vaccination even though they may have been initially dubious about its value.

The introduction of vaccination on an ever-expanding scale definitely reduced the percentage of those dying from smallpox. The decline, while slow at the start, was nevertheless detectable. For example in Paris before 1789, smallpox was responsible for nearly 30 percent of all deaths in the age group from one to four. Two decades later, as a result of vaccination, that figure was definitely falling.[63] The same trend could be seen developing in London. There, in 1806, for the first time in 150 years, a whole week passed without a single individual dying from this disease.[64] This decline did not mean, of course, that smallpox was being eradicated. It only suggests that there were now some areas in Europe, specifically those that were introducing programs of vaccination, where the population was increasingly being protected from the threat of smallpox. This was especially true of London where death rates from the disease were being dramatically lowered. Epidemics still took place, but the numbers perishing were much lower than they were before. Moreover, only once, in 1831, did the total number of deaths from an epidemic even approximate the average heights attained during any of London's all-too-frequent epidemics of the 18th century.[65] The disease was, in fact, relentlessly being subdued in the British capital. By the 1850s, deaths from smallpox were only half of what they had been fifty years earlier at the turn of the 19th century.[66] And on a per capita basis, deaths were even lower than before, taking into account the fact that London's population had nearly doubled during that time when deaths from the disease were being halved.

During the second half of the 19th century, an extremely virulent form of smallpox continued to decimate the younger portion of the European population. It was only checked in those places where governments had conscientiously vaccinated their own citizens. In spite of legislation in several countries that made vaccination mandatory, protection was still wildly uneven. This happened because compliance was, for the most part, voluntary and, as a result, often neglected. While the general situation was, at best, spotty, the Prussian military did take steps to make vaccination compulsory.[67] This program guaranteed the emerging Prussian army of the 1860s a degree of immunity and protection that, by contrast, the French army did not possess. It is true that Napoleon I had introduced the practice earlier in the century, but by mid-century, the French High Command no longer considered it necessary. This negligence badly hurt the French. For as chance would have it, the Franco-Prussian War of 1870-1871 was fought right in the midst of Europe's last great pandemic of smallpox. The Prussian army was virtually untouched by the disease. But, the French army, left unprotected, lost nearly 20,000 men, both sick and dying, to an epidemic among its troops.[68]

The epidemic of smallpox that stuck the whole of Europe in 1871 and 1872 proved that this disease was just as contagious and the pathogens just as deadly as they had ever been. From the evidence, there was no let-up, whatsoever, in the toxic character of the virus responsible for the smallpox. If anything, the disease may have been more virulent than it had been in the past. In Great Britain, Europe's last pandemic of smallpox took some 42,000 lives, while another 30,000 died of it in Belgium.[69] Yet another 30,000 perished in the Netherlands at the very same time that the toll in Prussia was climbing past 40,000. Not only did hundreds of thousands lose their lives, but the total number of those contracting the disease may have been as high as 10 million. It was the numbers affected that finally convinced many Europeans of the value of vaccination. For the statistical evidence gathered on this epidemic certainly favored those who had been protected ahead of time. Improved record-keeping showed that in countries like England, Scotland and Bavaria, all of whom had mandatory programs of vaccination, the death-rate during the epidemic from smallpox per 1 million inhabitants was respectively 1,012, 428 and 1,045. Whereas, in countries such as Prussia, Belgium and the Netherlands, which had not protected their civilian populations, the rates were, in turn, 2,432, 4,168 and 4,355. The differences were anywhere from two and a half to four and a half times greater.[70]

While various national governments and the public at large were finally beginning to place greater emphasis upon vaccinations, the actual technical procedure for injecting the vaccine was still, unquestionably, uneven and sometimes even unpredictable. Many, because of neglect, were, of course, not protected at all. But, contrastingly, large numbers of those who received the vaccine were either not fully immunized or, in many instances, definitely needed to be revaccinated. In truth, the actual process of vaccination was right into the 1890s, oftentimes, a rather arbitrary one. This disquieting fact about vaccination was brought to light all over again during the London epidemic of 1884-1885. Here, many who thought they were protected suddenly discovered that they were coming down with the disease. Indeed, as the records of the West Ham Hospital in London revealed soon after this, vaccination could provide some measure of protection against the disease. But, since the process of giving the vaccine was still in an imperfect state technically, vaccination was not necessarily a guarantee. This reality was obvious from the report of the West Ham Hospital which ran:

> Of 1,211 cases treated in the West Ham Board of Guardians Hospital . . . , twenty-six of the cases were said to have been revaccinated, and one of them died, but the death was owing to pneumonia. . . . Of those not revaccinated but with three or

more good vaccination marks [usually given in the first time] 4 percent died; with one or two marks [also given the first instance] 15 percent, in the case of the imperfectly vaccinated 29 percent, of those said to be vaccinated but without evidence 44.6 percent; and of the unvaccinated 56.22 percent died; 132 unvaccinated males were admitted with 76 deaths, and 101 unvaccinated females with 55 deaths, a total of 233 unvaccinated with 131 deaths.[71]

Interpreting the results of this report, Dr. John Moir pointed out what European society had already known for several decades about vaccination procedures. He declared: "I have no hesitation in saying that the protection against death by smallpox afforded by vaccination is in exact ratio with the efficiency of the operation, and that vaccination confers practical immunity from confluent [extreme] small-pox, or from death from small-pox."[72]

It is historically impossible to gauge the exact potency of the small-pox antigens that were still murderously attacking Europeans in the last half of the 19th century. This can not be done because such a large part of the European population was being vaccinated that the overall effect of this disease was actually being blunted. One thing is certain, however; never again would the continent experience another pandemic of smallpox of a type or kind that would match the intensity of the one that struck in the early 1870s. With smallpox now on the wane, the true virulence of the disease still operating at this time can never be determined, since increased vaccination was demonstrably subduing the toxic effect of these antigens in the majority of the population. However, if the figures produced by the West Ham epidemic of 1884-1885 are to any degree illustrative, then it could be argued that vaccination was overpowering a disease whose virulence was continually expanding. For, in that particular outbreak, the death-rate rose at times to an astonishing 50 percent of those taken ill. Taking this and other facts into account, the decline of smallpox after the 1870s may have come at the exact same moment in time when the antigens involved here were biologically the most toxic. Putting this particular point aside, by 1914, vaccination was unquestionably the most widely accepted medical procedure in Europe. Its ultimate value was put to the test during the First World War. By the end of the war in 1918, certain diseases such as syphilis, typhus and influenza were raging uncontrollably in certain parts of Europe. Smallpox, on the other hand, was almost completely contained. In 1919, there were a total of 300,000 cases of smallpox reported from various scattered pockets in Russia, Rumania, Czechoslovakia, Yugoslavia, Germany, Spain and Portugal. In actuality, this was a rather minor outbreak in comparison with smallpox's somewhat free-wheeling past.[73] Smallpox became all but extinct in Europe over the course of the next two decades. As of 1929, medical teams from the League of Nations were able to discover no more than 25,000 cases of the disease in the whole of Europe.[74] By then, its few remaining focal points on the continent were being progressively mapped and eventually eliminated. By 1938, public health authorities in Europe reported the existence of a mere 800 cases of smallpox.[75] As of the late 1930s, Europe's long-standing nightmare with the disease had come to an end. Like plague, smallpox's devastating path through European history was about to become little more than an historical memory.

The fact that smallpox was being overcome in the late 1800s meant that both the cities and the countryside were now being spared this disheartening experience. By then, most were convinced that smallpox was, if anything, a universal disease affecting all parts of the continent equally. But, prior to these decades, the impression of most observers who thought about it was that this disease was primarily urban in origin. The famous English epidemiologist of the 17th century, John Graunt, certainly found this to be true. He even produced figures which cogently demonstrated that rural mortality from smallpox was generally lower than that which was found in the cities.[76] This widely-held belief about smallpox was the result of the fact that most English towns and cities harbored the disease endemically from a very early date. Its constant presence in the larger population centers of the time led rather naturally to the belief that smallpox was basically an urban affliction.[77]   The evidence for this conclusion was everywhere. However, it should be pointed out that in time the disease became so ubiquitous that death-rates in the cities of Europe were only marginally higher than they were in the countryside. That it attacked the cities with great regularity can not, on the other hand, be denied. Municipal records for the city of Lyons show that smallpox was present in that city long before it became prominent elsewhere.[78] In some of the larger population centers like London and Geneva, smallpox was present decade after decade, uncompromisingly taking the lives of a set percentage of the population each and every year.[79] Moreover, it was in the cities where the truly virulent form of smallpox seemed to predominate. The pathogens at work here evidently needed numbers in order to survive and they found them in the more crowded areas of pre-industrial Europe. Whether or not the cities of Europe were the actual geographic home for smallpox is a question that can only be settled as a result of more study. One thing, however, is certain, this disease was effectively limiting the growth of urban populations. If smallpox had continued to kill up to ten percent of the young, its dampening effect upon urban growth would have been obvious through much of the 19th century.   Instead, the very opposite began to happen; the urban population began to swell with the coming of industrialization. The disappearance of plague coupled with the progressive conquest of smallpox went a long way towards making urban development a distinct historical possibility.[80]

Vaccination, that striking medical technique which eventually saved Europe from the ravages of smallpox, was discovered by an English country doctor, Edward Jenner, in the late 1790s. The life-saving ability of this medical practice was recognized very early on by a number of Jenner's devoted disciples throughout Europe. Even more importantly, within a decade of Jenner's unprecedented insight into the value of this process, the Royal College of Physicians in London was backing the procedure, declaring almost prophetically:

The College of Physicians feel it their duty to strongly recommend the practice of vaccination. They have been led to this conclusion by no preconceived opinion, but by the most unbiased judgment, formed from an irresistible weight of evidence which had been laid before them. For when the number, the respectability, the disinterestedness and the extensive experience of its advocates are compared with the feeble and imperfect testimonies of its few opposers . . . the College of Physicians . . . [think] that the public may reasonably look forward to some degree of hope to the time when all opposition will cease, and the general concurrence of mankind shall at length be able to put an end to the ravages at least, if not to the existence, of the smallpox.[81]

The Royal College of Physicians believed at the time that there was ample evidence to support Jenner's rather boastful claim "that the Cow-pox protects the human constitution from the infection of Small-pox."[82] However, while the medical profession was becoming increasingly convinced of the value of vaccination, it would be long decades before the general public looked so positively on this procedure.

The idea that lay behind Jenner's somewhat extraordinary belief that cowpox could protect against smallpox dated back more than 100 years to the practice of inoculation. Neither the medical profession nor the public at large had any real insight into the working of plague or syphilis prior to the 19th century. By contrast, at least something was known about smallpox. For it had been observed early in the overall history of the disease in Europe that a mild case of smallpox conferred long-lasting immunity against a further attack. This realization led a few doctors to begin to advocate "the buying of smallpox" for the purpose of inoculating oneself. This procedure became known in the 18th century as variolation. The earliest reported cases of variolation took place in the German-speaking areas of central Europe in the 1670s[83] As it turned out, the notion of using pus from a smallpox abcess to give oneself a mild case of the disorder did not win much popular approval. As it was, the majority who heard about this procedure came to look upon it with disgust. Nonetheless, there were a few courageous types like James Jurin who strongly favored the process. Jurin predicted great things for variolation, insisting that: "If upon a fair and exact Balance of the good and ill Success of it, it appear in the main to be beneficial to Mankind; [inoculation] will in Time, in spite of clamour and unreasonable Opposition, be reckon'd among the many Blessings."[84] Jurin's hope was never realized. Despite this, the basic idea behind variolation did win out. For, it was Jenner who in the 1790s capitalized on the novel medical assumption that lay behind variolation that disease could be used to fight disease.

Although Jenner could not possibly have known it, the cowpox vaccine that he used in his experiments contained antigens that were anatomically similar to the virus that is responsible for smallpox. The antigens located on the outer membrane of the two viruses are, in fact, very close to one another both in structure and chemical composition. While the two seem very much alike, they react somewhat differently both in the body and in the laboratory. Those differences are so subtle, however, that a trained eye is needed to detect them. For example here, the two antigens will react distinctively in both the blood stream and other bodily fluids. Beyond this, the lesions that the two viruses produce can be distinguished, one from another, by color, size, appearance and length of time the accompanying pustules need to attain maturity. The lesions produced by the two will also apparently haemorrhage at different intervals. Another striking difference between these two viruses is that they respond to temperature changes, meaning that the toxic materials that they contain become more active at different temperature readings. Modern biochemistry has in recent times likewise proven that the two viruses grow at separate rates when they are placed in the same type of tissue culture. All of these rather sophisticated findings about the two viruses have come, of course, only in more recent times. While they are intrinsically interesting they have not altered the fact that an injection of cowpox antigens will protect against the invasion of a smallpox virus.[85] Having said all of this, it is still not clear whether the followers of Jenner were using a pure form of cowpox vaccine or not. The vaccine that the World Health Organization has been administering of late to stamp out smallpox around the globe has itself passed through so many generations that its actual content and origins are now obscured.[86] It is conceivable, that the vaccine now being used is, in actuality, a mixture of both cowpox and smallpox antigens, although no one seems to be quite sure on this point. Jenner's own experiments undoubtedly involved the use of what he called pure "cow-pox lymph."[87] However, his followers do not seem to have been as careful and meticulous as he was. For, very early on, some physicians evidently got into the habit of increasing the potency of the original cowpox vaccine by adding to it a certain amount of lymph taken from smallpox patients.[88] This practice presumably developed because the illness produced by the cowpox virus in humans was so slight that it was not clear to many doctors that an adequate level of protection had actually been established.[89] The addition of small quantities of the virus responsible for variola major evidently heightened the clinical response of patients to the original injection. This growing practice also tended to produce a vaccine which was by the 1820s and 1830s a kind of hybrid, falling somewhere in between cowpox and smallpox.[90] Evidently, experimentation combined with carelessness had early in the 19th century produced this somewhat unexpected result.

Throughout the course of the 19th century, vaccination itself remained a rather imperfect process. It unquestionably cut down on smallpox mortality, but it did not necessarily safeguard all of those who had been vaccinated. Whenever and wherever vaccination was introduced there was an almost immediate statistical decline in the number of deaths due to smallpox. Sometimes, the disease was even made extinct. This happened in Glouchestershire in south-western England in the early 1800s. Indeed, one grateful doctor wrote to Jenner enthusiastically reporting that: "It is now fourteen years since smallpox has been subdued in this place except in solitary instances, in paupers occassionally passing thro - so that young mothers know nothing about the disease and consequently feel no fears for their offsprings."[91] As encouraging as these remarks may have been, vaccination did not always produce such perfect results. For almost always, a very small number of those vaccinated either became ill or died soon after the operation had taken place. This happened periodically, for example, in the Ansbach region of western Germany. Records, scrupulously kept for the period from 1801 to 1817, showed that a total of 149,371 individuals had been vaccinated during that era. Of that group, 28 people died soon after they had received the vaccine. Local physicians, themselves personally convinced of the value of the operation, laid the blame for these untimely deaths on an impure mixture of cowpox and smallpox. This may have been the case. But, it is much more likely that these people died from an allergic reaction, since most of them went into either a spasm or a convulsion before they finally expired.[92] In actuality then, the campaign in favor of widespread vaccination was surrounded by a good deal of insecurity during much of the 19th century. In certain instances, fear of causing death made some physicians increasingly timid. In numerous cases, to prevent mortality and to quiet the public outcry from those who were still suspicious of vaccination, dosages were significantly weakened by physicians, all of which made revaccination an increasing necessity during much of the last half of the 19th century.[93]

The eventual conquest of smallpox within European society was the result of a long and sometimes uneven evolutionary process. In those countries before 1914 where vaccination had been legally adopted, both the morbidity and mortality from this disease fell precipitously. But, not every country bothered to make vaccination mandatory. As a result, some areas on the continent were hit hard by the disease, while others were obviously able to contain its impact. In the south German state of Bavaria, which had a compulsory program, death-rates during the smallpox epidemic of 1871 were only a quarter of what they were in the Netherlands, which had no such policy.[94] The evidence in favor of vaccination, thanks to better recordkeeping, was there for all to see. After the lessons of 1871, vaccination was on its way towards being legislated all over Europe, and smallpox, in turn, was on its way to extinction. The disease that was progressively being overcome everywhere in Europe was still, however, a very virulent and a very toxic disorder. Historically, it is now possible to look back and see this ever-expanding disease gaining more and more strength from one century to another. One of the key turning points here was the decade of the 1690s when the rather mild form of smallpox, variola minor, began to give way to its much more vicious successor, variola major. This sudden upsurge in the disease's toxicity must have been the result of mutation. For there is no evidence from the times to suggest that the overall level of immunity within the general population dramatically dropped. No conspicuous changes in levels of nutrition have, for example, been noted for the period.[95] What, then, is far more likely is that the microorganism at work here underwent such a precipitous mutation that its toxicity suddenly became overwhelming.

The innate capacity of microorganisms to mutate within a very short period of time represents one of the more fascinating aspects of the study of epidemiological trends. There is, it is true, no first-hand biochemical evidence that this process has actually taken place. As was mentioned previously, the microorganisms of the past have not left behind any evidence of their former presence in the form of microfossils. In spite of this lack, there is still plenty of symptomatic evidence, described in the literature of pre-industrial times, to suggest that rapid mutations have taken place. The sudden transformation of smallpox from a truly simple childhood disease, somewhat akin to modern-day chicken pox, into a highly deadly disease represents one of those moments. This particular metamorphosis was not the first which had taken place. It had happened before, apparently in the case of plague and unquestionably with syphilis. Mutating organisms have in the European past taken a tremendous human toll. For not only have these tiny substances measurably increased their toxicity, they have also apparently become much more plentiful. Singling out populations that have concentrated in urban areas historically, the sheer quantity of those poisonous microorganisms has evidently gone shooting up right at the moment when they have begun to mutate. As in the case of other diseases, the spread of smallpox may conceivably be explained in terms of two biological concepts. It could be explained by the rising virulence within the microorganism involved here, <u>Treponema pallidum</u>. It could also have happened as a result of a truly dramatic proliferation in the number of viral agents associated with this disease. Both of these biological phenomena may have been at work in the early 18th century when smallpox turned into the most uncompromising killer of the young that Europe had ever seen.

CHAPTER 4

TYPHUS AND CHOLERA

> **It is not always the case that in every place where typhus can be found one can inevitably also find cholera, but it is a frequent experience that in those places in which typhus is periodically epidemic, a good part of the time cholera will likewise find a home.**
>
> **--Max von Pettenkofer, <u>Was Man Gegen die Cholera thun kann</u> (Munich, 1873), p. 21.**

In comparison with the overall impact of plague, syphilis and smallpox, typhus and cholera must be regarded as secondary diseases. The reason why one set of diseases was so much more influential historically than the other was undoubtedly because of the variation in virulence between them. From the evidence, accumulated so far, it is safe to say that the pneumonic form of plague along with malignant syphilis and variola major were caused by intensely virulent microorganisms. They were so powerful, antigenetically, that they easily overwhelmed large numbers of people, most of whom proved to be extremely susceptible to the toxic influences of these highly potent diseases. Human efforts over time to contain these diseases, such as improvements in public sanitation and quarantine, were usually woefully inadequate to stop their advance. What is more, they were only subdued in the end by discoveries such as vaccination and antibiotics, medical breakthroughs that had an almost miraculous character. In comparison with plague, syphilis and smallpox, typhus and cholera were less damaging diseases. They claimed fewer victims, their geographic sweep was much more limited and their death-dealing impact was confined to a smaller portion of the population, largely the poor and downtrodden. Even their gradual elimination in the latter part of the 19th century was more the consequence of public campaigns than it was of scientific discoveries, for typhus and cholera were in the main, diseases of human squalor and once public sanitation became a reality they began to lose their grip on certain sections of the European population. Those reformers who were conscientiously advancing the cause of cleanliness in the 19th century actually went a long way towards eliminating typhus and cholera. Prior to this, the presence of both of these diseases seemed, if anything, to be inversely proportional to the ability of public health authorities to disinfect the environment in which the masses found themselves.

Like smallpox, typhus made its way into European society slowly. It first appeared on a regular basis sometime during the 15th century, functioning mostly as a local disorder. Generally-speaking, when it did occur, it only produced an endemic. Still, once in a while it did take on epidemic proportions, but that was a rarity during its early years in European society. More than likely, typhus did exist during the Middle Ages. But in the midst of the plethora of fevers, boils and spots caused by other diseases, its existence as a separate and distinct affliction was only periodically suspected.[1] Nosology, or the scientific classification of diseases, was in its infancy during the Medieval period. Because of this, it was especially difficult at the time for medical men to distinguish one febrile disorder from another. As a result, if typhus did exist, its presence would not have been easily detected. Even though typhus was lacking in truly unique symptoms, it seems probable from the literary evidence available that the disease was, at least, occasionally present during part of the Medieval era. Bohemia, or what is today western Czechoslovakia, was, for example, definitely hit by a typhus-like disorder in the year 1095.[2] However, after this, actual reports of this disease were so infrequent down to the era of the Renaissance that one leading expert still insists that typhus did not, in fact, enter Europe until 1489. Whatever its origins, a spectacular outbreak of typhus did occur in 1489 among Spanish troops which were then besieging the Arab stronghold of Granada in the southern part of the Iberian peninsula. The Spanish chronicler Luis de Toro who reported on the epidemic described it, in unmistakable terms, as "malignant spotted fever."[3] From Spain, typhus next moved into southern Italy. And from there, it advanced up the Italian peninsula, taking the historic route of both plague and syphilis. Soon after this, it was appearing here and there in various isolated spots on the continent.[4]

The epidemic which decimated the Spanish army and took some 17,000 lives in 1489 and 1490 was, as far as this age was concerned, yet another new and frightening affliction. Its symptoms in the late 1480s and early 1490s must have been similar to those that were described a few decades later by an eye-witness to an epidemic in Antwerp. Typhus in that city was regarded as a very depressing disease, a state of mind which was brought on by a whole host of oppressive symptoms. This characteristic feature of typhus was observed in Antwerp, where it was noted that:

> There were rarely any . . . [forewarnings] to an outbreak of the disease; it mostly set in abruptly and usually in the night time, with chills followed by heats; the patients complained at the same time of oppressive palpitations, headache, want of breathe, a sense of pressure or tightness in the region of the stomach and sickness. As the symptoms rose in intensity, a . . . sweat broke out . . . , accompanied by a spotted, papular or vesicular exanthem [eruption].[5]

While typhus struck Europe at about the same historic moment that syphilis did, Europeans did not see cases of typhus with anything like the same frequency that they witnessed syphilitic attacks. For an extended period after 1500, typhus broke out only randomly, usually occurring during war time. This happened so often that the disease came to be identified in the public mind with the movement of troops. Military camps were highly vulnerable largely because they had notoriously poor drainage for both urine and faeces. That along with the filthy state of the soldiers themselves were usually just the conditions that typhus needed in order to proliferate and grow.

The well-documented historic connection between typhus and the movement of armies across the European continent continued right into the 16th and 17th centuries. Moreover, at certain critical moments, the course of both political and military history was unquestionably changed because of the presence of this disease. Acting quite arbitrarily, typhus attacked a French army fighting the Spanish for control of southern Italy in 1582, leaving the Spanish troops virtually untouched. What was left of the French army after it was singled out in this way was then forced into a humiliating retreat.[6] This story was repeated a few decades later when typhus ravaged the army of the Austrian Emperor Maximilian II, forcing him to terminate his campaign against an encroaching Turkish force.[7] The second half of the 16th century was relatively peaceful. But in the first part of the 17th century, Europe was engulfed by the Thirty Years War. That seemingly endless conflict produced untold human suffering, with typhus breaking out repeatedly. When it did, it added to the already heavy toll of life that was being taken in certain war-torn areas such as central Germany.[8] The sight of thousands of troops dying from what this age called spotted fever undoubtedly drew a great deal of attention. But, much less noticeable was the fact that typhus was now progressively creeping into the civilian population, where in certain locales it was becoming endemic. When it struck endemically, typhus was, of course, a relatively mild disease, picking off one or two victims here or there but never producing either high morbidity or high mortality. Operating as it did in a kind of subdued fashion, typhus has been exceedingly difficult to trace historically, for not only did it sometimes not spot, but, all too often, contemporaries confused it either with typhoid or with one or another of the half dozen febrile disorders prevalent at the time.[9]

One thing here is, however, certain. The military was, beyond question, the vehicle by which typhus kept penetrating the general population. Epidemics of typhus were, for example, reported among civilians in Italy in 1505, 1528 and 1535-1537, in particular during the Franco-Spanish campaigns for control of the Italian peninsula.[10] Given this kind of start, typhus had by the early 1600s located itself in certain key areas on the European continent, including such far-flung locations as Ireland, France and Russia. A major outbreak of the disease also occurred in England in 1623.[11] Prior to that date, typhus had attacked England so sparingly that when it did invade, it was immediately labelled as an entirely new disease.[12] The word typhus was used at this time to describe the disease because it literally meant coma or stupor. The term turned out to be more than appropriate especially when one considers that the disease usually prostrated its victims to the point of delirium. This peculiar symptom was noticed almost instantly by the English physician Edward Greaves. For, in addition to a rapid pulse, spotting and a characteristic fever, the disease, according to Greaves, seemed to take over the whole body, producing:

> A great weakness without any manifest cause appearing which hath been, and is still very apparent in this Disease, in so much that strong men, in a very short time, have so much lost their vigour, as they have not been able to walk, or scarce to stand, without the help, and assistance of those about them.[13]

The renowned English poet John Donne, who was taken ill by typhus, described even more graphically what it was like to be attacked by the disease. Remembering his own experience, he recalled: "In the same instant that I feele the first attempt of the disease, I feele the victory; In the twinckling of an eye, I can scarce see, instantly the tast is insipid, and fatuous; instantly the appetite is dulle, and desireless; instantly the knees are sinking and strengthlesse."[14]

Sometime during the course of the 17th century, typhus settled into a number of additional spots on the European continent, including the Baltic littoral, eastern Germany and the Hungarian plain. By the 1620s, in certain parts of Hungary, typhus was continually present claiming anywhere from six to 20 lives in one village after another. The disease, always functioning locally and endemically, never seemed to take a large number of lives. On the other hand, it remained curiously mortal in these areas year in and year out and decade after decade.[15] Given this limited impact, typhus obviously never had the same kind of deadly sweep that at one time or another had characterized plague, syphilis or smallpox. For some still unexplained reason, then, typhus remained throughout this period, geographically self-limiting.   Decades after this trend first developed, the Englishman Thomas Bateman perceived this somewhat subtle tendency of typhus, declaring: "Circumstances [favorable to typhus] are perpetually recurring, which give it a local and partial experience."[16]   Whether it functioned endemically or was proliferating epidemically, typhus definitely located itself for long periods in certain well-defined geographic areas.   Parts of Italy and France were repeatedly subject to epidemics of typhus in the late 17th and 18th centuries, but they were always purely regional in scope.[17]   The same was true of the epidemic of 1789-1790 that hit Manchester.   Other areas in northern England close to Manchester remained mysteriously free of the disease.[18]

As a regional rather than a continental disorder, typhus was unquestionably spreading towards the end of the 18th century. During these critical decades, some of its previous foci were now enlarging to the point where most of Ireland, much of northern and western France and a substantial part of European Russia were all beginning to know this disease more or less constantly. Trying to detect the presence of typhus over long periods has been a very difficult thing to do historically. It was not a dramatic disease. It never killed large numbers of people as plague and smallpox did, nor did it disfigure the face and body in the way that syphilis had. Moreover, as already mentioned, its early history in Europe has been so irretrievably confused with the course of other febrile disorders that its actual presence in European society up to the late 1700s is still shrouded in mystery. However, by the end of the 18th century, from all appearance some kind of change was definitely beginning to occur in typhus. The disease was either being detected much more often or it was becoming much more widespread, or both. By the 1770s, typhus was definitely expanding in northern France, especially in the area of Normandy.[19] Here, the disease was suddenly and justifiably becoming notorious. From Normandy, the disease spread right into neighboring provinces, a major epidemic of typhus breaking out in the Vendée in western France squarely in the midst of a peasant revolt against the new revolutionary government in Paris.[20] On the other hand, warfare was apparently no longer needed to help spread this accelerating disease. For, by the turn of the 19th century, typhus was also spreading through the chronically-poor rural areas of Ireland. There, the disease even took on epidemic proportions during the disastrous Irish crop failures of 1817.[21] Besides France and Ireland, typhus was also beginning to saturate much of western Russia by the 1790s. Russian physicians were not only noting the disease's spreading influence, they were also becoming increasingly alarmed by the number of victims the disease was claiming.[22]

By the early part of the 19th century, European society, for one reason or another, was becoming much more conscious of typhus. Typhus, it is now known, is caused by a tiny organism which is generally referred to as a rickettsia. Rickettsia, primarily because of their size, are normally ranked half way in between bacteria and viruses.[23] The particular microorganism involved here Rickettsia prowazeki is transmitted from one victim to another by infected body lice that are known, somewhat revealingly, by the Latin term Pediculus hominis. Because the lice that spread this disease survive best in conditions of human filth and squalor, typhus has historically been identified by a number of names, including camp-fever, famine-fever, putrid-fever and jail-fever.[24] The cause of typhus and the vector responsible for spreading it were finally discovered as a result of studies done just before and during World War I. The bacteriologist who finally uncovered the microorganism responsible for this disease was a Brazilian, one Henrique da Rocha-Lima. Da Rocha-Lima made his monumental breakthrough while he was working in Germany among Russian prisoners-of-war, many of whom were already suffering from typhus. He first identified the microorganism in 1916. It was at that particular moment when he decided to name it eulogistically after two fellow scientists, the American Howard T. Ricketts and the Austrian Sanislaus von Prowazek, both of whom had died investigating the origins of the disease.[25] There was no question in da Rocha-Lima's mind, or that of the scientific community, that he had the right organism in 1916. For, rather convincingly, he had found the Rickettsia prowazeki in a full 95 percent of the cases that he examined in the Cottbus prisoner-of-war camp outside of Berlin.[26]

Da Rocha-Lima's unexpected discovery of this microorganism led almost directly to the conquest of typhus. Scientists already knew a number of years before the war that typhus was transmitted by a vector. That fact about typhus had been uncovered in 1908 by a leading French bacteriologist, Charles Nicolle of the Pasteur Institute in Tunis.[27] A year after da Rocha-Lima published his findings, a Polish biologist by the name of Rudolf Weigl was able to come up with a workable vaccine against the disease. It was historically the first effective vaccine against a major European disease since the introduction of cowpox vaccine more than a century before. However, unlike Jenner, Weigl did not use a related substance. Instead, he developed his vaccine directly from the microorganism that was naturally housed in the intestine of the infected lice.[28] The perfection of this vaccine came too late to subdue the last great epidemic of typhus that began to rage out of control in the eastern parts of Europe at the end of the war. Nevertheless, by the late 1920s, thanks to the widespread use of Weigl's vaccine, the disease was virtually extinct in most of Europe.[29] The introduction of antibiotics, which proved just as effective against rickettsia as they were against bacteria, also helped to guarantee in the 1940s that typhus would never return. The victory of medical science over typhus, historically-speaking, was a swift one. Prior to this, of course, the cause of typhus, like the cause of so many other infectious diseases, had been an epistemological mystery. More often than not in the historic past, typhus had not even been seen as a unique disease. In fact, for long periods of time it was simply classified as just one of a whole series of barely perceived diseases that included a fever. When the medical profession finally did begin to see that typhus was, indeed, a distinctive disease, it, nonetheless, continued to view the fever that inevitably accompanied this disease as its most outstanding feature.

The Scottish physician William Cullen, for example, certainly believed that the initial chill and subsequent fever were critically important to understanding the pathological course of this disease. Focusing in minutely on the disease's very first symptom, Cullen described it, by saying:

> At the same time, the face and extremities became pale; the features shrink; the bulk of every external part is diminished; and the skin, over the whole body, appears constricted, as if cold had been applied to it. At the coming on of these symptoms, some coldness of the extremities, . . . may be perceived by another person. At length, the patient himself feels a sensation of cold, commonly first in his back, but, from thence passing over the whole body.[30]

This initial chill soon gave away to an extremely high fever, one which came and went. As far as most physicians were concerned, this particular syndrome, featuring first cold and then heat, was the most conspicuous characteristic of typhus and the one they looked for most often. After this beginning, typhus usually lasted for another two weeks, sometimes spotting its victims, sometimes not. Rather acutely Thomas Bateman noticed in the 1810s that typhus took an entirely different course in various individuals. It affected some people mildly, while others were made desperately ill. Discussing the milder form of typhus, he described its rather uncomplicated impact by saying:

It commences with lassitude, shivering, and headache, which
are soon followed by heat and dryness of thirst, aching pains
in the loins and limbs. . . . Occasionally, nausea and vomiting
occur at the beginning; the appetite is lost; and the tongue is
covered with a thin white mucus. Even when neglected these
symptoms frequently subside spontaneously after a week or
ten days.[31]

The much more extreme form of typhus that Europe was beginning
to know over an extended geographic area by 1800 was also described by
Bateman.   Complicated typhus, as he referred to it, was both more
disabling and more deadly. According to Bateman, it acted much more
violently than the milder form did, causing extreme drowsiness, parched
skin and a delirious rambling among those it attacked. Those who were
unfortunate enough to come down with complicated typhus were in the
words of Bateman, struck "as late as the 12th [day] . . . [with] a
considerable increase of langour and debility . . . . The voice became
feeble and the speech slower, the tongue dry, with a brown streak in the
center . . . [with] the pulse smaller . . . [and] the eyes dull."[32] More often
than not, complicated or, more exactly, malignant typhus wound up killing
a fair proportion of those that it infected. Although Bateman was not on the
Continent at the time, he could just as easily have been describing scenes
from the pandemic that struck Europe in the wake of Napoleon's military
adventures, for in 1806, just after the battle of Austerlitz, typhus broke out
among Russian prisoners-of-war. That beginning rapidly produced what
was probably Europe's greatest epidemic of typhus ever. Starting in
Bohemia, the disease spread relentlessly into southern Germany, northern
Switzerland and eastern France. After that, it turned southward, affecting
parts of Austria, Hungary and Russia. In Moravia, which bordered on
Bohemia, highly accurate records were kept by public officials of the
number of victims claimed by the disease. Those records revealed that
there were a total of 13,262 cases of typhus in 1806 in this one Austrian
province alone. And of those who came down with it, some 1,171 died.[33]

A few years later in 1812, Napoleon's Grand Army went marching into Russia with little or no suspicion that they were invading one of the disease's main geographic focal points. Retreating from Moscow in the following year, typhus began to spread through Napoleon's army drastically decimating its ranks. According to one French eye-witness the disease that was spreading so alarmingly through the French troops was indisputably a form of malignant typhus. His report stated that "the typhus that showed up was for the most part the malignant form with very pronounced symptoms."[34] At Vilna, in Lithuania, meanwhile, Napoleon suddenly decided to leave behind some 30,000 sick and dying soldiers, those who obviously could not keep up with his regular units. Most of them were hospitalized under the most primitive conditions imaginable. According to the memoirs of one French observer, Count Gasc, the suffering among these troops reached absolutely startling proportions. Writing after these events, he recalled:

> The disease broke out in its most severe form causing wild delirium, very large petechial abcesses and gangrene. Many patients succumbed within twenty-four hours . . . . The corridors and courts [of the hospital] were filled with dead bodies and with refuse of all kinds, while in the rooms themselves there was no less filth, since nobody removed the excrements. The courts and corridors were so covered with dead bodies that it was necessary to walk over heaps of them in order to enter the rooms.[35]

The precise mapping and recording of incidences of typhus proceeded more scientifically with each passing decade during the 19th century. By then, the medical profession and public health officials had all been trained to look upon typhus as a truly distinctive disease. Either because it was growing in virulence or because it was detected more often or both, typhus now seemed to be blanketing larger and larger areas on the European continent. Without, of course, ever really knowing why it was happening, the military still found itself constantly harassed by this disease. One of the worst disasters associated with typhus occurred at Torgau in Silesia in the 1810s. Here, a local epidemic of typhus wiped out a garrison of 25,000 men in a matter of a few weeks.[36] While the military was still being affected, the widespread presence of typhus in the general population was being confirmed both by better diagnostic techniques and by improved record-keeping. Documents, for example, compiled by the British Registry Office for the years 1837-1843 proved that during this time period 112,072 individuals died of typhus. Since the death-rate from typhus during these decades usually hovered at about seven or eight percent of all those taken ill, it is relatively safe to conclude that nearly a million Britishers had this disease during this short six-year span.[37] Even more distressing was the fact that the sheer scale of the morbidity and mortality being reported meant that typhus was now occurring in Britain at about the same rate as smallpox. London, moreover, definitely seems to have been a focal point for disease, with the city averaging 2,500 deaths from typhus each and every year during the 1850s. In addition to this, a full eight percent of the patients treated at the London Fever Hospital in the 1860s, while the disease was on a downward swing, were typhus patients.[38] All of this information raises the rather intriguing question of just what percentage of those dying from the seemingly innumerable fevers of a bygone age in London were, in actuality, the victims of typhus. Those often ill-defined fevers were, of course, an all-too-common cause of death in 18th-century London. The same was true a hundred years earlier. For in the 17th century, 3,000 Londoners a year were dying from fevers, a certain number of them presumably from typhus.[39] Given the state of medical knowledge in these earlier periods, it is impossible to tell whether these people were dying from typhus or from some other febrile disorder such as malaria, tuberculosis or influenza. The truth can never be determined largely because of the past's persistent inability to separate one type of fever from another.

As in the case of syphilis, the 19th century's growing penchant for keeping more precise records than ever before revealed that a truly astonishing amount of typhus was present in European society. Hospital records, in particular, tended to bring this fact out into the open. For example, death-certificates compiled at the Berlin Charity Hospital, the medical facility for the poor and indigent in the German capital, proved that tuberculosis was the principal cause of death among the hospital's patients. That particular bit of information was not all that surprising, considering that tuberculosis was by the last third of the 19th century taking one out of every three adults lives. What was remarkable, however, was that of all the post-mortems done for 1875, typhus turned out to be the second leading cause of death in the hospital wards.[40] Even more fascinating were the statistics published by the Munich General Hospital for the years 1865 to 1875. They proved conclusively that typhus was, again somewhat surprisingly, the second leading cause, after tuberculosis, of hospital admissions.[41] Typhus was not only operating more extensively than had been previously thought in such major urban areas as London, Berlin and Munich, it was also evidently present in the countryside as well. A highly significant study of family records accumulated in Hüttenheim, a small village in the eastern part of France, for the late 18th and 19th centuries has brought to light a very consistent pattern of typhus mortality. Decade after decade, this disease persistently stole the lives of seven percent of those who were unlucky enough to come down with this illness.[42] All of which raises, once more, the still unanswered question of just how much undetected typhus there actually was in Europe before the coming of the Industrial Revolution.

The endemic typhus of the 19th century, seen so often in certain parts of the European continent, was more than likely the geographical pool from which Europe's last great pandemic was to emerge. That horrifying pandemic broke out right in the midst of World War I. It just began raging out of control on the eastern front during the summer of 1916. The medical descriptions of the disease that was then spreading so quickly over the fighting area are highly reminiscent of previous reports on typhus that had occurred much earlier historically. In fact, the following analysis of the disease's symptomatic course is in itself a rather telling reminder of certain 18th-century descriptions which emerged at the very same time when typhus was first being recognized as a separate disease. The kind of typhus that was soon to engulf all of eastern Europe was described by two Allied doctors. According to them, this disease was:

> ... characterized by a continuous fever, lasting ... a fortnight, and by morbid symptoms which are chiefly nervous and respiratory. One of its symptoms, and the most constant, is the appearance, during the first days of the disease, of a characteristic exanthem [rash] .... . It commences on the trunk ... first of all under the armpits, on the shoulders, then in the region of the epigasstrium [abdomen] .... The appearance of the eruption coincides with an aggravation of the intensity of all the morbid symptoms. The nervous disorders and the delirium are aggravated. The eye is haggard, the face now pale, now flushed. The temperature oscillates between 104 and 106 ; the pulse small and feeble.[43]

From this and other descriptions, it was becoming more and more apparent that a very malignant form of typhus had broken out in the trenches of eastern Europe. Moreover, it was soon coursing its tortuous way through large segments of the civilian population, with the Russians being especially hard hit. Inside Russia, the disease raged on, almost uninterruptedly, from the later part of 1918 right into 1922. During that time, an estimated 25 million Russians, nearly a quarter of the country's pre-war population, came down with typhus. Of those affected, some 25,000 died, a miraculously low figure when one considers that this represents a mere one percent of those taken ill,[44] for, if this epidemic had anywhere near the death-dealing effect of earlier episodes of the disease, up to 2 million Russians would have perished. The epidemic that was to ravage Russia for the next four years first broke out in November and December of 1918, right in the midst of the growing food shortages and political chaos associated with the Russian Revolution. By the early part of

1919, the newly established People's Commissariat of Public Health was reporting that a fresh 250,000 cases of the disease were occurring each month.[45] The situation was even worse for the Red Army, which was then engaged in fighting against White forces during the Russian Civil War. For whole units of Red Army troops were being immobilized by the disease during the crucial spring and summer of 1919.[46] This already far-reaching epidemic grew even more intense during the famine of the early 1920s, with more than 850,000 cases of the disease occurring in a single month, specifically February of 1920. Even after reaching this peak, it still took two more years before this disease finally loosened its grip on Russia. For that matter, as late as March, 1922, 280,000 new cases of typhus were being reported in the country.[47] Over the course of the next six months, the epidemic, at long last, subsided. When it did, it marked the very last time that an epidemic of typhus would ever go racing through any part of the European continent. After this, typhus just faded from European history. Thereafter, the Health Section of the League of Nations was systematically able to monitor its declining impact upon European society. By 1929, most governments were reporting that typhus was now totally absent from their countries.[48] By then only a half a dozen cases could be found in the whole of Europe. The final elimination of typhus was made possible a few years later in the mid-1940s by the introduction of antibiotics, which proved to be highly effective against rickettsial disorders, especially typhus.

As in the case of so many other diseases, the actual number of people who died from typhus in the historic past is virtually impossible to determine. This disturbing disease, with its characteristic fever and spotting, turned out to be even more perplexing to the medical profession than plague and smallpox had ever been. For typhus was rarely seen as a separate and distinct disease. Nosologically, it was not even separated from typhoid, which is caused by a bacteria, until 1837.[49] As far as can be estimated from the much-improved record-keeping of the 19th century, death-rates from typhus were normally in the range of seven or eight percent of those who were clinically affected. Statistical studies done on the Moravian epidemic of 1813 demonstrated rather conclusively that death-rates there hovered at just below 10 percent.[50] Other evidence also exists to substantiate this figure. For example, in eastern France, where the disease seems to have been present indigenously, the death-rate during the epidemic of 1864 was exactly seven percent of those who were made ill.[51] Half a century later, the League of Nations estimated that during the Russian epidemic of 1918-1922, one-tenth of those who came down with serious typhus infections were, in fact, killed off.[52] Typhus, on extremely rare occasions, could be a lot more fickle and much more murderous. A prime example of this occurred in Serbia in 1915, where a full 60 percent of those suffering from the disease were to die of it.[53] An examination of what statistics do exist on typhus further reveals that this disease was primarily a killer of young adults. This pattern held true, rather mysteriously, whether typhus was operating endemically or epidemically, all of which raises the truly puzzling question as to why children and older adults were spared the more serious consequences of this disease when it did strike.[54]

Typhus, when it attacked the civilian population anywhere, was pre-eminently a disease of the poor and downtrodden. As the Scottish physician William Alison explained in the case of Edinburgh: "I hold it to be fully ascertained that at this moment the unemployed and destitute poor, although they must be a very small minority, probably 1 in 20 of the population of Edinburgh and its neighborhood, furnish a large majority -- usually three-fifths to two-thirds -- of the fever population."[55] Pharmaceutically, typhus was virtually ignored down through the centuries. Vomiting, purging and bleeding, the classic remedies employed for handling most disease, were, in turn, normally prescribed up to the early 19th centuries in cases of typhus. One or several of these techniques were used all in an attempt to help "Nature endeavoring to expell the morbifick matter."[56] It is true that during the middle and later parts of the 19th century, a few drugs such as opium and aspirin were used, but they were mostly employed to ease some of the disease's more disquieting symptoms.[57] In comparison with plague, syphilis and smallpox, which were at times in the European past highly visible diseases, typhus went relatively unnoticed for long periods. It was not a disease that worryingly attracted the interest of the medical profession, primarily because its symptoms were so difficult to sort out from a variety of other ailments. Over the long haul, then, typhus operated more or less surreptitiously. It remained for untold centuries, a disease whose influence was so subtle that it usually went undetected. Even though it was unrecognized, typhus was not an uneventful disease, for it was apparently killing off Europeans with a kind of muffled efficiency long before it was finally recognized. Once that identification took place in the 19th century, it often seemed as if typhus was operating with about the same impact as smallpox. It may be that typhus had always operated to this degree. The truth in this case is difficult to determine, largely because the overall history of typhus has been dimmed by a lack of knowledge of the disease.

Unlike typhus, which penetrated European society almost silently, the coming of cholera in the early 1830s was not only noticed, it was literally heralded by health officials. A great deal was already known about cholera and its disturbing consequences to the body long before it first arrived in European Russia in 1829. British doctors, working in the Indian subcontinent, knew well that one of the disease's main focal points was in Bengal in the eastern part of India.[58] Beyond the knowledge that the medical profession already had of this disease, medical cartography was so advanced by the early 1830s that both governments and public health officials could literally watch cholera gaining ground from one country to another.[59] Cholera itself began to spread out of its Asian homeland in the late 1810s and bleakly started to make its way towards the major population centers of the Middle East and Europe. Very few people in Europe had ever seen this disease before. As a result, the general population was, from a biological point of view, completely unprotected against the disease, with levels of immunity obviously quite low. Cholera invaded the European continent with about the same intensity as plague had in the 1340s and malignant syphilis had in the 1490s. Although less deadly than its real Medieval predecessor, plague, cholera was still an extremely frightening disease. Before it finally exhausted itself in most of

Europe towards the end of the 19th century, it wound up taking somewhere in the neighborhood of 10 million lives.[60] Most Europeans were, at the time, terrified by cholera, especially as one pandemic began to succeed another. That fear was bound to be there, considering the fact that cholera whenever it struck took tens of thousands of lives almost instantly.

Asiatic cholera, as it was called, first penetrated Europe proper in August of 1829, attacking the Russian city of Orenburg on the Ural River. Russian physicians on the spot were very much surprised by a set of symptoms the appearance of which they had never seen before. Even more astonishing to them was the way in which the disease acted so suddenly and so violently, sometimes killing in a matter of hours. Europe's very first case ever of cholera struck a young Russian soldier by the name of Andreas Ivanov. On August 26, he was admitted to the local military hospital suffering from "bilious vomiting, diarrhea, unbearable pains in the abdomen, shrunken features, blue lips, a slimy tongue, cold extremities, . . . weak pulse and extreme anxiety."[61] He died within a few hours. Russian medical teams could do little else than watch helplessly as more and more soldiers and civilians began to succumb to the disease. More often than not, these first Russians died exceedingly painful deaths. Actually, a rather full and complete record still exists of the disease's third victim in the city of Orenburg. Obviously resigned to the final outcome of this disease, his attending physician wrote:

> The disease began at two in the morning, with a dreadful purging, which returned every minute. About five o'clock he was without feeling, quite powerless, and affected with constant cramps. At six I found him again sensible, but with sunken pale-blue cheeks, dimness of the eyes, coldness of the feet and hands, and bedewed with clammy sweat. He was tossing about and complaining of trembling in the hands, a sense of oppression at the pit of the stomach, and intolerable thirst. The vomiting . . . commenced much later

than the purging . . . . The exhausted, powerless conditions of the patient, in particular his completely imperceptible pulse, . . . left me no hope for his recovery . . . . soon afterwards the man expired.[62]

Within months of these initials cases, millions of Europeans would be coming down with similar symptoms, with up to half of them dying from this new and seemingly unstoppable disease.

Like two other of Europe's great deadly and disabling diseases, plague and smallpox, cholera was, in fact, a very ancient ailment. But it differed from the other two in that for long centuries it was confined to those areas that bordered on the Delta of Ganges River. Alexander the Great and his marauding army may possibly have come in contact with cholera in the western portion of India. If he did, he never returned it to present-day Europe. A millenium after the time of Alexander, Tibetan records spoke descriptively of a disease which was then called nja. The symptoms of this disease were unmistakably similar to cholera. Even at that moment, cholera was a disease that quickly exhausted its victims. The Tibetan records suggest this, speaking as they do of a disorder that "suddenly destroys the vigour of life and changes the warmth of the body into cold, but sometimes this changes back into heat. The various vessels secrete water so that the body becomes empty . . . . The nja kills invariably. Its first signs are dizziness, a numb feeling in the head, then most violent purging and vomiting."[63] For hundreds of years after this, beginning with the age of exploration, Portuguese, Dutch, French and English adventurers and settlers all described the disease. But even though Europeans were constantly coming into contact with cholera, the disease still remained enigmatically confined to the Asian littoral. Then suddenly and without warning, cholera began in 1817 to spread out from its Asian homeland, penetrating the Middle East and reaching Russia by the later part of 1829. Meanwhile, back in British India, cholera was taking on a virulent character, and it was this extreme form of the disease that was just about to descend upon Europe.[64]

After gaining a foothold in the eastern and southern parts of European Russia, Asiatic cholera moved steadily westward reaching Moscow in the autumn of 1830 and St. Petersburg in June of 1831.[65] Right after the epidemic had peaked and had passed on to central Europe, government officials inside Russia placed the number who had died at more than a quarter of a million. Beyond this, death-rates from the disease were discovered to have been around 50 percent of those clinically affected. Moscow and St. Petersburg and the rural areas surrounding them were hit very hard, with nearly half of the country's confirmed cases and up to 100,000 deaths taking place in these two regions alone.[66] After ravaging parts of Russia, the disease next attacked Warsaw and its environs. Cholera also operated here epidemically, with German observers reporting that "the number of sick was so large . . . the hospitals were so crammed with sick that they were virtually brought to a standstill."[67] From Poland, the disease was soon spilling over into Prussian territory. The unrelenting advance of this disease, from east to west, frightened the French government into sending a medical team to Russia, Poland and Prussia to study cholera's intensifying virulence. The two French physicians from the Royal Academy of Medicine who were part of that team, Auguste Gerardin and Paul Gaimard, were so startled by what they saw that they immediately grew pessimistic. They wrote back to Paris saying that: "The progressive march of cholera from east to west can not be presently arrested by any power known to man."[68] Their conclusions were accepted almost fatalistically, for nothing seemed capable of stopping cholera as it steadily made its way into western Europe.

By the summer of 1831, most of the major cities and ports of central and eastern Europe had been overwhelmed by the disease. Only Italy, France, and the Low Countries and Great Britain had, up to this point, been spared. The British, for a short while at least, were hopeful that the disease might be confined to the Continent, the king telling Parliament in June of 1831 that: "It is with deep concern that I announce to you the continued progress of a formidable disease . . . in the eastern parts of

Europe. ... I have directed that ... precautions should be taken ... against the introduction of so dangerous a malady in this country."[69] The king was speaking of imposing a quarantine. But, administrative measures of that kind proved woefully incapable of arresting the disease's growth. This became apparent when shortly after this cholera progressively invaded the Netherlands, France and England. The horrifying sights produced by so many of the disease's victims were almost too much for some to bear, many turning to panicky flight. Not only were secondary symptoms such as headaches, blue lips, stomach pains, tremors and ringing in the ears a frightening spectacle, but the sheer quantity of the vomiting and purging, all coming on so suddenly, was distressing to watch. These later symptoms were described, somewhat dispassionately, by a British physician, who observed that in most cases:

> The stool became extremely frequent and watery, of a peculiar unnatural smell, and greyish white colour, so as exactly to resemble ... barley water in appearance; vomiting comes on, and after the common contents of the stomach, a clear watery fluid, interspersed with flakes of mucous is discharged; copious sweat breaks out; and anxiety and debility rapidly increase.[70]

In western Europe, as well as elsewhere, cholera singled out the poverty-ridden elements within society. As was the situation with typhus, those living in destitution and squalor proved to be the most vulnerable. In the city of Paris, mortality among well-to-do elements actually declined during the epidemic of 1832, partially because some of the rich had already fled. By contrast, among poorer elements especially those in artisan society, death-rates often doubled and tripled.[71] The escalating intensity of the disease's impact in the French capital was from all accounts psychologically overpowering. During the week of April 1st, there were 79 reported deaths from cholera, by the 8th the figure had jumped to 861, and within another week it was up 7,000.[72] Very often the faces of those who were dying from the disease were visibly transformed. Within hours, youthful vigor gave way to the cragginess of old age. Many in Paris saw the familiar features of friends and relatives literally change overnight. This obviously disquieting metamorphosis was described in one case in the following way:

> The countenance assumes a peculiar appearance; by which alone the disease may generally be distinguished. This is so remarkable as occassionally to render servants recognized with difficulty by their masters, even in the early stages of the disease. It is difficult to be described, but it bears a striking resemblance to age; and seems to arise from the paleness, wasting and shrinking of the features, and the depressed and disturbed state of the mind, conveying into the countenance a strong expression of care, anxiety and alarm.[73]

After taking some 15,000 lives in Paris, cholera made its way to London where it soon claimed another 7,000 lives.[74] Death-rates from the disease in western Europe, however, did seem to be significantly lower than those that had been chalked up in eastern Europe. But, given the ferocity of the disease along with its painful symptoms, these statistics were not particularly comforting to those who came down with cholera. As it turned out, the population of London proved to be just as jumpy as any other once cholera invaded. For here, as elsewhere, victims of the disease were made ill "from nausea . . . [and] an acute attack of pain, either in the stomach or colon, . . . [with] an irritable condition of the bowels or actual diarrhoea, varying in its intensity and duration from one hour, to two, three or more days."[75] After passing through the British Isles, this first great pandemic of cholera next moved on to Italy where it finally exhausted itself in 1837. In Italy, the disease proved almost as punishing as it had been in Russia and the rest of eastern Europe. For here it took over 100,000 lives, attacking all parts of the peninsula more or less evenly.[76] The speed with which cholera had struck the European continent in the 1830s amazed both government authorities and public health officials. Nothing like this had happened since the now all-but-forgotten plague epidemics of the 17th century. But, once cholera had passed through Europe, little trace of it could be found in the late 1830s and early 1840s. The same could not be said of the late 1840s, when Asiatic cholera returned in pandemic form, only to stay on after that as a recurring epidemic disease.

After an absence of nearly ten years, cholera enigmatically returned to Europe in 1847. Once again, it entered Europe by way of Russia. As in the early 1830s, the disease positively punished Russia, this time far more seriously than before. With record-keeping significantly more advanced than during the first epidemic, public health authorities recorded a staggering total of two and half million cases of disease and over a million deaths.[77] Just as during the first pandemic, cholera swept across Europe from east to west. It then moved on to France and Great Britain, before eventually hooking south into Italy, where, as it had before, it finally came to an abrupt end, this time in 1855.[78] Some of the major population centers in western Europe were again singled out for attack, with Paris losing 19,000 lives and London, 14,000.[79] Not only did cholera follow the same geographic path that it had travelled in the early 1830s, it showed a very similar level of intensity. For, again, it turned out to be considerably more virulent in the east than it had been in the west. Moreover, it was during this second pandemic that cholera began to settle permanently into parts of Poland and Russia. After this, from 1847 down until 1902, Russia was to experience endemic cholera continuously. During this entire period, she was only free of the disease for one year.[80] Meanwhile, Poland, which had suffered the loss of 24,000 lives during the epidemic of 1848, would likewise know the disease year after year.[81] Even worse for the population of these two countries, cholera kept reasserting itself epidemically, leaving an additional 48,000 dead in Poland in 1852 and killing another 131,000 Russians in 1855.[82]

By the late 1840s, Europeans had become fatalistically accustomed to the rather gory symptoms produced by Asiatic cholera. A good deal of that fatalism was the result of the medical profession's inability to stop the ever-increasing vomiting and purging that characterized this disease and which ultimately led to the death of so many patients. The following medical report on a 21 year old Englishman, suffering from cholera, was typical of the way in which this disease struck countless others. This young man entered the hospital on August 22, 1847. The report on him at that moment disclosed that: "He was vomiting to-day about two quarts of fluid, and has been purged so often that he cannot tell the number of times, but says he has had seven stools in the last five hours." The symptoms persisted for the next seven days, so exhausting the patient that by August 29, he was, the report now read: "Comatose, breathing hurried and labourious . . . sometimes ceasing for more than a minute, and then there is long gasping inspiration; skin of head and trunk warm; of extremities icy cold; pulse intermittent; eyes sunken and fixed."[83] He died on the next day of a disease which the medical profession still considered to be highly perplexing. The actual symptoms of cholera were so exaggerated, that unlike typhus, it was relatively easy to identify right from the start. But, the etiology of cholera and the precise way in which it was transferred were for several decades really quite baffling. As it was, however, the age of medical discoveries, based on microscopic studies, was about to begin and cholera would not remain a mystery for too much longer after the 1840s.

Cholera itself is caused by a water-borne bacterium known as Vibrio cholerae.[84] The survival of this rather fickle microorganism is almost totally dependent upon environmental conditions. Outside of the body, it is extremely fragile and easily dies off. But, inside of the body, it is extraordinarily destructive. Within the body, it normally attacks the walls of the intestines. When this occurs ingestion is effectively curtailed, causing, in turn, the vomiting and purging that is so characteristic of an attack of cholera.[85] It is now known that the actual infection is caused by either one of two microscopic agents. The first is the older or more classic type, which was evidently rampant during the European pandemics of the 19th century, and the second is the El Tor variety, which is presently quite common in both Africa and Asia.[86] The specific microorganism that caused the more classic type of cholera was for a very long time thought to have been discovered by the noted German bacteriologist, Robert Koch in 1882.[87] However, more recent research strongly suggests that the Italian biologist Filippo Pacini was, in fact, the first to identify this microorganism some 28 years earlier in 1854 through its ubiquitous presence in the intestines of its victims.[88] Pacini called the organism he had discovered miriadi di vibrioni and very early on proved that it did, indeed, have a corrosive influence on the walls of the small intestines.[89] However, writing in a language that was not international, his important breakthrough was obviously lost to a medical profession that was desperately searching for the disease's etiology.

The coming of cholera produced a great deal of confusion among medical men. During its onset, French physicians, working among the sick in Poland in 1832, could only compare this disease to either dysentery or simple diarrhea, even though its actual pathological consequences went far beyond those two individual illnesses.[90] Among others, the French physician, Ferdinand Foy immediately noticed that Asiatic cholera was an extremely fast-acting disease, especially the more virulent form that was now rampaging its way through the eastern part of Europe. Reporting on its all-too-obvious alacrity, Foy commented: "The duration of cholera is ordinarily very short, many subjects succumbing to the disease in four, six or twelve hours; while others are able to resist for twenty-four or thirty-six hours, rarely more than forty-eight."[91] Watching cholera in action, Foy was extremely skeptical about the medical profession's ability to help those who were already ill. Almost hopelessly, he remarked: "If there is one disease whose lack of therapy has spread despair and discouragement among the friends of medicine, it is cholera."[92] As lethal as cholera was to many of its victims, many others seemed to escape it completely. Doctors and nurses were, for example, rarely touched by the disease even though they were in close proximity to many patients suffering from it. This led the Scottish physician William Ferguson to say about the cholera that: "No one . . . can be warranted utterly to deny the existence of contagion, but . . . if contagion do exist at all, it must be the weakest in its powers of diffusion, and the safest to approach of any that had yet been known amongst disease."[93]

Modern autopsy, which was just about to reveal the long concealed third stage of syphilis, was likewise used in an attempt to pinpoint the physiological damage that cholera was capable of doing. At first this was almost impossible to determine, largely because cholera soon developed into a constitutional disorder that finally damaged widely-separated portions of the body, including the sinuses, the brain, the venous system as well as parts of the intestines. Even into the 1840s, highly detailed post-mortems still failed to locate the disease's true center of attack.[94] Initially, it was thought that cholera might be a blood disease, largely because of the rather extensive haemorrhaging that cholera always caused. The well-known Italian physician Antonio Gambin was an early exponent of this theory. He kept encouraging others to investigate the blood for more active signs of the disease's presence.[95] This avenue of inquiry was, however, soon exhausted, and by the early 1850s anatomical studies from all over Europe were pointing unmistakably to the intestines as the real center of the disease's attack. The Royal College of Physicians in London, strongly persuaded by the work of both German and French pathologists, unanimously agreed in 1854 that "the mucous membrane of the small intestine was constantly a rose tint . . . we almost always found intense capillary hyperaemia."[96] It was this discovery that kept fascinating Pacini and which led him towards his monumental discovery of the germ involved here in the same year.

While the medical profession was moving closer and closer to a true description of cholera's pathological course in the body, speculation still abounded as to just how the disease was spread. The well-known German medical thinker, Max von Pettenkofer, believed that the disease was being carried invisibly in the form of seeds. These seeds were, he thought, passing from the human alimentary tract to the ground where they germinated simultaneously giving off an infectious gas.[97] This highly imaginative variation of the much older miasmatic view of the origin of disease won a considerable amount of backing. One of Pettenkofer's leading disciples went on to explain this point of view even further, saying that the "disease is induced by some deleterious vapor or gas perhaps proceeding from the bowels of the earth, which mixing with our atmosphere and applied to the body, or inhaled . . . exerts its deleterious influence on the blood and vital organs."[98] Given the prevailing miasmatic interpretation of the origins of disease, only one lone anonymous voice was heard in London in 1832 arguing instead that the disease was most likely water-borne.[99] It took the work of two Englishmen, the statistician William Farr and the physician John Snow to finally point the medical profession in the direction of the more accurate idea that cholera was indeed carried by water and not by corrupt vapors in the air.

Farr and Snow, working independently, both came up with rather convincing evidence that cholera was primarily a water-borne disease. Farr was by training a statistician who probably never fully realized the medical implications of his findings. Nevertheless, functioning as a governmental investigator, he demonstrated, using statistical evidence, that cholera was linked to water. Proceeding from the facts that he had accumulated, he was able to conclude that: "Cholera was three times more fatal on the coast than in the interior of the country."[100] Snow, by contrast, was a physician who approached the question of cholera's origins, not environmentally as Farr had, but as one might expect diagnostically. Snow was convinced as early as the late 1840s by evidence from post-mortems that cholera primarily attacked the alimentary tract. From that information he deduced that the only way it could have gotten there was as a result of being swallowed.[101] This led him to assume that contaminated water must, of necessity, be the source of the disease. Publishing his conclusions, he wrote in 1854: "there is often a way open for it [cholera] to extend itself more widely and to reach . . . [all] classes of the Community; I allude to the mixture of cholera evacuations with the water used for drinking and culinary purposes."[102] Snow's argument that a person had to swallow "the peculiar poison or morbid matter," rather than breath it in, was not readily accepted by other physicians, most of whom were still intellectually tied to the miasmatic view.[103] Snow's ideas were not finally accepted until decades later. Even as late as 1874, medical men from all over the continent, meeting in Vienna for the Fourth International Sanitary Conference, still voted unanimously that the air was the sole means by which cholera was spread.[104]

An estimated 10 million people died of cholera during its stay in European society. Not since plague had a single major European disease produced such high mortality in such a short period of time. For cholera did kill up to 50 percent of those that it infected, primarily, as Farr had so rightly seen, those who lived in either river towns or in port cities. Because it definitely was a water-borne disease, cholera kept singling out commercial centers for attack. This pattern first became obvious in the early 1830s. Moscow, St. Petersburg and Budapest, all on major river systems, were extremely hard hit by the disease, with death-rates consistently in the neighborhood of 50 percent. For example, in Russia alone between 1829 and 1834, there were a reported 236,715 deaths out of a total 553,743 cases, a majority of them in and around the major urban areas of northern Russia.[105] Hungary was just as badly mauled, with Budapest and its surrounding area taking the brunt in 1831 of a national epidemic which ultimately claimed some 237,614 lives.[106] As Asiatic cholera moved towards the west, both its fury and its death-dealing effect seemed to diminish. The French port of Bordeaux, however, proved to be a conspicuous exception. Here the disease turned out to be unexpectedly virulent, with a full two-thirds of those infected dying.[107] Everywhere else in the west, death-rates fell off in comparison to what they had previously been in the east. In England, there was strong evidence that the disease had, indeed, lost some of its virulence. For in York, in northern England, the overall death-rate among those infected was only 40 percent, while in Exeter to the south and west, it was only 35 percent.[108]

DEATH TOLLS IN SELECTED EUROPEAN
CITIES FROM CHOLERA, 1830-1892[109]

City	Date	Number Killed
Moscow	1830-31	4,588
London	1832	6,800
Paris	1832	14,592
London	1849	14,000
London	1854	10,700
London	1866	5,918
Rotterdam	1866	1,242
Naples	1884	5,000
Hamburg	1892	8,200

After two great pandemic sweeps, one in the early 1830s, and the second in the late 1840s and early 1850s, cholera returned to Europe in pandemic form for a third time in the middle of the 1860s. As in its two previous visits, cholera once again travelled from east to west before finally turning south into Italy. This time around, however, Russia was treated much more leniently than she had been in the past. Other areas, as it turned out, were not as fortunate. Bohemia and Moravia, both staging areas for troops fighting during the Austro-Prussian War of 1866-1867, were severely attacked with more than 80,000 civilians in the two provinces perishing from cholera. Unusually widespread epidemics of the disease also occurred in Italy, where another 130,000 people died in many instances, it was reported, extremely painful deaths. Most other parts of Europe were spared, including France which this time around only lost some 10,000 lives.[110] Although, the third pandemic of cholera was much more subdued than earlier ones, the cities were again made to feel its sting. In the Netherlands, as an illustration, such major urban centers as Gronigen, Utrecht, Leiden and Rotterdam all quickly reported deaths in the hundreds or thousands.[111] Like the previous pandemics of cholera, this one also began to wane. When it did, it turned out to be the last time that Asiatic cholera would ever spread itself across the whole of the European continent.

Cholera returned to Europe in pandemic form for the very last time in 1892. It sped quickly across the length of Russia and northern Germany before inexplicably coming to an abrupt halt. In the early 1890s then, cholera did not move across the entire continent. Instead, it turned into a purely localized disease.[112] Even though the cholera epidemic of the early 1890s was limited as never before in its geographic sweep, it was, nonetheless, just as deadly as it had ever been. Inside of Russia, the death-rate hovered, as it always had, at about 50 percent of those actually infected. During the course of 1892, 145,000 Russians would die from cholera, a figure that is just under one-half of all those known to have been taken ill.[113] After punishing Russia, cholera next raced across northern Germany, where it took a truly frightening toll of those living in the port city of Hamburg. There, the disease wiped out nearly 16,000 people in a matter of just a few short weeks.[114] After this somewhat pronounced pandemic, cholera settled down to become a peculiarly Russian disease, lingering on in that country endemically. Here, over the following four years, it would tragically claim yet another quarter of a million lives. But in the ensuing decade and a half, cholera seemed to be diminishing inside of Russia. That decline proved to be more apparent than real, what with major epidemics of cholera flaring up all over again in 1910 and 1921.[115] Finally, as of the early 1920s, cholera was definitely gone from Europe. Historically-speaking, cholera's stay in Europe had been much shorter than that of most other diseases. Moreover, by comparison, it never did claim anywhere near the total of lives that plague, smallpox and tuberculosis would eventually take. Still, its symptoms were so ghastly and its death-rate so high, that its very presence in industrial society seemed to be some kind of ghostly reminder of what life had been like in Europe when plague was still rampant.

The cholera that was now passing from the European scene had long since been identified by Koch as a bacterial disorder. But it was not a disease that could be easily cured. In actuality, during most of the 19th and early 20th centuries, this disease was simply left untreated. This happened in numerous cases largely because physicians dealing with the disease had very little time in which to act since death usually ensued in a matter of hours. Most doctors, moreover, were personally helpless to prevent the massive loss of liquids containing such life-giving substances as potassium salts and water.[116] When one considers the number of nutrients being lost to both vomiting and purging, what is truly remarkable is that up to half of those who were afflicted actually recovered on their own. Fortunately for most Europeans, cholera was not a particularly contagious disease. The very fact that the microorganism involved here was not capable of being air-borne obviously limited its impact. The only way that it could be taken in was if someone indigested food or water already contaminated by germ-laden human faeces.[117] Quite obviously then, personal hygiene along with a relatively clean supply of water could and did steadily reduce the spread of this disease in the 19th century. For like typhus, cholera needed both filth and squalor if it was going to perpetuate itself.

Although cholera went unchecked during its stay inside of European society, today it is a disease that can be easily controlled. In fact, in areas of the globe such as Africa and Asia where it is still known, cholera has been repeatedly overcome. This is largely the result of the fact that antibiotics, in particular the tetracyclines, have proven to be so effective against the disease. In addition to the use of drugs, the World Health Organization has come up with other useful measures. Most of these new techniques have been developed to stop the excess loss of liquids which frequently lead to death by dehydration. When they care for the sick, teams from the World Health Organization normally make use of a treatment which they refer to as rehydration. This highly specialized approach requires, first of all, that the patient take in large quantities of a solution containing both glucose and salt. This is done in order to increase the patient's level of physical energy and to restore some lost electrolytes. If the case is especially severe, the victim is next treated with a special solution of sodium chloride, sodium acetate, potassium chloride and glucose, all designed to restore lost nutrients.[118] These modern techniques, along with an ever-improving system of public sanitation, have, of course, gone a long way in recent decades towards taming this disease.

Although they are caused by entirely different microorganisms, both typhus and cholera were routinely bred by squalid living conditions, especially in the larger cities. If anything, these diseases just seemed to aim for those areas where human waste simply lay in stagnant pools, never being flushed away. Still, when everything is taken into account, both typhus and cholera must really be regarded as secondary diseases. They neither lasted as long as plague, syphilis or smallpox, nor did they take anywhere near as many lives as the other three did. They did add, however, sometimes dramatically, to the growing number of illnesses that seemed to beset 19th-century European society. Europe as a whole was becoming more prosperous during this advancing industrial age. Her overall population doubled between 1800 and 1900. Food was both more nutritious and more plentiful. And it was fast becoming more available to all levels of society. Improving levels of nutrition were soon reflected in an increase in longevity, with average life-expectancy rising during this century from 28 to 50 years.[119] The great anomaly in all of this was that Europe's growing prosperity was significantly marred by the presence of so many deadly and disabling diseases. For even as the century moved along, smallpox was still common, so was tuberculosis, which by the 1880s was taking one out of every three adult lives, and so also were syphilis and typhus. In actuality, of course, these last two diseases were being discovered by record-keepers in quantities that made them, indeed, seem more prevalent than ever before. Add to this already alarming total, the death-dealing effects of cholera and Europe would certainly appear to be what it had always been, still essentially a disease-ridden society.

The age of truly infectious disease, which had been such an integral part of the European past, was about to end. Modern sanitary conditions along with the use of microbiology and chemotherapy would together soon end the grip which certain microorganisms had on the European population. More importantly, during the 19th century, the continued presence of these microorganisms inside of European society did not conspicuously limit either the growth of population or the increase in life-expectancy. The irony of it all was that they continued to exist and do damage in a society that was growing healthier and more prosperous with each passing decade. The question might be legitimately asked at this point then -- why were these diseases so prevalent at a time when the population of Europe was biologically stronger? The answer may very well lie in the fact that Europe was now undergoing a process of urbanization. Unquestionably, microorganisms need numbers in order to survive. Apparently, they found them in the burgeoning populations that were making their way into nearly every European city during the 19th century. Those populations, obviously, improving their living standards, were, nonetheless, still evidently lacking in truly effective levels of immunity. As a result, many of them proved susceptible to one or another of these crowd diseases. Among other considerations then, the sheer act of crowding can go a long way to explain the continued existence of smallpox, the flare-ups of syphilis and typhus and the epidemics of cholera that were taking place in 19th-century Europe.

CHAPTER 5

TUBERCULOSIS

Among the imminent Symptoms ushering in Acute Consumption, must . . . be reckoned an Haemopotoë or spitting of Blood, which sometimes happens on a sudden, and in large Quantities, without any previous Cough, but is accompanied with Pain and Heat of the Breast.

--Benjamin Marten, A New Theory of Consumptions, More Especially of Phthisis, 2nd ed. (London, 1722), p. 8.

Of all the diseases that were prominent in European history, tuberculosis was undoubtedly one of the most widespread and worrisome ever to occur. Rising in importance as time went on, tuberculosis first came to public attention during the 17th century. From there on in, it started to claim a higher and higher percentage of those dying until, by the end of the 19th century, it was taking the lives of one out of every three adults. Not only was the mortality being caused by tuberculosis steadily rising, so also was the morbidity. The result of all of this was that by the last quarter of a century before World War I, tuberculosis was becoming as universal as smallpox had been a hundred years earlier. Before the coming of the Industrial Revolution, no one ailment had ever claimed the lives of more than 20 percent of the population at any one time. The only exception to this rule was, of course, when a particular area was unlucky enough to be hit by an epidemic. Tuberculosis was to change all that. Historically, tuberculosis has always been listed as an epidemic disease. The fact that few in the past ever spoke of tuberculosis in pandemic terms is really quite confusing, especially if one considers that by the late 1800s tuberculosis was fast becoming the most serious health problem that Europe had ever encountered. Tuberculosis may have been described as an endemic disease, but it was by then killing in truly pandemic proportions. It has been estimated that tuberculosis would ultimately take the lives of some 350 million Europeans, a large number of them during the 19th century. Hundreds of millions of others also had the disease, but they were fortunate enough, it seems, to overcome it.

Even though the medical profession was growing decidedly more confident as the 19th century went on, it was justifiably fearful of the growing presence of tuberculosis. The well-known German bacteriologist, Robert Koch was among those who were fully conscious of the public health problem that tuberculosis was now beginning to pose for everyone. Placing the problem in historical perspective, Koch commented: "If the number of victims that a disease claims is a measure of its significance then all diseases particularly the most dreadful infectious diseases such as bubonic plague ... [and] Asiatic cholera, must rank far behind tuberculosis."[1] One of the keenest minds ever to work in the area of medical science, Koch was himself responsible for two gigantic breakthroughs in the area of tuberculosis detection. For not only did he discover the microorganism responsible for tuberculosis, he also devised a technique, known as tuberculin, for uncovering the presence of the disease in those who were still alive. Armed with tuberculin, the medical profession beginning in the 1890s could easily determine just how prevalent tuberculosis actually was. The results were often shocking for investigators. For example, in Vienna in 1927 and 1928, one study conducted with tuberculin proved conclusively that a full 61 percent of the six year olds in that city had already been infected by the disease.[2] It was clear from both this and countless other studies that tuberculosis was, indeed, saturating a major part of European society.

Tuberculosis normally produces both internal and external symptoms that make it, at least in its final stages, a disease that is relatively easy to identify. Constant coughing along with the spitting of blood were in the historic past definite signs to others that the disease had taken hold. There were also some internal signs of the disease's presence, but they were not discovered until much later on. But by the 1700s more and more autopsies were revealing the fact that in advanced cases of pulmonary tuberculosis, nodules were forming and embedding themselves in lung tissue. It was from this last symptom that the name for tuberculosis was eventually drawn, since the word tubercle in Latin originally meant nodule.[3] There are, rather curiously, no outstanding references whatsoever to some of the more obvious symptoms of tuberculosis in biblical times.[4] On the other hand, modern-day anthropologists working with mummified remains in Egypt have reported tell-tale spottings on lung tissue as well as spinal lesions.[5] Both of these pathological findings are symptoms of very advanced cases of tuberculosis. While there is, then, rather convincing evidence that tuberculosis existed in Egyptian times, there is no proof that the disease was in any way universal. Rather, what traces of the disease anthropologists have discovered indicate, at the most, that tuberculosis was probably only marginally present in Egyptian society.[6] Among the ancient Greeks there were some literary hints that tuberculosis may have existed at that point in history. Homer, for instance, did fleetingly refer in his writings to a "grievous consumption that separated soul and body." Shortly after the time of Homer, yet another pre-Christian writer may have been thinking about tuberculosis when he declared, somewhat angrily: "The Lord shall smite thee with a consumption, and with a fever, and with an inflammation."[7] Whether these somewhat cryptic remarks were actual references to tuberculosis is, of course, not all that clear. More than likely they were, since very few other diseases in history have acted in the same debilitating and all-consuming way that tuberculosis has.

Outright evidence that tuberculosis existed on a large scale in Roman times is just as difficult to come by as evidence for its presence in ancient Greece. Medical literature is, in this connection, a rather accurate barometer of a disease's dominance. The reason for this is that physicians in the past tended to focus their attention on those illnesses that they came across most frequently. With the single conspicuous exception of Galen, most of the medical literature from Roman times is completely silent on tuberculosis and its symptoms. By contrast, Galen did produce an extraordinarily detailed account of a disease that was unmistakably a case of tuberculosis. Perhaps, Galen was more perceptive than some of his contemporaries, or conceivably he just stumbled onto a number of isolated cases of the disease. Either way, his account stands virtually alone, indicating that the disease was more than likely not all that prevalent in Roman times. The only consideration that might possibly qualify this particular conclusion is the fact that autopsies were not all that common during the Roman period. And it is true that tuberculosis is sometimes difficult to diagnose unless a post-mortem has actually taken place. Still, the evidence mustered up to this point strongly suggests that the disease was only marginally present both during the Classical period and then thereafter during the Medieval era. It was there, however, often enough in the Middle Ages to give rise to the recurrent myth that Medieval kings were endowed by the divinity with special powers to drive away the symptoms of tuberculosis.[8] The so-called King's touch was suppose to be able to produce this kind of miraculous result. While tuberculosis existed, here and there during the Medieval period, it was never seen as a truly worrisome disease, for the society of the times was troubled, not so much by tuberculosis, but by a series of other diseases such as scabies, leprosy and plague, and, towards the end of the period, syphilis. In the medical literature of the age, all of them overshadowed tuberculosis.

Tuberculosis, which for a long period of time was better known as phthisis, did not burst forward as a truly major disease until the 17th century. By then, it was systematically claiming a number of royal victims, including Louis XIII of France and William of Orange. Almost inevitably, these deaths, along with others, began to give to this disease a notoriety that had not been previously attached to it.[9] Meanwhile, during the latter part of the 17th century, the medical profession, after centuries of neglect, was finally beginning to focus in on this disease. Among those who were proving to be leaders in this field of inquiry was the Dutch physician Sylvius de la Boë. Watching the disease claim more and more victims in the upper reaches of society, Sylvius consciously turned to autopsy in the 1670s in a determined bid to learn more about phthisis and its anatomical effects. What he discovered turned out to be both new and revealing. For it was Sylvius who firmly established in the medical mind the connection between phthisis and the damage it was capable of doing to lung tissue. Focusing his attention on the pulmonary form of tuberculosis, the only kind which was then known to exist, he immediately discovered in one victim after another the disease's characteristic pitting. Commenting on his findings, he declared: "I found more than once larger and smaller tubercles in the lungs, which on section were found to contain pus. From these tubercles I hold that not infrequently phthisis has its origin. . . . Only the wasting originated by an ulcer in the lung is to be called phthisis."[10] These strikingly original studies by Sylvius started to take on greater significance primarily because of the growing mortality that was being attributed to the disease. What Sylvius discovered was, of course, one of the most conspicuous features of pulmonary tuberculosis, nodules forming on the lungs. What he and his contemporaries did not perceive was that tuberculosis could and did act even more subliminally than this, for tuberculosis was just as capable of affecting other parts of the body. That fact was lost to the medical profession for the next century and a half. Indeed, even in some cases of pulmonary tuberculosis, the lungs are not all that noticeably affected. Even though many cases of tuberculosis were in this era being missed by doctors, tuberculosis was, nevertheless, still killing according to official reports, up to 20 percent of all those dying, for example, in the city of London in 1700.[11] The so-called "White Plague" of the late 17th and early 18th centuries had evidently already begun.

This unprecedented growth in the number of cases of tuberculosis inevitably captured the attention of others within the medical community. One of the most famous studies done on the disease at this time was published by the English physician Robert Morton in 1689. His work became so well known that it was soon regarded as a classic. It was widely used both in England and on the Continent for nearly a century after it had first been published. As it turned out, however, Morton's work was flawed. He evidently went astray when he accepted without question the assumption of the Roman writer Galen that the lungs were somehow regulated by invisible glands. These glands, according to Morton, were what were actually being attacked when tuberculosis first struck. Elaborating on this theory, Morton pointed out: "The glands of the lungs which in natural condition are imperceptible are immensely increased and stimulated into aposthemes [ulcers], when they become abnormal, . . . an apostheme is the whole immediate cause of consumption."[12] Combining this notion with the prevailing miasmatic view of disease, Morton went on to declare at another point: "An Original Consumption is that, which arises purely from a Morbid Disposition of the Blood, or Animal Spirits, which reside in the System of the Nerves and Fibers."[13] Not all of Morton's studies were based upon misconceptions. For example, he was among the very first to notice that the pleura, the rather thin, protective membrane that surrounds the lungs, was, in fact, consistently inflamed by this disease.[14] For the next century and a quarter, the medical profession did not make much headway beyond the original discoveries of Sylvius and Morton. Totally unable to check the advance of this disease, tuberculosis was fatalistically listed in most medical lexicons as a constitutional disorder, one that was incapable of being cured.[15]

As the 17th century moved along, tuberculosis began to affect more and more Europeans. By the 1630s, the English epidemiologist John Graunt was able to report that, as of that moment, tuberculosis was the leading cause of death in the city of London. It was, according to his figures, responsible for a full 15 percent of the mortality in the English capital.[16] Given the fact that this age tended to identify this disease exclusively as an infection of the lungs, his calculations were, if anything, more than likely too low. Graunt's figures for the city of London are also a bit suspect because they do not take morbidity into account. And undoubtedly, some people who had the disease did somehow manage to recover from it. Even so, from the middle of the 17th century on, tuberculosis remained London's most persistent killer, claiming anywhere from between 35,000 and 45,000 lives each and every decade down until the 1750s.[17] By then, of course, hundreds of thousands of Englishmen had become melancholily acquainted with tuberculosis of the lungs. The onset of this disease in a growing number of people was graphically described in the early part of the 18th century by one Benjamin Marten, who wrote:

> A Consumption of the Lungs is often introduced in the following manner: The patient . . . is . . . first seiz'd with a Defluxion of thin Rheum from the Nostrils, a Soreness of the Palate, Throat, Breast and Lungs, which is soon attended with Hoarseness, a troublesome Coughing up of Matter, at first thin and white, then bluish, but in a short time yellow or green, resembling the Pus or Matter commonly found in external Ulcers . . . . The symptoms are . . . often accompan'd with the Head-ach, and almost universal Disorder of the Body, and always with a slight Fever.[18]

All over England in the 18th century, both in the capital and in the provinces, there was a relentless increase in deaths from tuberculosis. Statistical evidence accumulated at Chester, in the northwestern part of the country, proved that by the early 1770s a full 22 percent of the deaths in that city were directly attributable to consumption. Lagging far behind the figures for tuberculosis as a cause of death were a series of secondary ailments including old-age, cancer, cough, ricketts and tooth-decay.[19] The impression that was gaining force among medical people that tuberculosis was fast becoming the nation's number one health problem was confirmed by statistics brought together by John Bateman. Drawing upon published material, Bateman cogently pointed out that in London in 1669, tuberculosis was unquestionably responsible for 1 in every 6.2 deaths. By 1749, the same figures had climbed to 1 in every 5.5 mortalities, and by 1808, they were a horrifying 1 in every 3.6.[20] Just as apparent as the mounting death-rate were the symptoms that were tormenting a larger and larger percentage of the population. Tuberculosis was in the historic past among the most quixotic of all killers. In some cases, it would run its course in a matter of weeks, while in other instances it would linger on for up to twenty years or more.[21] Unfortunately, for most, the ever-increasing pain and suffering that this disease brought to them hung on for an excruciatingly long period of time. The English physician Thomas Beddoes described for later generations the agonizing symptoms that those who were terminally ill had to put up with. Writing in an almost mournful tone, Beddoes described the painful symptoms that some had to endure, saying that they consisted of:

> [a] hard rendering cough, attended sometimes by retching and vomiting . . . ; the expectoration sometimes nauseous, always offensive to the eye and harrassing when it is not free; the languor with which the patient finds himself overpowered . . . the extremes of cold and heat through which he is carried by the daily returns of hectic [fever]; the sweats in which he repose by night drenches him; the breathlessness on motion or without motion, arising by degrees to a sense of drowning and terminating in actual drowning when there is no longer strength to bring up the fluids, secreted by the chest.[22]

The coming of the 19th century also saw the number of deaths from tuberculosis start to proliferate on the Continent. By then, tuberculosis was spreading so dramatically, that in the words of one historian it was now beginning to appear on nearly every street.[23] Prior to the 19th century, consumptives, still virtually the only recognized form that this disease took, were not normally hospitalized. They did not warrant hospitalization because it was universally assumed that they were incurable. The practice of excluding consumptives from hospitals declined at the beginning of the 19th century. This change came about because most physicians were now convinced that tuberculosis was a constitutional disorder, a disease which was not in the least bit contagious. Since it was taken for granted that consumptives were not dangerous to others, the admission of those with tuberculosis to local hospitals was increasingly being seen as a charitable gesture, and something that should be done. In actuality, of course, tuberculosis was a contagious disease, so that the admission of consumptives to the wards of the Hôtel-Dieu, the principal charity hospital in Paris, did have the immediate effect of spreading the disease.[24] The admission of consumptives to hospitals and other types of institutions did help public health authorities, on the other hand, to assess just how much tuberculosis there was in European society. For example, by the late 1830s, the Strasbourg City Hospital in the eastern part of France was regularly reporting that 10 percent of its patients were now dying of pulmonary tuberculosis.[25] Shortly after this in the early 1840s, a check of the children in Lisbon's only public orphanage proved that 30 percent of them were already suffering from consumption.[26] By mid-century, tuberculosis was so commonplace that it could be readily found anywhere. Even the mental wards of the Bethlem Hospital in London knew the disease. For by the 1850s, one of every three of its patients who died succumbed to symptoms that were recognizably those of tuberculosis. Even more revealing were the statistics that were gathered at the Royal Naval Hospital in Malta. Here, crewmen were treated over a long period of time by doctors who had an excellent opportunity to observe certain diseases run their course. Of those dying in this Maltese hospital, between 1829 and 1838, an astonishing 40 percent of them, after carefully-conducted post-mortems, were found to have died from pulmonary tuberculosis.[27]

During the early part of the 19th century, most physicians sincerely believed that tuberculosis was an incurable disease. Among others, Dr. Antoine Portal, professor of medicine at the College of France, simply assumed that the victims of tuberculosis had been singled out ahead of time for the disease by their own weak constitutions. Writing in a somewhat despairing tone, Portal summarized this kind of thinking in 1809 when he argued: "There is no more dangerous disease than pulmonary phthisis and no other is quite so common. For the most part it carries off individuals who are destined for it by birth by a bad constitution of their organs."[28] Because this disease was thought to be, in the words of the well-known French pathologist G. L. Bayle, "nearly always . . . fatal,"[29] very few drugs were ever prescribed for it.[30] Without any hope of relief whatsoever, most victims of tuberculosis simply had to endure the pain that was nearly always with them. In this regard, the widely read English novelist Robert Louis Stevenson has left behind a rather gripping account of what life was like for those suffering from tuberculosis. Describing his own situation, he wrote:

> I lie awake troubled by a hacking, exhausting cough, and praying for sleep or morning, from the bottom of my little shaken body. I have written in bed, and written out of it, written in haemorrhages, written in sickness, written torn by coughing . . . the Powers have so ordained that my battle field should be this dingy inglorious one of the bed.[31]

The long standing mystery as to what caused tuberculosis was finally cleared up in 1882 when Koch discovered the microorganism, Mycobacterium tuberculosis, responsible for its spread. Koch not only isolated the bacteria at work here, he was also able to reproduce the disease in certain laboratory animals.[32] Koch's evidence was so convincing that his findings were almost immediately accepted by the rest of the medical profession, without significant rancor or debate taking place. But, for decades before this, the medical profession had been struggling to understand just what caused this highly debilitating disease. For the most part, its thinking had been bogged down by the belief that tuberculosis was, strictly speaking, a constitutional disorder. It had just been assumed in the past that tuberculosis had been inherited by those who had a feeble disposition to start with. In these types of individuals, the disease would eventually reveal itself by directly attacking the lungs, if not sooner then later on in their lives.[33] Beyond this, unless the lesions caused by tuberculosis were there on the lungs and discovered by means of an autopsy, the disease was thought to be totally absent from the system. The rather rudimentary state of the profession's knowledge about this disease was summed up in 1814 by the English physician Henry Southey. He clearly explained that post-mortems on the victims of tuberculosis would unfailingly produce certain results. Reporting on what he inevitably found, he declared:

> On examining the lungs of those who have died of strumous phthisis, a number of vomicae [tubercles] are . . . found of different sizes; a whole lobe, and sometimes the entire lung of one side will be found filled with them, small portions of lung in a sound state intervening. It is sometimes impossible to make an incision without cutting into an abcess.[34]

These readily observable clusters, ordinarily scattered over the lung, remained in the early 1800s the only recognizable internal sign that death had taken place as a result of consumption.[35] In this respect, then, the medical profession had barely advanced beyond what it had already known a century and a half earlier.

By the decade of the 1830s, medical knowledge about tuberculosis was finally beginning to advance. Even though the notion that certain emaciated individuals were predestined for tuberculosis still hung on, there was an increasing awareness by medical men that this disease could affect the whole of the body and not just the lungs. In spite of this discovery, physicians continued to be highly pessimistic about the outcome of this disease. Among those who were still not convinced that tuberculosis could be cured was the pioneering French physician E. C. A. Louis. Pointing to the chronic character of this disease, he said somewhat bleakly: "From the nature of the causes, the universality of the disease, and the variety of organs in which tuberculosis deposits take place, it [tuberculosis] cannot be regarded as a specific, but an almost physiological and necessary consequence of the more or less prolonged application of influences."[36] Even though he himself was among the legion of doctors who despaired of ever finding a cure for tuberculosis, Louis was, nevertheless, among the very first to understand that tuberculosis could affect the whole of the human body. This, in itself, was a rather significant advance over previous medical thinking. Gains would also be made in other areas. For instance, modern autopsy, which was so instrumental in revealing new facets about syphilis and typhus, was soon to break down some of the false thinking that had surrounded tuberculosis up to this point. Much more minute studies of lung tissue, making use of the microscope, were, for example, by the 1840s proving that tuberculosis could not only kill more quickly than earlier suspected, but that a good deal of pulmonary tuberculosis was, indeed, going undetected. The English coroner, William Addison reported on just such an eye-opening experience in 1843. Still somewhat startled by his own discovery, he told of one highly revealing post-mortem that he did in the following way:

> Case I - A girl, six years old, making no complaint whatever of the chest, was taken with vomiting and fever, succeeded by pain in the head, drowsiness, dilated pupils and insensitivity, in which state she died. On examining the lungs they appeared to be quite healthy, . . . of the normal light pink hue; no tubercles could be detected by the touch, and all the sections that were made swam in water. After two days' maceration [soaking], the sections were slightly extended, and examined by lens, when a great many minute tubercles were discovered.[37]

Although the true pathological course of tuberculosis through the human body remained a rather deep mystery, more and more was being learned about the symptoms of this disease. For generations before this, medical attention had focused in on the so-called hectic fever that usually accompanied an attack of tuberculosis. By the middle of the 19th century, the tendency of this fever to go up and then down no longer seemed to be as diagnostically significant as it had once been.[38]   While the medical profession was slowly changing its mind as to what was and what was not an important symptom of this disease, the strongly entrenched belief that tuberculosis was a constitutional disorder still dominated medical thinking right into the 1850s. Bodily weakness, often symbolized by poor appetite, inevitably predisposed a large group of individuals to the disease, according to Dr. Henry Ancill. What else could explain, he and others asked, the fact that so many who were in daily contact with consumptives never came down with the disease. Far from being contagious, Ancill argued, logically in his own day, there were those in society who were unfortunately destined for the disease by heredity. These types could be easily identified, he pointed out, because their whole manner was characterized thus:

> A deficiency of vital power, corresponding with the low vitality
> of the blood, and the structural imperfections of the tissues
> and organs, is the most general expression by which the
> state of the functions of life in tuberculosis subjects can be
> characterised; and this is measured by a greater or lesser
> degree of constitutional debility. This debility is exhibited in
> the organ functions especially, and has already been
> exemplified by the weakness of cell-growth in the ultimate
> nutrition of the body.[39]

This time-honored view of the disease's origins was being challenged, at least in part, by mid-century. Critics were beginning to point out that apparently healthy individuals were likewise coming down with tuberculosis. Along with others, Dr. John Hogg, still clinging to the idea of predisposition, did give in some and grudgingly admitted that "an exciting cause, such as a cold, a damp residence, or an unhealthy occupation may [also] induce . . . [tuberculosis] in a person of robust frame, descended from healthy parents."[40] In spite of this concession, the general feeling persisted among medical men that the disease was, in most instances, inherited.

While new insights into the pathology and etiology of tuberculosis came very slowly, progress was being made much more often in the area of detection. Developments in this field were measurably aided by two rather dazzling discoveries both of which were made by the noted French physiologist René Laennec. In the year 1816, Laennec discovered, almost by accident, that if he used asculation he could often determine the presence or absence of pulmonary tuberculosis in one of his patients. The wooden cylinder that he developed for testing sounds in the area of the chest was, of course, the forerunner of the modern-day stethoscope.[41] Armed with this device, physicians could now literally listen to the lungs and determine, by differences in tone, whether or not a patient had tuberculosis. Asculation, as this process was originally called, did improve the ability of physicians to diagnose advanced cases of tuberculosis. But it hardly saved any lives, for that would have depended on much earlier detection. Still, the use of asculation proved what some had already suspected, that tuberculosis could make some of its victims terminally ill not over the course of years, but rather in a matter of weeks or months. Just such a case occurred in Dublin at the Meath Hospital. The patient in this case was a young Irish woman, one:

> Bridget Doyle . . . 28 years, a servant, [who] was admitted on the 29 of September, stating that five weeks previously she had been attacked with cough, . . . accompanied by febrile symptoms. She was much relieved by bleeding . . . , but early in November, the voice [through asculation] could be heard indistinctly issuing through the cylinder . . . . The expectoration began now to assume the tuberculosis character and we concluded that a cavity was beginning to form.[42]

According to the French physician Laennec the traditional assumption that everyone who came down with tuberculosis died of it was not necessarily true. Challenging older beliefs about this disease, Laennec became more and more convinced that some patients were naturally overcoming tuberculosis. Laennec's own work in the area of post-mortems proved, at least to his satisfaction, that the scars on some people's lungs were, in actuality, a kind of pulmonary tuberculosis that had already been healed. Writing about his highly unorthodox discovery, he optimistically reported that:

> After I was convinced of the possibility of cure in the case of ulcerations of the lungs, I began to fancy that nature might have more ways than one of accomplishing this end, and that, in certain cases the excavations [tubercles], after the discharge of their contents, by expectoration or absorption, might cicatrize [heal with a covering scar] in the same manner as . . . in other organs . . . . In consequence of this idea I examined these productions more closely, and came to the conclusion that, in every case, they might be considered as cicatrices.[43]

Laennec's rather astonishing discovery here was not generally accepted by his fellow physicians. Instead, as has already been mentioned, tuberculosis continued to be viewed, rather darkly, for decades after this as a disease that could not possibly be cured.

Right up to the decade of the 1850s then, the medical profession was still unaware of the actual pathological course that tuberculosis was capable of taking inside of the body. Most still passionately believed that it was a disease that was exclusively confined to the lungs. In this kind of atmosphere, novel ideas about the disease put forward by such enlightened thinkers as Laennec did not get very far. Meanwhile, tuberculosis was fast becoming a disease that nearly everyone was thinking about.[44] For death rates were rising very precipitously. By 1900, at least three million Europeans a year were dying from the various forms of tuberculosis.[45] What had once been regarded as a mere endemic disease was quickly turning into Europe's most fearsome pandemic ever. Not since the terrifying days of the Black Death in the 1340s had any one disease acted to take the lives of so many Europeans. The heavy death tolls being chalked up by this disease even convinced some medical observers, especially after the discoveries of Koch in the early 1880s, that tuberculosis was actually gaining in virulence. In most places in the 1890s, tuberculosis definitely appeared to be more toxic than it had ever been.[46] Tuberculosis was either becoming more dangerous or it was being detected more often, or both. By the end of the 19th century, the medical profession certainly knew a great deal more about the disease. By then, it understood, all too clearly, that the microorganism at work here was just as capable of attacking nervous, abdominal, intestinal and bone tissue as it was of destroying the lungs.[47] Once that realization took place, it soon became apparent to Koch and a host of others that tuberculosis had, indeed, become the most serious health problem that Europe had ever confronted.

In the second half of the 19th century, no part of Europe was spared the ravages of tuberculosis, with the single exception perhaps of Great Britain. The British Isles were still experiencing the disease on a wide scale, but proportionally in this area of Europe at least tuberculosis had evidently peaked and was by the 1850s now starting to decline. London was an outstanding example of this particular trend. During the period right after 1800, London was losing about 5,000 lives a year to consumption.[48] Four decades later, the figure was up to 7,000. But, in relation to London's exploding population, which had nearly quadrupled in the interim, the proportion of Londoners dying from tuberculosis had long since begun to decline.[49] These figures, while they seem to be representative, are marred by the fact that only those dying from tuberculosis of the lungs were actually included in the statistics. Beyond this highly revealing information for London, there is additional evidence that the disease was on the downswing elsewhere in Great Britain. For example, figures gathered for such major urban centers as Liverpool and Ipswich also showed that by mid-century death-rates from tuberculosis were first stabilizing and then declining. To begin with, tuberculosis was not all that common in the rural areas of Britain. By the middle of the 19th century, however, it was occurring there almost as frequently as it was in the cities.[50] Starting in the 1850s, death-rates from tuberculosis, particularly in England and Wales, began to fall sharply. By the 1870s, deaths from this disease in relation to overall population were just half of what they had been two decades earlier, and, by the 1890s, they were one-third.[51] Meanwhile, in neighboring Ireland, death-rates here were also beginning to stabilize and by the 1870s would likewise be dipping downward.[52] This does not mean, of course, that tuberculosis was releasing its hold on these three areas of the British Isles. For even as late as the 1910s, tuberculosis was still the leading cause of death in Britain, albeit, less often than before.[53]

The decline in the number of deaths attributed to tuberculosis in Britain, perhaps due to a loss of infectivity on the part of the microorganism involved here, was not matched by developments on the Continent.[54] There, if anything, the age-old symptoms of this disease were being seen with greater, not lesser, frequency. Moreover, the disturbing sights and sounds produced by tuberculosis were just the same as they had been before. In the words of one physician, they remained:

> . . . a dry hacking cough, dyspnoae [shortness of breath], . . . increasing emaciation and exhaustion, with intermitting febrile attacks, and great depression of spirits, the cough on a sudden becomes loose, and the expectoration copious, and altogether changed . . . to a thick yellowish, homogeneous fluid, or to ash-coloured, light-greyish, flocculent, ragged-edged globular masses, or the same somewhat thinner, with little white masses like boiled rice in it, or streaked with white striae, with somewhat of a peculiar, faint disagreeable odour.[55]

In the decade of the 1910s, hundreds of millions of Europeans were being personally tormented by these nightmarish symptoms. For by then, it has been conservatively estimated a full 50 percent or more of the European population had this disease. Some were lucky enough to have it in its relatively mild primary stage, while others were terminally ill from a disease that they were physically unable to throw off.[56]

Tuberculosis deaths evidently peaked on the Continent sometime during the 1880s and 1890s. The German-speaking areas of central Europe were especially hard hit by a disease which up to this point was seemingly growing more infectious and more contagious all the time. Knowing all of this, few people were surprised when officials attached to the Rudolphean Hospital in Vienna announced that, between 1879 and 1888, 46 percent of the hospital's patients who had died had succumbed to tuberculosis.[57] A few years later in 1895, government officials in Germany were publicly warning about the menace of this disease. At the same time, they revealed that in Germany one out of every three adults between the ages of 15 and 70 was dying from some form of tuberculosis.[58] As it turned out, this terrifying trend did not continue. By 1900, death-rates on the Continent from tuberculosis, for one reason or another, were beginning to decline. This happened even as the disease was being more broadly defined by scientists to include other forms of tuberculosis besides the one that attacked the pulmonary system. The disease was obviously still prevalent inside of Europe, but its killing effect was being lessened. None the less, even as late as 1908, 33 percent of all the autopsies being performed in Paris showed unmistakable signs of the presence of tuberculosis. In Munich, it was 29 percent, and in Geneva it was 25.[59] Moreover, these figures taken from the Continent must be judged against the fact that some cases of deep-seated tuberculosis, involving the bones and certain organs, were still not being uncovered.[60] In spite of this unforeseen factor, it is safe to say that tuberculosis after 1900 was statistically on the decline in Europe. Never again would it regain the deadly prominence that it once had. Tuberculosis deaths declined most rapidly in those two countries, Britain and Germany, that were the most highly urbanized. That fall off tended to amaze most contemporaries, for people believed that the disease was primarily of urban origin, the result, as one observer put it, "of the intemperance and vices of the great city."[61] Whether the city was all that guilty or not, tuberculosis was definitely declining in the urban areas of Germany. Here on the eve of World War I, death-rates had collapsed fortunately to about one-half of what they had been.[62]

In the middle of the 1890s, medical science was handed an extraordinary device for detecting the presence of tuberculosis among the living. That fascinating new technique was, of course, tuberculin. Tuberculin is a protein extract that can be easily derived from tubercular baccilli. This particular substance was originally discovered by Koch in the 1890s. He hoped to use it as a vaccine against tuberculosis. In that regard, tuberculin was both a failure and a disappointment. But, as a diagnostic tool it turned out to be an extraordinarily useful device.[63] For, just by injecting small quantities of this sterile liquid into a person, physicians could readily tell whether the disease was present or not. An inflammation, or positive reaction to the injection, clearly indicated to the attending doctor that the subject had already built up immunity either to a past or present infection.[64] At first, tuberculin was used only hesitantly as a diagnostic tool. As of the early 1910s, however, that reluctance had vanished and it was by then being widely administered. The insights that tuberculin gave into the sheer volume of tuberculosis that was present in European society were absolutely astonishing to many. In 1907, for instance, 55 percent of all the children in Vienna who regularly visited a clinic were found to have either a latent or active case of tuberculosis. In the very same year, in Hamburg, among those who were 11 to 14 years of age, rather alarmingly 94 percent of those tested responded positively. Meanwhile, in the Austrian military just prior to World War I, 76 percent of those troops that were recruited from Bosnia and 39 percent of the young men conscripted in Hungary either had the disease in the past or still had it. And even as late as 1927, one out of every three children entering the school system in Vienna already had this disease.[65] By the decade of the 1910s, tuberculin was proving for all to see that, while the death-rate from tuberculosis was unquestionably falling, the amount of tuberculosis in European society that was subliminally present was still extraordinarily high.

By the turn of the 20th century, tuberculosis was no longer being viewed as an incurable disease. In fact, just the opposite was now true. Medical thinking in regard to this disease had undergone a complete turnaround. Almost everywhere, clinics, sanitaria and national programs were springing up all dedicated to bringing about a cure for tuberculosis. Many of their programs were helpful. The therapy that they nearly always encouraged included greater cleanliness, a constantly improving diet and the benefits of fresh-air.[66] While many of these considerations proved to be useful, tuberculosis was also, in all probability, declining on its own. Around the time of the First World War, deaths from tuberculosis were conspicuously falling off both in the more advanced industrial states of Europe and in those countries that were still overwhelmingly agricultural. This fact was confirmed immediately after the war by studies that were done both by the Health Secretariat of the League of Nations and by certain national bodies. In the more highly industrialized areas of western Europe, including England, France, Belgium and Germany, deaths from tuberculosis per 100,000 inhabitants in each country fell precipitously by about 40 percent between 1911 and 1935.[67] The same trend was observable in countries that were still principally agricultural, such as Spain and Italy. Here, death-rates started to peak around 1900 and then, they too, began to decline.[68] While the death-dealing effects of tuberculosis were less noticeable in most of Europe, a few countries like Greece and Rumania continued to be punished by this disease, for unlike the rest, they had continually escalating death-rates right into the 1930s.[69] This overall downward trend naturally affected the way in which both the medical profession and the public-at-large looked upon this disease. By the 1920s, it was increasingly being seen as both a less fatal and a less fearsome disorder.[70] This fall in deaths was probably the result of rising levels of immunity within the general European population. As people grew stronger biologically, fewer were dying from tuberculosis, although just as many seemed to be suffering from its morbidity.

Once Koch discovered the bacteria that was individually responsible for tuberculosis, the medical profession suddenly realized that this disease was, indeed, highly communicable.[71] Beyond this, doctors, who were able to trace the social impact of this disease, soon learned that tuberculosis was primarily a disease of young adults living and working in an urban environment. This widespread impression was soon backed up by hospital records which proved beyond all doubt that those who were dying from tuberculosis were overwhelmingly between the ages of 25 and 35.[72] And when these young adults perished, they did so much more frequently in the city than in the countryside. Precise statistics being kept for such major urban areas on the Continent as Berlin, Munich and Vienna all showed that death-rates in these cities were significantly higher than the national average.[73] Along the same lines, almost every study done in Great Britain likewise demonstrated that over the long run death-rates in the cities from tuberculosis exceeded those for rural areas.[74] Some physicians in Britain, obviously struck by this dichotomy, went on to explain that farmers, ploughmen and shepherds who worked in the out-of-doors inevitably developed an immunity to tuberculosis. Actually, this was not the case. For large numbers of those living in rural areas of Britain did develop tuberculosis. This was especially true in the 1880s and 1890s when this disease seemed to be spreading out of its urban bastions.[75] In spite of this all-too-apparent development, it was popularly believed that fresh-air possessed a special curative power, one that was capable of overcoming the microorganism responsible for the various forms of tuberculosis.[76]

PROVEN AND PRESEMPTIVE VICTIMS OF TUBERCULOSIS
WITH THE AGE OF DEATH.[77]

Balzac	52	Goethe	83	Poe	40
Chekhov	44	Gorki	68	Rousseau	66
Descartes	54	Kant	80	Schiller	46
Dostoevski	60	Locke	72	Spinoza	44
Gibbon	57	Molière	51	Voltaire	84

By the early part of the 20th century, tuberculosis was no longer the baffling disease that it once had been. Ever since the 1860s, the medical profession had been steadily accumulating fresh insights into the exact functioning of this disease. Gradually, over the course of decades, medical men were finally coming to an understanding of the physiological affects of this disease upon the various parts of the body. Physicians were progressively steered onto the right path by a number of key discoveries. Among them was Laennec's earlier contention that tuberculosis was an autonomous disease, not one that had to be first triggered by some other infection such as bronchitis or pneumonia.[78] Two of Laennec's contemporaries during the early 1800s added even further to the profession's growing speculation about this disease. One of them was G. L. Bayle. After performing more than 200 autopsies on patients who had died of pulmonary tuberculosis, Bayle came to the conclusion that the disease had three readily discernible stages. The first, he argued, was relatively harmless, but the second and third were characterized by a growing infection that was, by its very nature, irreversible.[79] Portal, the second of Laennec's contemporaries, advanced the notion that there were several types of tuberculosis, all of them in tune with accepted medical thinking for that time, involving the lungs. Most of the new assumptions being put forward about tuberculosis in the 1810s and 1820s were really quite elementary. But, many of the newer ideas did help to break down some of the fossilized thinking that had previously been associated with the study of tuberculosis and its effects.[80] While some medical men were probing for new answers, overall progress in this area was being stymied by a lack of hard physical evidence concerning the course that tuberculosis was taking inside of the body. As late as the 1850s, innumerable autopsies performed by Laennec, Bayle and Portal, and their students, had still not revealed the fact that tuberculosis could act destructively in other parts of the body outside of the lungs. The very idea that tuberculosis could attack and inflame the glands, the larnyx, the meninges and the intestines was a concept that was still beyond the understanding of the best pathologists that this age had produced.[81]

The ability of tuberculosis to spread insidiously to the furthest recesses of the body was finally brought to light by the great French pathologist J. A. Villemin. Working rather unconventionally with rabbits, and not with cadavers, Villemin suddenly discovered that tuberculosis was capable of engulfing one part of a rabbit's body after another. Writing about his findings, Villemin in one memorable passage literally wiped away centuries of myth and misinformation about the true pathological course of tuberculosis. Summarizing the results of his experiments, he declared:

> Death [in rabbits] from tuberculosis is due to a variety of causes, but can be primarily explained as the result of asphyxiation, the direct consequence of tubercles accumulating in the lungs. Beyond this, the digestive disturbances caused by this disease are the consequence of the tuberculization of the nerves in both the stomach and intestines, all of which tends to produce intestinal haemorrhaging. Factually, death may be said to occur from the general effect that tuberculosis has on a whole series of organs. Tuberculosis is indeed consumptive, it involves the entire body.[82]

Villemin's amazing discovery, along with his often-expressed conviction that tuberculosis could be passed from animals to man and was therefore contagious, revolutionized the medical profession's thinking about tuberculosis.[83] For the first time in nearly two centuries, physicians now had a clear idea where to find tuberculosis in the human body.

In the years after this intellectual breakthrough, subsequent anatomical studies verified over and over again his original argument that tuberculosis actually did involve the whole of the body. By the end of the 19th century, the ability of tubercular baccilli to find any number of hospitable areas inside the body was an accepted medical fact.[84] Among the most disquieting and continually painful forms of this disease to be uncovered was tuberculosis of the bones. Here the disease normally attacked and deformed either the spine or the bones in the legs leaving the hapless victim either stooped or crippled.[85] Carefully-analyzed autopsies were by the late 1800s also proving that a variety of organs in the body, in particular the spleen, the kidneys and the liver could just as easily be pock-marked by this disease as the lungs.[86] Of the all-too-numerous forms of tuberculosis that were being discovered in the 1890s and thereafter, the most vicious was unquestionably tuberculosis meningites. That form of tuberculosis was considered both then and for decades to come absolutely incurable.[87] By the period of the 1920s, anatomical studies had even progressed to where it was clear that tuberculosis was having a very deleterious effect upon the heart, inevitably producing rather severe arterial tension. It took nearly half a century for modern medical science to finally unravel the mysterious affects of tuberculosis. Most of those discoveries were made only after medical men knew what to look for. In this respect, they were, of course, aided immeasurably by the work of Villemin and Koch. For together, they had produced the two critical insights from which all subsequent research was to flow.[88]

The introduction of first tuberculin and then X-ray in the 1890s proved to the satisfaction of most doctors that tuberculosis was truly a long-lasting disease.[89] These means of detection continually demonstrated that tuberculosis usually began in childhood. After that, it would hang on for years before finally killing its victim, death often occurring during the young adult years. This did not mean, of course, that the young necessarily escaped death. They too were seriously affected, usually dying of tuberculosis of the lungs.[90] Even though some deaths occurred in the younger years, far more commonly the disease just lingered year after year. The slow development of this disease in the vast majority of instances, led the famous German doctor Franz Hamburger to describe this ubiquitous disease in the following way:

> One can define tuberculosis as a chronic process of infection, that effects almost every cultural level from childhood on . . . . This chronic process of infection cannot be seen simply as an illness, however. It is much more subterranean than that. For one can say assuredly that tuberculosis can only be understood, for what it actually is, if tuberculosis is seen as a special dilemma of childhood.[91]

By the 1920s, the medical profession had accumulated a fair amount of knowledge concerning tuberculosis. It had pinpointed its etiology, it knew the time of life when an attack would occur and just who was most likely to prove susceptible to it.[92] On the other hand, none of this painstakingly acquired knowledge was actually bringing the profession any closer to a cure for this disease.

True, Koch's discovery of the bacteria responsible for tuberculosis in 1882 had created a great deal of optimism in this direction. But as the years unfolded, a cure for tuberculosis continued to elude the medical profession. As it turned out, the immediate impact of Koch's monumental breakthrough was more psychological than it was physiological.[93] Virtually overnight, the rather stultifying pessimism of the past that had surrounded this disease suddenly evaporated. Few believed right away that tuberculosis might be wiped out, but many now began to put forward the notion that tuberculosis was a treatable disease and that recovery was, in many instances, a possibility. More directly, Koch's discovery encouraged others to try entirely new approaches in order to bring about a cure. In Germany, the idea began to develop that surgery could be used to cut away those parts of the body that had been infected by tuberculosis.[94] In Edinburgh, an even more promising prospect was soon being explored by Dr. Robert W. Philip. Philip was absolutely convinced in the 1890s that early detection, along with a clean and healthy environment, could do a lot to defeat the disease even in those who had already been touched by it.[95] Beyond this, all kinds of self-help books were appearing by the 1890s, suggesting that a judicious combination of fresh air, wholesome food and the right environment would inevitably arrest the impact of this disease. Some of these cures worked, others did not. But what was most astonishing was the extraordinary optimism that was now being expressed by the medical profession, a group which just a few decades before had almost universally adjudged tuberculosis to be incurable.

Tuberculosis was finally conquered in the first half of the 20th century by two rather amazing scientific advances. The first was the development of BCG and the second the discovery of antibiotics. BCG was the title that was given to the vaccine that was first developed to combat tuberculosis. The co-discoverers of this vaccine were two French researchers Leon Calmette and Camille Guerin. Over the course of two decades, these two men laboriously attenuated a strain of tuberculosis to the point where it was no longer toxic to man.[96] After many trials and a few notable failures, BCG was increasingly used during the 1920s and 1930s, especially on the Continent, with good results. Like other vaccines, it tended to produce a minor infection which in turn gave to those who were inoculated a certain level of immunity.[97] In truth, tuberculosis was only partially subdued by BCG, for the disease was not finally eradicated until the 1940s and the discovery of antibiotics, in particular streptomycin. The discoverer of this drug, the American Selman Waksman, knew by 1946 that his antibiotic was definitely effective against virtually all forms of tuberculosis.[98] The widespread use of antibiotics led almost immediately to the elimination of tuberculosis in European society. So much so, that by the 1950s incidences of tuberculosis were being looked upon as an oddity.[99]

Tuberculosis was unquestionably the greatest bacterial killer that Europe had ever experienced. But unlike other bacterial diseases, such as plague, syphilis and cholera, a great deal was known about tuberculosis even at the time when it was raging out of control. In the case of other bacterial diseases, the medical profession had been continuously groping against an unknown attacker. The same was not true of tuberculosis. For after 1882, it knew exactly what to look for. The pioneering efforts of Villemin and Koch obviously helped because they proved that tuberculosis was both infectious and contagious. Moreover, by the eve of World War I, it was generally agreed that man was the principle reservoir for this disease and potentially the source of most future contagion. The more people who were infected, the more, it was now assumed, the disease would spread to others.[100] Fear that there would be higher and higher incidences of tuberculosis in the general population led to a series of public health campaigns all designed to combat its growth. Families where tuberculosis already existed were carefully watched for further outbreaks. Sanitaria were also erected at a record rate in a determined bid to bring about more cures.[101] These public health campaigns undoubtedly helped. So did even more direct attacks on the bacteria causing this disease such as pasteurization, for it was now becoming obvious that tuberculosis was just as much a disease of cows as it was of humans. Infants and children were by the early part of the 20th century thought to be picking up the disease from cow's milk that was contaminated by tubercular bacilli. Pasteurization, which was simply the act of boiling the milk, killed off these dangerous germs. Once this process was generally accepted in the 1920s, the incidences of tuberculosis among young people did begin to drop.

During the time when tuberculosis was most prominent, few men knew more about the social consequences of this disease than the Scottish physician, Robert Philip,[102] once called "The Captain of all these men of Death." Always a daring thinker, Philip was by the 1890s almost alone in challenging the long accepted notion that tuberculosis was somehow hereditary. While he accepted the fact that this disease did run in certain families, he suggested, rather intriguingly that the real cause of these infections was not heredity, but a reduced state of resistance among certain individuals.[103] This concept, which is actually the more modern idea of levels of immunity, had also been advanced by a few others, including the Silesian physiologist Hermann Brehmer in the 1860s.[104] It was not, however, until the 1890s that this notion gained any kind of acceptance at all. Obviously somewhat ahead of his time, Philip put forward the highly challenging notion that tuberculosis was not really all that contagious, its ability to infect being dependent on an individual's power to resist.[105] In the decade of the 1890s, before the idea of immunity became a popular biological concept, Philip was, in fact, only dimly aware that there was such a thing as immunity. But, over the course of time, he and the rest of the profession came to understand this life-giving process better. Forty years later in the 1930s, a much more knowledgeable Philip could declare: "Varying degree of resistance to the infection was offered by different individuals. The resultant of the infection depended on the amount of the infecting dose and its repetition, and on the resistance offered by the individual."[106]

As early as the 1890s then, Philip had perceived one of the major reasons why the death-rate from tuberculosis was in actual decline. Right up to the 1930s, tuberculin and X-ray were both proving that there was just as much tuberculosis present in European society as there had been, but fewer people were dying from it.[107] Two equally plausible reasons have been put forward to explain just why this was so. The microorganism at work here, Mycobacterium tuberculosis, may conceivably have lost some of its virulence. The microorganism, in this regard, could have been both more widespread and less toxic at one and the same time. The overall history of other diseases strongly suggests, of course, that the virulence of other microorganisms has fluctuated over time. Arguably then, a less virulent strain of the disease may have been functioning just before and just after 1918. While this explanation stands up, other considerations must also be taken into account, including the question of immunity. For the first time since the onset of plague, European society when it confronted a bacterial disease was not entirely helpless, for, in truth, the strength and stamina of the average European was much greater than ever before. Rising levels of nutrition were, in all probability, producing higher levels of immunity. All of this suggests that the killing effect of tuberculosis was being blunted, as Philip perceived somewhat vaguely, by advancing rates of resistance within the general population.[108]

By the decade of the 1950s, tuberculosis was just about to pass out of European society. It was, of course, the last serious bacterial disorder to harass the whole of European society. The age of the great bacterial killers, plague, syphilis, cholera and tuberculosis had now come to an end. While these diseases had been prominent, they had sealed the fate of hundreds of millions of people. While they had existed, they had caused death, separated families, dislocated lives and punished people both physically and psychologically. What is clear from the history of these diseases is that millions upon millions of people had proven to be too weak to fight off the toxic effects of these microscopic parasites. The question that logically emerges at this point is why? Was it because of the potency of these deadly microorganisms or was it because the mass of men and women in the past lacked sufficient levels of immunity to ward them off? The history of tuberculosis, its declining ability to kill at the very moment when it was apparently most widespread and most infectious, strongly suggests that the poverty and malnutrition of the past account to a significant degree for the prolonged presence of the great bacterial diseases in European society.

CHAPTER 6

INFLUENZA

> In sundry places it began with a weariness, heaviness and painful sensation; heat and horrours seized the whole body, chiefly the breast and head, with a dry cough, hoarseness, roughness of the jaws, difficulty of breathing, weakness and langour of the stomach.
>
> --Thomas Short, <u>A General Chronological History of the Air</u>, <u>Weather</u>, <u>Seasons</u>, <u>Meteors</u> (London, 1749), p. 9.

For an extended period stretching from the early 1600s to the late 1800s, influenza was present in European society, killing few but inconveniencing many. Operating locally, rather than on a continental scale, it eventually became known to the medical profession by a series of purely regional names. In England, during the 16th century, it was popularly known as the Sweat, later on in France it was called la grippe and in Germany it was referred to as the Blitz-Catarrh. While in eastern Europe, it was known somewhat derisively as the Russian Catarrh.[1] Unlike most other epidemic diseases, influenza was rarely a deadly disorder. Quite obviously a tame disease, its transitory symptoms in the bulk of those that it made ill failed to intrigue most medical men historically. Because it was, by and large, neglected in most medical books, influenza, even as it passed from one century to another, was often regarded as a disease that did not have a history. Each new outbreak often seemed to be the first that had actually taken place. This mistaken assumption about influenza arose because the disease would normally appear here and there only after long periods of time had elapsed. If influenza had murdered people on a truly massive scale and had occurred with greater frequency, it would, of course, have drawn a lot more attention. But, since the disease was only mildly distressing to those who had it, it remained in the minds of most just a secondary disease, one that came and went, for the most part, uneventfully. Realistically, influenza could hardly have been considered all that terrifying, especially at a time when other diseases constituted a much more serious threat to one's existence. For centuries, then, influenza lived on as a relatively harmless disease. It was barely noticed except for those extraordinary moments when it suddenly and inexplicably turned vicious and became pandemic. There were two times when this happened, once in the early part of the 16th century and then once more at the tail end of World War I.

Because influenza was such a random disease during most of its history, memories of its attacks obviously faded rather quickly. And since its presence often went unnoticed by chroniclers, it actual course through European history has been somewhat difficult to trace. Influenza was present, more than likely, in the period before 1485, the date that is usually given for its arrival on the European scene. Evidence in favor of this hypothesis is convincing largely because the basic symptoms of this disease have not varied from one time period to another. Making use of this characteristic feature of influenza, some historical epidemiologists have been able of late to pinpoint the presence of this disease throughout the whole of the Medieval period. In Italy, for example, no less than 355 separate chronicles from this era have been discovered, all mentioning a disease that surely must have been influenza. All together, they speak of 43 different epidemics, some of them dating as far back as the 4th and 5th centuries A.D.[2]   Russian researchers, meanwhile, have traced the presence of influenza in their country to the year 1173.[3]   The influenza which was apparently common to this period was the milder form of the disease.[4]   Moreover, most of the epidemics that did occur during the Middle Ages and later on in early Modern times came so infrequently that some historians have taken it upon themselves to refer to influenza as "the ephemeral pestilence."[5]   However, once historians began to make a conscious effort to identify it in the European past, their task was made extraordinarily easy by the fact that the symptoms of this disease were so remarkably uniform from one century to another.   In most of these instances, according to the German historian Otto Leichtenstein, the symptoms were the same, for:

> Typical influenza consists in sudden fever which is initiated by a chill or frequently chilly sensations, and lasts from one to several days, is associated with severe headache . . . pain in the back and legs, disproportionately severe prostration, and loss of appetite.   Often ten to twelve hours of perspiration ensues, and in twenty-four to forty-eight hours the fever has usually subsided in many of the patients, leaving them with great weakness and with pains in the muscles and joints which disappear within a few days.[6]

Even though there is now fairly reliable evidence that a mild form of influenza was present, at least locally, in the Middle Ages, the date 1485 is still being given by some for the onset of this disease in Europe. In that year an unusually virulent form of influenza struck England.   The chroniclers of the time certainly believed that they were dealing with an entirely new disease, one that attacked suddenly and caused profuse sweating before it killed off its victim. Far from being a mild disorder, the English sweat, as influenza came to be called, turned out to be an extraordinarily lethal disease. Writing in startled tones about its arrival, John Caius noted that:

> In the same year [1485] a new kind of sickness came suddenly through the whole region . . . , which was so sore,

so painful and sharp that the like was never heard of to any man's remembrance before that time. For suddenly a deadly and burning sweat invaded their bodies and vexed their blood with the most ardent heat . . . so that, of all of them that sickened, there was not one among a hundred that escaped.[7]

According to Caius' account, all of the symptoms that modern science has come to identify with influenza had become intensified. Caius, reporting further on the arrival of what he regarded as a new disease, even compared it unfavorably with plague, declaring that:

In the year of our Lord God, 1485, shortly after the 7th day of August . . . , their chanced a disease among the [English] people, lasting the rest of the month and all of September, which, for its sudden sharpness and unwonted cruelty surpassed the pestilence [plague]. For [the plague] commonly gives 3 or 4, often 5, sometimes 9, sometimes 11, and sometimes 14 days respite to whom it vexes. But . . . [the sweat] immediately killed some in opening their window, some in playing with children in their street doors, some in one hour, many in two it destroyed, and, at the longest, to them that merrily dined it gave a sorrowful supper.[8]

As an apparently mild disease during the Middle Ages that produced only transitory symptoms, influenza was relatively easy to ignore. After all, it could very easily be seen as just another minor ailment in an age when physical suffering was almost universally accepted as inevitable. Then, at the dawn of the Modern era, influenza was suddenly transformed into a highly dangerous disease. By becoming more deadly, it also became much more noticeable and this consideration undoubtedly accounts for the mistaken belief that influenza initially penetrated Europe in the year 1485.

After first invading England epidemically in the middle of the 1480s, influenza kept springing up over and over again in that country right down until the 1550s. Actual death-rates during England's initial epidemic in 1485 can only be guessed at. But, when the disease struck again in 1499, it swiftly took the lives of some 30,000 people in the city of London alone.[9] The disease attacked again in 1510. This time it spread out of its apparent geographic focal point in England and began to cover the whole of the continent. In the words of one contemporary English student of pandemic trends, Thomas Short: "It attacked at once, and raged, all over Europe, not missing a family, and scarce a person." The excruciatingly painful symptoms that all reports said accompanied this disease in 1485 were now repeating themselves. According to Short's account, they consisted of: "A grievous pain of the head, heaviness, difficulty of breathing, hoarseness, loss of strength and appetite, restlessness, watchings, from a terrible taring cough. Presently, succeeded a chilness, as so a violent cough, that many were in danger of suffocation." The profuse sweating from which this disease had originally drawn its name in 1485 was not present in 1510, nor was the disease particularly deadly this time around. For as Short went on to point out: "None died, except some children."[10] The pandemic of 1510, demonstrably milder than the ones that had come before it, was followed in 1529 by yet another outbreak. For some enigmatic reason, this one turned out to be just as deadly as the one that had occurred in the 1480s. This particular pandemic moved out from England, still evidently the disease's geographical center, to other parts of Europe. It quickly jumped the Channel, spreading to France, the Low Countries, Germany and Scandinavia before finally moving eastward into Poland, Lithuania and Russia. Wherever it struck, it filled local populations with both dread and worry.[11] Once again, the disease was characterized by profuse sweating. Even though local chroniclers reported that large numbers were being felled by this disease, more precise information about death-rates was not being recorded. However, it has definitely been established that in the south German city of Augsburg there were some 18,000 cases of the disease and of that total 1,420 died.[12]

At the dawn of the modern era, the European continent was seemingly being inundated by what the age regarded as a whole series of new diseases. For, in rapid succession, influenza, typhus and syphilis had all penetrated the continent, bedevilling a population that was already subject to the periodic return of bubonic plague. Malignant influenza appeared to most to be an added form of punishment. While the symptoms of this disease in 1529 were amazingly similar from one part of Europe to another, influenza itself acted in a very arbitrary and confusing manner. In some places, such as Amsterdam, it killed swiftly taking some 400 to 500 lives in just a few days. In Stuttgart, on the other hand, the disease acted in an entirely different way. There, thousands fell gravely ill, but only six persons actually perished from the disease.[13] The sweating sickness, as influenza was often called, almost always made its victims grievously sick. This was true both of the minority that died from it and that vast majority who successfully overcame it.[14] By the early 1530s, most Europeans were either personally or indirectly acquainted with the symptoms of flu. The onset of those symptoms was usually so sudden that it literally jolted the victim, leaving him in a state of complete exhaustion. The writer Casticus described just such an attack at Antwerp. Referring to the symptoms that were fast becoming all too familiar in Europe, Casticus recorded that:

> There were rarely any prodormal symptoms to an outbreak of the disease, it mostly set in abruptly and usually at the night time, with chills followed by heats; the patients complained at the same time of oppressive palpitations, headache, want of breath, a sense of pressure or tightness in the region of the stomach and sickness. As these symptoms rose in intensity, along with general turgescence of the skin, a profuse sweat broke out over the whole body.[15]

After the decade of the 1520s, influenza returned to punish the European continent on numerous occasions before finally exhausting itself in the later decades of the 16th century. The malignant form of influenza vanished first of all in England, its original homeland.[16] It visited there for the last time in 1551. According to Caius, the disease that struck the city of London in that year was just as toxic as it had ever been. He reported that those who were terminally ill were seized "by a heavy dull pain in the head, by insane raving and delirium, and after this langour and an unconquerable necessity for sleep. For the disease was as violent as the poison of noxious air, because the mind was seized with fury and overcome with torpor. Then came a violent death."[17] After this, influenza, at least in its more dramatic and virulent form deserted England. It did, however, live on in the remainder of Europe, occasionally as a deadly disorder, but more often than not growing tamer with each passing decade. After sweeping across Europe, then, in one pandemic after another from the late 1510s to the early 1550s, influenza lost much of its force and evidently a good deal of its toxicity. Thereafter, it settled down to become a purely local affliction, preying, for example, on parts of France and Italy, but only once in a while and only in certain small areas. For centuries after this, influenza lived on in France. But it was almost entirely confined to isolated focal points from which it inevitably took on a number of new names, including the Picardy sweat.[18] In the main after the 1550s, influenza only inconvenienced people. It might make thousands in one locale or another ill in a single stroke, but it rarely took many lives. There were a few exceptions. One of them occurred in Rome in 1580. Here, several thousands were killed, those dying being afflicted with a "heat . . . , a dry cough, hoarseness, roughness of the jaws, difficulty of breathing, weakness and langour of the stomach, [and] vomiting."[19] In the 20th century, these symptoms would have been clinically diagnosed as primary uncomplicated influenza. That form of the disease was apparently the one that had ravaged Europe for the better part of a century, only to settle down thereafter and become a disabling, but not a particularly deadly, disease.[20]

If the evidence can be believed, influenza was, to begin with, an exceedingly tame disorder that grew more tempestuous and violent beginning in 1485. For several decades after this, its pandemic force was so great that it ranked with plague and syphilis as one of the more demoralizing experiences that Europe then had to confront. But, by the second half of the 16th century, influenza, probably because of a mutation, grew milder. It still operated epidemically, but it was no longer capable of producing a high rate of mortality. Through all of these twists and turns, the symptoms of influenza remained remarkably uniform.[21] Returning after the 1550s in a much more subdued form, influenza was now barely recognizable to those who had previously known it to be highly lethal. In time, of course, memories of this once powerful killer faded. So much so, that by the 17th century, renewed outbreaks of influenza were thought by many to mark the advent of a brand new disease. By then, with its history all but forgotten, it was being identified by a whole series of new names, including "the hot agues," "the new sickness," and "the strange fever."[22] Epidemics of influenza, moreover, did continue to occur from that point right through to the 18th century. The epidemic that took place in 1693, for instance, did spread from Ireland into the west of France and from there further east. But, the number of deaths that it caused was absolutely minimal, although those who were ill were, in fact, confined to their beds for up to a week or ten days.[23] Symptoms recorded during the French epidemic of that year had an extraordinarily familiar ring, except that there was no intense sweating whatsoever. Describing that particular epidemic, the French observer Molyneux remarked that:

> Some were more . . . affected, so as to confine awhile to their beds, those complaining of feverish symptoms, as shivering and chilness all over them, that made several returns, pains in many parts of the body, severe head-aches, chiefly about their foreheads so any noise was very troublesome; great weakness in their eyes, that the least light was offensive . . . . When the cold was moderate, it usually was over in eight or ten days.[24]

Medical cartography, if it had actually existed during the 18th century, would have shown a map of Europe that was pock-marked here and there by outbreaks of influenza. In some isolated areas it was a fairly common disorder, but in most other places it was virtually unknown. The pandemic of 1712, which spread rapidly across the length of England, France and Germany was immediately identified, probably because of the disease's novelty to most, as some kind of new disease. It barely affected mortality at all, and it would have in all likelihood been ignored except that it was prevalent at the same time in three countries.[25] Epidemics of this kind of influenza were more commonly of a local nature, like the outbreak that took place in southern Italy in 1733.[26] While this disease did touch some communities during the 18th century, a much larger number of cities and towns, like Lyons in east central France, not only never experienced the disease, they did not know that it even existed.[27] The pattern of the disease's attack was, to say the least, wildly uneven. During the 18th century, Italy, in apparent contrast to nearly every other country in Europe, was struck by influenza over and over again, indicating that it was now in all probability, the new geographic center for influenza.[28] The classic symptoms that were reported on here were pains, headaches, fever and cough, all of which were normally followed by a rather quick recovery.[29] Those who were ill were simply confined to their beds for two or three days with symptoms that were relatively subdued. This was because the influenza of the 18th century was hardly the virulent disease that it had been centuries before.[30] On rare occasions, influenza in this era was capable of turning into a murderous disease, but predominantly it just came and went with its muffled impact barely causing a stir.[31]

Influenza was not a disease, like plague or smallpox, that continuously fascinated the medical profession. Its attention was usually rivetted on those disorders that had a much more spectacular affect. At best, a disease of only secondary importance, influenza succeeded in drawing medical attention only at those moments when it acted virulently. Medical interest in this disease was sparked at long last by two major pandemics, the first occurring in 1890-1891 and the second in 1918-1919. During the second of those two pandemics nearly two million Europeans lost their lives. For an extended period from the 1890s to the 1930s, it was generally believed that influenza was a bacterial disease. That well-established myth was suddenly exploded in 1933 by the discovery of the virus that was actually responsible for the disease. The virus was isolated by an English medical team headed by Dr. Wilson Smith. The big breakthrough came when Smith and his colleagues, working with ferrets, proved conclusively that Type A virus, as it came to be called, was directly responsible for the transfer of the disease from one animal to another.[32] This initial discovery that viruses existed was soon followed in 1940 by the discovery of yet another tiny microorganism. This virus, hereafter christened Type B virus, was likewise specifically implicated in the transmission of the disease. This time, an American scientist, Dr. Thomas P. Magill was the principal investigator involved in this pioneering work.[33] Shortly after this, yet a third kind of virus, Type C, was isolated. But, in actuality, it has been Types A and B which have been linked to the pandemics that have seemingly come and gone every ten years or so since World War II.[34]

Modern research in the field of biochemistry has repeatedly shown that any attempt to study influenza's actual pattern of attack can be a very bewildering one. Although the precise symptoms produced by this disease have been amazingly similar over the centuries, this fact about influenza has only served to camouflage the highly fickle character of the microorganisms that cause this disease. Over the past few years, Type A virus has been evolving at such a heady pace that it has now managed to distinguish itself from almost every other known microorganism in existence. On its own, it is perfectly capable of mutating within an extremely short period of time. And these constantly changing characteristics are what are so difficult for modern medical science to combat. The cause of one epidemic after another over the course of the last four decades, Type A virus has been dramatically changing its antigenic structure. Each year, it seems to produce a new strain that is once more toxic to man.[35] This truly indefatigable virus changes its antigenic structure so often and so fast that the human body has a tremendously difficult time producing enough antibodies to keep up its own protection. It will, of course, never be known whether or not Type A was, in actuality, the virus that attacked Europe so unpredictably through much of the Medieval and Modern periods. But, making use of antibodies drawn from some modern survivors of influenza, medical science has been able to deduce that every major outbreak of this disease in Europe since 1890 can be traced to the influence of this one particular microorganism. Serological studies of those who managed to survive the devastating epidemic of 1918-1919 have definitely established a close relationship between the influenza of that period and ensuing pandemics.[36] In the pandemics that have been so frequent since the end of World War I, however, Type A virus has definitely changed its antigenic character. Sometimes, those changes have been rather limited, while at other moments they have been truly dramatic. The more spectacular changes have inevitably resulted in increased toxicity for the microorganisms and more serious epidemics among the general European population.

The unprecedented ability of Type A viruses to keep producing a radically different antigenic structure sharply distinguishes this microorganism from nearly every other toxic organism that is currently known. The truly unique ability of this microorganism to give birth to new and potentially dangerous strains finally came to light during the 1950s. This happened during the Asian flu pandemic of 1957-1958, when British laboratories successfully isolated more than a thousand different strains of this disease.[37] Both individual immunity and the development of a satisfactory vaccine for general use against influenza have been extraordinarily difficult to develop, largely because of the tendency of this microorganism to change, often within a matter of a few hours. In order to keep up with this virus, the body's immune system must be constantly monitoring the new antigens that are invading it. After that, it must produce, if it can, new and more appropriate antibodies in order to be able to protect itself.[38] Vaccines against this disease have also been difficult to come up with because they must necessarily have a range great enough to encompass the ever-changing character of both Type A and Type B virus.[39] By comparison, then, the conquest of the smallpox virus with its relatively stable antigenic structure has proven to be a much simpler task historically than the conquest of influenza. Considering the ability of influenza to mutate almost uncontrollably and the fact that it has proved difficult to control, the European continent has been fortunate. For, in truth, it has had a relatively lenient experience with this historically unpredictable disease.

Unlike the malignant form of influenza that has been so prevalent in recent decades, the more uncomplicated form of this disease that broke out now and again in the period leading up to the 1890s was, generally-speaking, harmless. Major pandemics did take place in 1803, 1830, 1837 and 1847. But they were followed, in turn, by long intervals during which the microorganism seemed to be relatively inactive.[40] However, after a lull of nearly 44 years, the disease suddenly burst forth once more, this time in the years 1890 and 1891. When it did, it produced the most virulent pandemic of influenza that Europe had seen since the first part of the 16th century.[41] Up to the early part of the 1890s, the disease that Europeans had known for several centuries was still a relatively mild one. Typically, patients who were affected by influenza in Vienna during the epidemic of 1837 were rarely if ever in danger of dying. Those who did come down with this ailment still experienced the disease's classic symptoms, but according to the Viennese physician Dr. Franz Seitz fevers were relatively mild and those who were ill were made only vaguely uneasy by an attack.[42] However, evidence was accumulating at this time that the disease was taking a new turn and was, in fact, attacking the gastro-intestinal tract. That symptom had definitely not been reported during earlier outbreaks of influenza.[43] Nonetheless, attesting to the continued mildness of influenza through the 19th century, the English observer Thomas Peacock, speaking of a case that he had encountered in 1847, remarked rather characteristically that:

> There was great difficulty of breathing, and the respiratory acts were performed quickly and imperfectly, the respiration in the minute varying from 30 to 40 to 50. The cheeks were much flushed, and the lips were of a purple colour.

Generally, there was no acute pain in the chest, but rather a sense of constriction and soreness; and the cough though frequent, and often occurring in paroxysms, was not usually severe.[44]

Prior to the 1890s, European society had accustomed itself to the rather innocuous comings and goings of influenza. Then, all of a sudden, it was literally invaded by a highly virulent form of this disease. Originally called the Russian flu in 1889 because it was thought to have come out of eastern Europe, this new and extremely dangerous form of influenza buffeted Europe in three separate but distinct waves during 1890 and 1891.[45] From here on in, every time that influenza entered Europe, it actually spread across the continent with momentous speed. The disease that invaded Europe in 1890-91 was, of course, a far more serious ailment than it had been in anybody's living memory. For not only was influenza much more common, it was simultaneously proving to be an extremely complicated affliction. As a direct result of this pandemic, for instance, deaths from pneumonia and bronchitis immediately leaped upwards. Their normally slower pathological course was obviously being accelerated by the presence of influenza. Tuberculosis patients, of which there were now literally millions, were also among those being threatened by the debilitating consequences of this disease. For one of the noticeable features of influenza at this time was its ability to compound and intensify already existing infections inside the human body.[46] In this regard, the report of the local Government Board of Great Britain in 1891 contained an important reference to just what was happening in this respect. The Report read:

> The winter of 1889-90 will be memorable for having witnessed the return in an epidemic form . . . of the historical disease known by the name of "Influenza," a disease not indeed very fatal, as an immediate cause of death (though the indirect cause of a considerable mortality), but of importance as occasioning much pain and disablement to

the considerable proportion of the community who becomes its victims.[47]

The reappearance of influenza, along with the fact that it regularly attacked those who were already suffering from a respiratory ailment, alarmed both health officials and the public-at-large. In Paris alone, some 5,000 people were killed off in an extremely short period of time. Of that total, only 216 deaths could be directly attributed to influenza. But, rather amazingly, an additional 1770 deaths occurred among those who were already bedridden by pneumonia, while another 1224 tuberculosis and 914 bronchitis patients also died after they too had come down with influenza. Beyond these deaths, hundreds of individuals suffering from heart disease, a growing phenomenon in 19th-century Europe, likewise died shortly after contracting the disease.[48] These obviously escalating death-rates among those who were already ill led some physicians to assume that the microorganism involved here, as yet unidentified, was actually attacking certain organs in the body. In the words of one Irish physician, "it slew its victims . . . by means of . . . affecting the breathing organs and the heart."[49] This widely accepted theory concerning influenza's actual pathological course inside the body existed side-by-side with yet another popular belief, that influenza was a form of meningites. This notion grew up as a result of a series of well-publicized autopsies all of which revealed the existence of an inflammation of the membrane that covers the brain, a substance which is better known as the pia. According the English neurologist Julius Althaus, the amount of blood accumulating in this part of the brain is "such as is never seen . . . in other cases, and this is particularly marked at the base of the brain, [the pia] being filled with blood to bursting, as if they had been injected with wax."[50]

Since influenza did not kill outright, but rather indirectly, precise statistics regarding its morbidity and mortality have been exceedingly difficult to come by.[51] Some information does exist, however, for the pandemic that took place in the early 1890s. In Great Britain, the disease probably claimed some 150,000 lives in the three year period stretching from 1890 to 1892. In all likelihood, death-tolls elsewhere in Europe during this same time span probably matched those that Britain was experiencing.[52] However, for some unexplained reason, children, during this epidemic, were being spared the punishing affects of this disease. But, in striking contrast, the adult population was being disproportionally singled out and attacked. In 1890, it was the age group from 40 to 60 and in 1891 those from 60 to 80 who were the ones who were most likely to die from an attack of influenza.[53] In London, for example, during the epidemic of 1890-1891, death-rates in these two age groups alone leaped forward by nearly 300 percent.[54] By the time that the pandemic of the early 1890s had waned, the medical profession had become fully conscious of the complications that this disease was capable of causing. In particular, physicians now had good reason to fear the onset of a secondary infection, especially during an epidemic of influenza. For by the year 1893, it was becoming abundantly clear to most doctors, thanks to autopsy, that influenza did, indeed, have a powerful propensity to pile an added inflammation onto lung, heart and kidney tissue that was clearly already seriously inflamed by some other disease.[55] In fact, the prevailing medical concept of a deadly secondary infection adding to damage already being done to the body was actually born during the influenza pandemic of the early 1890s. This line of thinking was the direct result, of course, of the medical profession's rather disillusioning experience with the secondary consequences of influenza.

The various influenza pandemics that occurred during the 19th century, that is up to the outbreak of 1890, were all marked by an extraordinarily high rate of morbidity. In nearly every instance, between 25 and 50 percent of the population caught in the disease's epidemic path finally came down with it. Yet, in spite of this, death-rates still remained extremely low.[56] The one conspicuous exception to this overall pattern was, of course, the pandemic of 1890 and 1891 which saw mortality go shooting up sharply. In all probability, some kind of mutation dramatically increased the virulence of the virus that caused influenza, turning what had been a tame disorder into something that was far more insidious.[57] The growing virulence of this disease inevitably attracted the attention of the medical world. However, medical thinking at this particular moment in time was rather thoroughly dominated by Koch's discovery of the bacteria that was directly responsible for tuberculosis. His discovery led other bacteriologists, including Koch's friend and colleague Robert Pfeiffer, to begin a feverish search for the unknown bacteria that was causing influenza. Influenza and pneumonia had occurred together so often in 1890 and 1891 that Pfeiffer was personally convinced for a short while that they might conceivably be the same disease. Correcting himself on this score in 1892, Pfeiffer confidently announced that he had discovered the bacteria that was responsible for influenza. [58] Insisting that he had found the same bacterium in every single one of the samples that he had investigated, Pfeiffer was able to convince a substantial portion of the profession that he had uncovered the microscopic agent responsible for this disease. Years later, it was shown that this particular bacterium, while it is often present in cases of influenza, was not the toxic agent that actually caused the disease.

Medical interest in influenza fell off sharply during the later years of the 1890s, especially as incidences of the disease began to decline. That flagging interest was suddenly revived in a rather spectacular way when the disease returned to Europe during World War I in its virulent form. What was truly frightening about this resurgence of influenza in the winter of 1915-1916 was that its mortality was so unbelievably high. Sometimes, it even reached 50 percent of those taken ill, a figure that could only have been matched during previous epidemics of plague and cholera.[59] Much more deadly than the disease which struck in 1890 and 1891, the reemergence of influenza in 1915 turned out to be just a prelude to the great pandemic of 1918-19 that ultimately took some 2 million lives. Exactly as it had in 1890 and 1891, the disease swept through the continent in three distinct waves, the first taking place in the spring of 1918. This initial attack was followed by two other major outbreaks, one in the fall of 1918 and a final one in the early part of 1919.[60] Just where this particular pandemic actually started is a question that is still partially unanswered. Both the Allies and the Central Powers, who were fighting the war, deliberately tended to suppress news concerning the spread of the disease. They did this, evidently, so as not to alarm their own populations. One of the few countries that did not try to hide the truth about the progress of influenza was neutral Spain. Here, the National Department of Hygiene dutifully issued public warnings in a deliberate attempt to prevent its continued spread.[61] The notoriety that was given to the disease by the Spanish government led, somewhat uncharitably, to the disease being labelled elsewhere in Europe as the Spanish flu.[62]

More than likely, the influenza of 1918 was a new strain of the disease that was brought to Europe by the American Expeditionary Force, which had landed in English and French ports. Once the first cases of the disease were reported in May of 1918, the disease spread rapidly from one army unit to another. To begin with, it was largely confined to the military. However, in time, it too began to affect the civilian population. The influenza that was now spreading proved to be extraordinarily contagious among the Americans. In one instance, it infected a full 90 percent of the soldiers assigned to the 168th Infantry Regiment. In another case, it affected the same percentage of the American naval forces stationed at Dunkirk in northern France.[63] Both sides in the war were eventually touched by the disease, the German commander General Erich von Luddendorff complaining that: "It was a grievous business having to listen every morning to the Chiefs of Staff's recital of the number of influenza cases, and then complaints about the weakness of their troops."[64] In many places, both the percentage of those taken ill and the percentage of those dying were distressingly high. Army units in neutral Stockholm were especially unfortunate. Here, the disease attacked producing scenes that were reminiscent of the Middle Ages and the era of the Black Death. According to one eye-witness who observed the impact of this disease in the Swedish capital, the situation was very unfortunate. He remarked:

> Not only the hospital but the gymnasium, the Chapel, the canteen, were crammed with sick and dying men. Even the

corridors were littered with stretchers placed head to toe - men whose end was fast approaching, cleared from the main wards to make room for new patients. Distraught relatives were everywhere; a Russian who knew no word of Swedish bent over her dying husband, beckoning pitifully to passers-by, frantic to communicate . . . . A father who had kept the final vigil over his son was hunched in a dark corner, sobbing like a child.[65]

Most experts are now generally agreed that it was the American army which introduced this highly infectious form of influenza to war-torn Europe. As soon as it started to break out among American forces stationed in Brest, in western France, cases of pneumonia and bronchitis ominously began to occur in those already sick with influenza. From the very onset of the epidemic then, the medical profession recognized that cases of influenza were being complicated by a series of "secondary bacterial invaders."[66] Just as it had done in 1890 and 1891, the disease moved through the population with alarming speed, infecting whole armies with symptoms that were a constant reminder of those that had also appeared in the early 1890s. The most conspicuous symptoms of the disease at the end of World War I were once again amazingly similar to those that had been reported in other epidemics, ones that reached far back into the historic past. One British army doctor, Adolphe Abrahams described those symptoms, saying of them:

A striking feature was the suddeness of the onset and the remarkable rapidity with which prostration occurred in a man who, whilst walking in the street or on duty, would be taken ill with aching in his back, head, and limbs to a degree that compelled him to lie down. At this stage it would be found that his temperature was raised, generally as high as 104 . . . . Gastro-intestinal disturbances were on the whole uncommon, although vomiting, was often encountered. . . . Epistaxis [the loss of appetite] sometimes of quite alarming degree, was unusually common . . . . In a large number of cases, too, the hearing was much impaired.[67]

After first establishing itself among American soldiers and sailors in their base camps in western and northern France, influenza was quickly passed on to other allied units. During the epidemic that occurred in the spring of 1918, a large number of soldiers fighting along the Western front were prostrated by influenza. However, the overall impact of this epidemic was relatively restrained in comparison to what was going to happen the following fall. For by then, deaths from influenza were soaring. Among American troops disembarking at St. Nazaire in northern France, deaths from influenza were now proportionally equal to those that were taking place on the battlefield.[68] Even more disturbing was the fact that for every one soldier dying there were ten to twenty others who were seriously ill. In the period stretching from September to November of 1918, some 100,000 American soldiers and sailors were hospitalized with symptoms of this disease.[69] Beyond this, it was reliably reported that there were tens of thousands of others who were ill, but were never treated for the sickness. Meanwhile, during the same three-month period in 1918, about 140,000 French soldiers were treated for flu in either army or civilian hospitals. And again, in the fall of 1918, in one six-week span, an additional 70,000 British soldiers were brought into field hospitals suffering from some of the worst symptoms of this disease.[70] After first appearing in the west, influenza soon began to engulf parts of Russia. Enough circumstantial evidence exists to prove that the Americans were again unintentionally responsible for the disease's transfer, now to the east. The first time that the disease was observed in Russia was in the port of Archangel, at the very same moment in September of 1918 when American troops were disembarking. Finally, after punishing the various armies that were fighting in the last stages of the war, the disease spilled over into the civilian population.

Civilian elements were initially inundated during the fall of 1918. The type of virus at work here, more than likely Type A, was as contagious as any virus that Europe had seen since the days when smallpox had raged out of control. In some areas of Europe, most notably Ireland, England, France and Germany, probably the disease's true epicenter, between 30 and 40 percent of the civilian population came down with influenza.[71] The disease spread so swiftly that it was immediately assumed by most that the infection was being transmitted by air-droplets, which were in turn settling into the respiratory tracts of new victims. Now more sophisticated than ever about how disease was transferred, public health officials were absolutely convinced that exposure, exhaustion, poor nutrition and overcrowding were all adding to the disease's electrifying advance.[72] The disease was everywhere. Even sturdy elements within the civilian population were quickly felled. One observer even pointed out that "apparently healthy people were suddenly overcome, and within an hour could become helpless with fever, delirium and chills."[73] Cities that were short of food because of the rationing that was introduced at the tail end of the war were extremely hard hit. They not only experienced numerous cases of influenza, but also a visibly accelerating death-rate. In the center of Berlin, actually one of the city's wealthier districts, death-rates in the fall of 1918 directly attributable to influenza went shooting up five or six times in a matter of just a few short weeks.[74] Overall death-rates, almost always difficult to determine in the case of this disease, probably hovered at around two or three percent of those actually taken ill. No one will ever know just how many people came down with influenza. An educated guess would place the figure at somewhere in between 50 and 100 million individuals during 1918 and 1919.[75]

Unlike the spectacular outbreak which occurred in 1957, the one popularly known as the Hong Kong flu, the elderly were not singled out during the epidemic of 1918-1919.[76] The greatest mortality of that time took place among those who were between the ages of 25 and 35. In London, for example, the statistics in this regard were amazingly consistent from one week to another in 1918. They proved that influenza was primarily a disease of young adults, children being mercifully spared just as they had been in the early 1890s.[77] The so-called Spanish flu of the late 1910s was the most murderous pandemic of influenza that Europe was ever to experience during the course of the 20th century. Its truly disastrous impact upon the population would never be repeated again, although public health officials for decades later still had lingering fears that it would, indeed, return with about the same degree of ferocity. In between the two World Wars, there were less dramatic outbreaks of influenza. They occurred more or less regularly in 1922, 1926, 1929, 1933, 1937 and 1940. However, each time that it did return, its fury was somehow lessened. Not only did incidences of the disease fall off with each subsequent revival, but the number of deaths associated with each epidemic likewise began to decline.[78] Influenza was, as it had done several times in the past, rather unpredictably changing its course. Moreover, those who were dying from this disease in this period when influenza was declining in intensity, were coming from a different part of the population. In both 1890 and 1918, young adults had been singled out by the disease. Now, however, in between the wars, influenza was mostly preying on older elements, the majority of those dying being in the age group 55 or over.[79] Beyond these considerations, the six pandemics that did take place in the inter-war period tended to be of a regional character. The era of pandemic influenza was obviously over at least until the 1950s.[80] The disease that was circulating in Europe during the 1920s and 1930s was according to health officials from the League of Nations a much milder form of influenza, one that rarely reached beyond two or more countries when it did attack.[81]

Although the actual cause of influenza was not discovered until 1933, the medical profession did know a fair amount about this disease even before that time. Most of the knowledge that doctors had accumulated was drawn from the profession's experience with the two great pandemics that had occurred in the early 1890s and the late 1910s. As a result of what had happened then, influenza was justifiably regarded as an extremely contagious disease. In fact, it was regarded as far more communicable than almost any other disease that might be mentioned. Not since the days of the Black Death had such a large proportion of the population been taken ill by any one disease in such a short period of time. Incidences of the disease during both pandemics multiplied so dramatically that physicians were often terrified by what might happen once it was introduced into some new area.[82] It is true that for several decades after 1892, a large percentage of medical men were convinced that the disease was probably caused by a microorganism that was known as Pfeiffer's bacillus. In time, however, this belief began to fade. More than at any time in its history, medical science was now empirically oriented. And, in point of fact, the bacillus was just not showing up often enough in autopsies to warrant its further acceptance as the incontestable source of this disease.[83] Even more importantly, in 1918, in far too many cases the bacillus simply could not be found in the sputum of those who were seriously ill. All of this led to the growing assumption that the real cause of influenza lay somewhere else.[84] Beyond the rather intense debates that surrounded the validity of Pfeiffer's bacillus, it was being strongly suggested by some that influenza came and went with a very high degree of periodicity. It was genuinely believed in some quarters that it would inevitably return every ten or eleven years. Actually, influenza, just like plague and cholera, seemed to come and go in a much more arbitrary fashion than the laws of periodicity would have ever allowed. Speaking historically, influenza has changed into a truly virulent disease so radically and so unpredictably that violent outbreaks of the disease have, if anything, been almost impossible to predict. The swine-flu fiasco of the mid-1970s seemed to demonstrate this point rather conclusively.

At those moments when Europe was hit by a truly virulent strain of influenza, health officials and physicians had a lot more to worry about than just the initial infection. For this type of influenza, as opposed to the simple uncomplicated variety, was, of course, inherently capable of producing all sorts of deadly complications. By the end of World War I, most medical men were conscious that the disease could, in up to 20 percent of those affected, so weaken the patient that pneumonia and bronchitis could set in all too easily.[85] In actuality, of course, deaths from these two bacterial diseases were often greater during an epidemic of influenza than the numbers that could be directly attributable to flu. Even during relatively mild outbreaks of the disease, such as those which took place in the inter-war period, deaths from pneumonia, evidently triggered by influenza, nearly always rose somewhat.[86] Since these two diseases accompanied each other so often in the same patient, it has been in many instances diagnostically difficult to determine which one was the actual cause of death. Indeed, by the 1920s, most physicians knew that they had an extremely fickle disorder on their hands whenever they were called in to treat a case of influenza.[87] It is now known that the rapidly changing antigenic structure of the viruses involved here is the real reason why this disease has such a quixotic character. Looking at the overall history of influenza in more modern times, it is easy to perceive that this disease grew much more virulent in 1890, 1918 and 1957 only to lapse in the periods thereafter into a much more innocuous disorder. Given the widely fluctuating nature of influenza over the past century, influenza must be ranked among the most unpredictable of all the deadly and disabling diseases. Its highly uneven impact is evidently a direct result of its swiftly changing antigenic character, the rhythm of which is still beyond the capacity of modern medical science adequately to foretell.[88]

Influenza is today the most widely reported disease in European society, accounting for an astonishing 23 percent of all recorded illnesses and a full 50 percent of all those known to be suffering from an infectious disease.[89] The problem of controlling this potentially dangerous disease is among the more formidable tasks that still confronts the medical profession. Fortunately, the disease is one that kills on a truly massive scale only every so often. Furthermore, it is well known that every new epidemic that does take place can be traced to a variation in either Type A or Type B of the virus.[90] Actually, the shifting nature of these toxic variations, along with modern overcrowding, have together virtually guaranteed that these viruses will continue to live on as a threat right into the foreseeable future.[91] The other great viral disorder from the past, smallpox, has proven to be much easier to control, largely because it is susceptible to a vaccine. The precise reason, of course, why it has been subdued is because the virus that causes smallpox has a much more stable antigenic structure than the one responsible for influenza.[92]

Influenza is the last of the great deadly and disabling diseases that still has some kind of upper hand. All the rest have been either significantly tamed or dramatically reduced to insignificance. Influenza still exists, but in the last part of the 20th century it is really no longer the threatening disease that it was earlier on. In point of fact, the aura, mystery and fear that once surrounded all of the major diseases of the past has now unquestionably evaporated. At best, they are only remembered as historical curiosities.

From the time of the Black Death of 1348 to the Spanish flu of 1918, Europe was consistently a disease-ridden society. There were, in actuality, a large number of diseases in the past that were the cause of Europe's very high rate of morbidity and mortality. People died from a wide range of ailments, most of which remained medical mysteries in their own age. This study has attempted to look at those seven that were the most prominent. Infectious disease was so rampant in former times that few ever bothered to cry out against them. Instead, they were just fatalistically accepted as part and parcel of this valley of tears. They almost had to be. For in previous generations, if people were not dying from one or another of the major European diseases, their enjoyment of life was being spoiled by some other ailment such as scurvy, leprosy, psoriasis and tooth-decay. Everywhere that one looked suffering and death were always present. Bacterial diseases, along with their first cousins, the rickettsial disorders, were the most dominant. These highly toxic agents which were responsible for diseases ranging from plague to syphilis and from cholera to tuberculosis undoubtedly produced the greatest amount of misery. It was only in time that the great viral disorders, smallpox and influenza, actually came into their own. Either way, life for the average European in the historic past was constantly being made uncertain by the presence of disease. Given all of this, the question might legitimately be asked at this point -- just why was Europe so disease-ridden? How did it happen that these toxic agents managed to reign over such an evidently helpless population for so long?

Part of the answer lies, of course, in the realm of microbiology, in the sheer potency of the toxic agents that kept invading the European population. But there is another consideration here, the condition of those who were infected. Here, one must take into account the gnawing poverty of the past and the depressing inability of one generation after another of Europeans to resist the successive waves of these diseases. Unquestionably, the age of infectious diseases in Europe was intimately tied to poor diets, mostly bread, that the majority of Europeans historically had to endure. The bulk of the men and women in the past never had the nutrients that they needed to build up antibodies. As a consequence, they were never able to fight off these highly dangerous microorganisms. The invading microorganisms of the past just ran through the European population, each time infecting that rather large pool of susceptibles who always seemed to be around whenever a disease struck. Presumably, the reason why there were so many victims was because poor diet deprived the majority of them of the ability to fight back biologically. Diseases do not operate on their own, they operate within a social environment. Given this fact, it makes sense to point out that a combined study of the social factors existing in the past and of biological considerations will together progressively help us to understand just why Europe was such a disease-ridden society for such a long period of time.

PART TWO

THE CONSEQUENCES

> The great majority of illnesses, whether they destroy the enjoyment of life for the many or only a small portion of mankind . . . are not the result of natural causes, but the consequence of existing social conditions.
>
> --Rudolf Virchow, quoted in Dieter Wagner, "Wandlungen der Begriffs Epidemie," NTM; Schriftenreihe für Geschichte der Naturwissenschaft, Vol. 9 (1972), 67.

From the Black Death in 1347 to the Spanish flu in 1918, Europe was unquestionably a disease-ridden society. Throughout this era, European society was repeatedly called upon to respond to the recurrent crises caused by the invasion of one disease after another. To a significant degree it failed. It failed because the crises brought on by the arrival of so many deadly and disabling diseases proved to be too much for it to handle. Europe's intellectual community simply did not know what to make of these diseases. As it turned out, medical diagnoses in this period were just as inexact as prevailing philosophical explanations were. It was only at the tail end of this period, with the coming of microbiology, that European society finally became conscious of what microorganisms were actually capable of doing to man. The mass of Europeans seemed, if anything, just as confused as the intellectuals were by the disillusioning presence of so much suffering and death. Their descriptions of symptoms, along with those of the medical profession, were highly accurate. But their explanations and solutions for these diseases were notoriously inaccurate and, to a significant degree, determined by their superstitions. As the second half of this study will attempt to show, most of the mistakes that were constantly being made at all levels of society concerning the potential causes of and cures for these diseases were the direct result of a lack of knowledge.

Except for the sudden onset of epidemics of plague and cholera, European society did not respond to the great deadly and disabling diseases either fearfully or apprehensively. In the main, previous generations of Europeans met them apathetically. There were, of course, some exceptions, but generally speaking, the fatalism of the past prepared the majority for a fate that many grew to maturity expecting. Religion, in particular a belief in the afterlife obviously saved many from the kind of psychological torture that might have made the physical suffering, so common at this time, even harder to endure than it was.[1] Still, there was so much pain in this society that it was difficult to endure, even in an age when most were taught to acquiesce to whatever fate came their way. This being the case, there was a constant search in the historic past for the kind of drugs that would either ease some of the pain or eliminate it all together. Most of the remedies that the past produced were ineffective; they neither reduced pain nor provided a cure. Still, this society, pressured from within by the presence of so much illness, kept searching for remedies. Those remedies, while often sought, were rarely, if ever, found. For just like the explanations for the presence of disease that were provided, the remedies and cures of the pre-industrial period were largely based on either misinformation or mistaken assumptions.[2]

Although the true cause of most diseases eluded the medical profession, physicians in a bygone era were amazingly precise in the way that they described the symptoms of these diseases. Whenever and wherever medical men saw a disease either fulminating or operating on the skin they looked at it carefully and described it minutely. They were trained to do just that, so much so that the entire profession became almost exclusively oriented towards symptoms, towards what modern medical science would now regard as externals. It is true that the Veronese physician Fracastoro did argue in the 16th century that disease was caused by tiny invisible organisms. But his ideas proved to be so novel that they were unable to overturn the more widely accepted view that disease was caused by foul air.[3] Finally, of course, in the latter part of the 19th century, this older attitude collapsed in the wake of Koch's monumental discoveries during the 1880s. Once he proved that microorganisms were, in fact, the cause of both tuberculosis and cholera, the medical profession at long last began to accept the much more modern notion that the origin of disease lay inside the body, not outside of it.

As the Middle Ages started to give way to modern times, governments emerged as the most significant institutions of the age. Instead of tolerating the presence of disease in their populations, governments deliberately tried to check their spread. Their efforts were not all that successful, in part because, like the rest of society, they really did not know what they were dealing with. Still, doing something was considered to be better than doing nothing. As a result, governments bought "drugs," built lazarettos, supported hospitals and even on certain occasions used troops, all in a desperate attempt to limit the affects of disease. Their periodic campaigns in favor of cleanliness or to establish quarantines in certain ports may have been momentarily successful. But, given the overall history of infectious disease in Europe, they hardly stemmed the tide of any one of these particular diseases for any length of time. Public health programs, supported by various central governments, did not begin to succeed until the 19th century.[4] They became beneficial largely because, by then, most public health officials knew what they were doing when they promoted vaccination or sought the elimination of pollution. For the first time, they were not operating blindly, but against an enemy that they increasingly knew how to control.

For the most part, those who are now living in the last half of the 20th century in Europe are relatively free from the affects of infectious disease. If diseases do strike with anywhere near the same intensity that they did in the past, they do so in the latter decades of life. The same could not be said of previous generations, for before the coming of industrialization, diseases actually attacked early and often, killing at every stage in life and taking proportionally a very high percentage of both infants and young adults. The great deadly and disabling diseases were then, of course, unsparing in the way they separated mother and child, broke up families and, in certain circumstances, even attacked whole social groups. When everything is taken into account, these diseases also appear to have been afflictions of the crowd.[5] It is true, for example, that diseases such as syphilis, smallpox, tuberculosis and cholera were known to the rural areas of Europe. But, the real demographic toll that these diseases took was among city dwellers. The great bacterial, rickettsial and viral parasites of the past apparently needed numbers in order to survive, and they found them among the more impoverished elements who lived in the urban areas of Europe.

It is immensely difficult for those who live in a society that has virtually conquered most of the infectious diseases to understand what life was like for those who were forced to live in a disease-ridden society. For most of them, disease and death were common everyday occurrences. While this last statement is historically accurate the burden of the past did seem to fall on some more than on others, for if the evidence of history can be believed, infectious diseases did seek out those much earlier in life who had less than they went after those who had more. Factually, this appears to be true and it suggests that the diseases of the European past were, in actuality, definitely linked to the existence of poverty. Once poverty, in all of its ramifications, including malnutrition and poor living conditions, was eliminated, the situation inside of Europe changed for the better. For, as the standard of living began to rise and new medical discoveries came in, Europe ceased to be what she had been for nearly 600 years, essentially a disease-ridden society.

CHAPTER 7

POPULAR ATTITUDES AND ACCEPTED CURES

> The appeal of folk medicine was built upon the conservative spirit of the people, their dependence on magic and mysticism, their religiosity . . . and their uncritical attitude towards false teaching.
>
> --G.A. Werhli, "Das Wesen der Volksmedizin und die Notwendigkeit einer Geschichtlichen Betractungsweise Derselben," in Charles E. Singer and Henry E. Sigerist (eds.), Essays on the History of Medicine (Oxford, 1924), p. 376.

The continuous presence of so many different diseases in the European past inevitably produced a great deal of stress within society. Human behavior in this era was undoubtedly subjected to an inordinate amount of tension.[1] Over the course of these centuries, both men and women did on occasion grow mad under the strain, with crowds sometimes venting their anger against either scapegoats or those who were in a position of authority. But, generally-speaking, the human response to the tragedy brought on by these diseases was considerably tamer than this.[2] Somewhat surprisingly, the response of the average European to these endemic and epidemic diseases was one of quiet acceptance, for, far from fighting back, most Europeans simply acquiesced in whatever fate came their way.

What saved much of Europe from the anguish of psychological torture and a desire for revenge was its long standing familiarity with death. Death was not seen in the pre-industrial period, as it is in more modern times, as a form of annihilation. Rather, it was viewed as just another stage in the overall development of one's destiny. Prior to the 19th century, an individual did not die. Instead, he or she was just put to sleep or laid to rest, all in preparation for the continuation of life that would take place once death had occurred. The belief in an afterlife, then, subtly helped to save Europeans. Otherwise, the mental torment being caused by unrelenting suffering and agonizing death, especially of loved ones, would have been too much for the vast majority of Europeans to handle.[3]

The diseases in the past that caused the greatest amount of fear and violence were, of course, those that killed without any forewarning whatsoever, in particular plague and cholera. In both instances, death often followed in a matter of days and sometimes in just a few hours. Even though both diseases killed swiftly, they never really claimed a majority of those who were in their path. Actually, they killed the few rather than the many, but this only compounded the fear that people felt. They were frightened because plague and cholera struck so unpredictably that no one really knew who was going to be next. It was exactly this kind of uncertainty that raised fears in London to a fever pitch when cholera first attacked during the 19th century.[4] Historically, the most infamous case of violence, obviously the result of collective madness, took place during the period of the Black Death. Convinced by wild rumors that Jewish elements had poisoned their wells and were spreading plague, half-crazed crowds set upon Jews in a series of cities, including among others, Basle, Freiburg and Strasbourg. Some were tortured, others were murdered.[5] Violence, of one sort or another, was always potentially close to the surface during any plague epidemic. While most victims of this disease simply surrendered to the suffering, others were apparently driven mad by the pain that inevitably accompanied the bursting of the buboes or boils. In England, there were numerous reports over time of those suffering from the disease either attacking people who were around them or actually committing suicide.[6] Violence of this type was almost impossible to predict ahead of time. During the plague epidemic that ravaged Moscow in 1771, the reigning archbishop, Ambrose, forbade the kissing of icons, a rather common religious practice of the time, purely as a sanitary precaution. Evidently fearing the loss of divine intercession, a rioting mob set upon the Archbishop and murdered him. After that, they started to attack others in a position of authority.[7] Similar acts of violence took place in Russia and Hungary during the cholera epidemic of the early 1830s. In these instances, peasant mobs evidently unaccustomed to the sight of so much death, turned against their priests and local noblemen, murdering a score of them before troops were able to restore order.[8]

Far more common than violence, however, were the superstitions and myths that always sprang up in the midst of an epidemic. Unable to explain the all-too-sudden appearance of plague in 1348, a popular superstition soon developed in several parts of Europe. It told of a pestilential wind that was supposedly carrying the disease from one spot to another.[9] Visions were also commonplace. In 1349, for example, a Plague-Virgin was seen by a large number of people in Vienna. According to this tale, every time she raised her hand another victim became infected.[10] One of the most enduring myths in the European past was the belief that Kings possessed the power to cure individuals of tuberculosis. All the monarch had to do was to touch someone who was suffering from this disease and he or she would immediately regain their health.[11] The difficulty for those who held this belief was getting close enough to the monarch to receive his healing touch. Superstitious practices also abounded. In Bulgaria, the peasants regularly plowed their fields either in the shape of an oval or a horseshoe as a way of protecting themselves against plague, smallpox and cholera.[12] Every epidemic that took place likewise encouraged quackery. Even as late as 1832, the cholera epidemic in England brought out hucksters all selling "Protecting belts, anticholera medicines, charms and bags to dispel infection."[13] Superstitious beliefs could easily reach into the highest levels in society. During the same epidemic, municipal authorities in Exeter in southwestern England spent nearly £40 on flannel belts, all in the expectation that they could somehow protect the local population from cholera.[14] Somewhat paradoxically, mass elements did not seem to fear smallpox even at that time in the 18th century when it was fast becoming the most universal disease in all of Europe. On the other hand, in certain parts of Prussia and Poland, peasant elements did take steps to protect themselves against this disease. They did it by purchasing "pox-pus" and injecting themselves so as to produce a mild case of the disease.[15] Peasants in this part of Europe, at least, obviously understood the value of inoculation even if most of their contemporaries did not. Not all of the remedies being pushed at this time were as sensible as inoculation. If anything, most of them tended to fall into the category of sheer folly. Even worse, the vast majority of trinkets and talismans that were sold during most epidemics were uncritically accepted by the desperate masses. Such practices were common during the epidemic of plague that struck London in 1665. Nathaniel Hodges, who watched with disgust the sale of these useless items, declared at the time that: "they were indefatigable in spreading their antidotes; and although equal strangers to all Learning and Physik, they thrust into every Hand some Trash or another under the Disguise of Pompous title."[16]

Not only did previous generations grow more desperate under the stress created by an epidemic, they also became much more fearful and much more suspicious. When an isolated epidemic of bubonic plague unexpectedly broke out in Siebenbürgen in eastern Austria in the 1710s, government officials, watching the death toll steadily rising, reported that: "the people were all afraid that no one would be left alive."[17] As it was, diseases that killed less dramatically, like smallpox, and more slowly, like tuberculosis, were historically less frightening than those which seemed to swoop down upon a population without any kind of advanced warning. As a result, of course, the greatest emotion tended to surround the incidences of plague and cholera, the two diseases that could literally attack in a matter of minutes.[18] As soon as one or the other of these diseases struck, the primary fear that most people felt was that the disease would be passed on to those who were still healthy. It was, for instance, commonly held that there were carriers in every population who were capable of deliberately spreading the sickness to others. "Spreaders," as they were called were regularly executed in the 16th century in Calvin's Geneva, and even as late as 1832 six Parisians were lynched during the cholera epidemic of that year for poisoning the wells and thus spreading the disease.[19] In the same vein, the fear that city dwellers would contaminate rural elements led to clashes in 1665 between villagers and those who were trying to escape the plague in London.[20] During a crisis brought on by an epidemic, anyone and everyone fell under suspicion, even the unfortunate bathkeeper in Brünn, who in 1568 was charged with poisoning the stew that he regularly served. His life was threatened as a result of a rumor which insisted that his stew was the origin of an epidemic of syphilis that was then overtaking the city.[21] What happened in Brünn in 1568 was rather typical. For, in the midst of most crises, far-fetched explanations readily replaced more reasonable answers, especially in the minds of those who were terrified by what they saw.

For untold centuries, the victims of disease could expect to be shunned by others. The sick and dying, far from being cared for, were usually ostracized both by their family and by their neighbors. This was especially true, of course, whenever an epidemic was raging out of control. The diseased were almost always accused of being the source of further contamination. As a result, virtually everything about the sick became the object of both scrutiny and suspicion. At one time, even the breath of those with plague was suspected of harboring the disease and being able to transfer it to others. The popular writer of the 18th century, Daniel Defoe referred to this widely-held belief speaking in one of his works of "distempered people . . . who conveyed the fatal breath."[22] The living were not the only ones who were mistrusted, so were the dead. In the German-speaking areas of central Europe, the bodies of plague victims were generally regarded as a health hazard largely because, it was said, they were corrupting the air and thus endangering others.[23] The Privy Council in London certainly shared their view. In 1625, it went so far as to order the deep burial of plague victims insisting that "the not burying of them deep enough have putrefied and corrupted the Air in such sort as the Plague have thereupon ensued."[24] Much later than this, in the 19th century, European society became even more conscious of the quantity of infectious material that might be floating around in the air. Tuberculosis patients, in particular, were thought to be adding to the total amount of contaminants in the air both with their phlegm and with their coughing. During the late 1800s, spitting up and coughing were increasingly being looked upon with revulsion and apprehension.[25] There was then in the historic past an every-present fear of contagion that might come out at any time. In an earlier age, large numbers of people were absolutely convinced, for example, that syphilis could be acquired simply by coming into contact with objects such as clothes and utensils that had already been touched by a syphilitic.[26] Such lasting fears were, of course, at least partially grounded in reality. They also revealed a kind of instinctive understanding of the fact that disease could be communicated from one person to another. The most persistent belief of all in pre-industrial times was the notion that the air contained certain foul and corrupt smells which were, in turn, the real origin of disease. In order to drive these offending odors from the air and presumably cleanse it, previous generations of Europe all went in for burning, fumigating and perfuming.[27] In so doing, they hoped to make the air more habitable than it had been before.

During the centuries when Europe was essentially a disease-ridden society, violence, superstition and fear were, in point of fact, the inescapable partners of fatalism and acquiescence. In truth, of course, neither the intellectual community nor the mass of Europeans really knew what was causing the diseases that were constantly threatening their lives. Most of the explanations that they came up with were little better than guess work. In this age of uncertainty, religion turned out to be a real solace. Almost inevitably, the prayers that were composed in this era spoke directly of the existence of disease and the very real threat that it posed to human life. Characteristically full of special pleading and self-denigration, the most commonly repeated prayer to St. Denis, the patron saint of syphilitics, begged that the supplicant be spared the horrifying consequences of this disease. This special prayer ran: "Protect me from the terrible disease called the French malady . . . Protect me from the wretched illness. O most gracious father Denis that I may make amends for my sin, by which I have offended my Lord, and that after this life I may come to the joy of eternal bliss."[28] A rather similar prayer, composed during one of the cholera epidemics of the 19th century, had the same imploring tone. It said: "Divine sweet Virgin Mary, consoler of the unfortunate, vouchsafe to preserve our lives for we know that you are our only real refuge."[29] In addition to prayers, processionals were also organized in an attempt to bring about divine intervention. During the terrifying days that characterized the outbreak of plague in Marseilles in 1721, there were almost daily processions. They all called upon God and the Virgin Mary to save the city from any more suffering.[30]

The explanations that were given in a previous age for the presence of various diseases would seem to a modern audience to be both strange and somewhat incomprehensible. The coming of plague and other diseases was considered for long centuries to be overwhelming evidence of God's disfavor for something that man had done.[31] Divine wrath, according to this belief, regularly operated through the air, taking the form of vapors, stenches, humors and poisons. For bad air, which smelled that way because it was foul or putrid, was still considered to be the basic means by which a disease was spread. What lay behind these ugly visitations was, of course, an avenging God, angered by the sins of man.[32] The Italian observer and commentator, Antero di San Bonaventura, even saw a blessing in these all-too-frequent displays of divine displeasure. According to him, they mercifully limited population in an obviously impoverished age, thus making it possible for others to survive. Dwelling on this point, he asked: "what would become of this world, if God did not periodically touch it with plague. How would it feed so many people. God would have to create other Worlds just to have enough to provide for this one."[33] Since God was the originator of disease, it seemed only logical in this day and age that he was also capable of mitigating its impact. This is why the population as a whole usually turned to prayers and processionals, thereby seeking his aid. When an epidemic did lift, a grateful population almost inevitably gave thanks. During the Middle Ages and early Modern times, the European continent was literally dotted with shrines and churches which were erected to express the gratitude of previous generations to a merciful and forgiving God, who had chosen, it was believed, to end one epidemic or another. Venice, which was punished over and over again by epidemics of plague, built four magnificent plague churches for this reason, the most famous of which was the Church of Saint Marie della Salute.[34] It was also a common practice throughout Europe that whenever an epidemic of any kind came to an end, Te Deums were sung in the local churches. This was done as a sign that the people were, indeed, grateful for having been delivered from the diseases.[35]

Ranking alongside the idea of divine wrath as a perfectly plausible explanation for the presence of disease was the notion of planetary intervention. Non-literate elements in European society before the coming of the Industrial Revolution seemed to be reconciled to the idea that diseases were sent by God either as a form of punishment or to test their faith. But, for some reason, educated elements seemed to require a more extensive and a more complicated explanation than this. They found the answer they were looking for in the movement of certain heavenly bodies. This kind of activity was so much in fashion that tracing the planets and stars and linking their movement to the appearance of both old and new diseases became for many intellectuals an extremely enticing experience. As a result of all this, astrological explanations for the presence of disease began to gain a wide currency especially around the dawn of the Modern era. They also produced all kinds of controversies, various astrologers being unable to agree on whether the arrival of syphilis had been caused by a conjunction of Saturn and Mars or by "Saturn when he entered into Aries."[36] In the late 15th and early 16th centuries, astrologers were constantly on the lookout for new diseases. They had plenty to discover what with typhus, syphilis and influenza all invading Europe at just about the same point in time, these diseases joining bubonic plague as outstanding examples of just how ferocious an epidemic could be.[37] The coming of so many virulent diseases, bunched together so closely in time, sparked an even greater interest in astrology than that which had previously existed. Disasters on such a monumental scale obviously produced a craving for some kind of explanation as to what was happening. These explanations, whether they involved the work of God, the movement of the planets or the actual composition of the air, were all of an external nature. What they did, of course, was to focus the attention of the medical profession on external causes, drawing it away from the more basic and scientific idea that the cause of disease lay inside of the body and not outside of it.

Because it did not attack suddenly and alarmingly the way that plague and the extreme forms of syphilis and influenza did, smallpox was viewed in an entirely different light by previous generations of Europeans. Smallpox, in the 18th century, because it was so universal, was often regarded as a natural disease, one that the majority of the population should have had. One French physician, who was perpetually unable to convince those around him that this should not be the case, kept railing against "the completely false but generally accepted idea that all the inhabitants have the germ of smallpox pre-existing in them."[38] So many Europeans were convinced of this that when vaccination was first put forward, it was approached by the majority both suspiciously and reluctantly. By the early decades of the 19th century, vaccination was, of course, being pushed by medical and public health authorities all over the continent. But, the public-at-large was so convinced that smallpox was inevitable and equally that vaccination might kill them that authorities met with a great deal of popular resistance to their programs. Beyond the fears that did exist, the very idea of trying to prevent a disease from occurring appeared to be incongruous to many. The idea seemed illogical to a generation of Europeans who had been brought up in a society where disease was not only constantly present but viewed as a natural and integral part of one's existence. A few decades prior to this in the 18th century, those who had supported the idea of smallpox inoculation could justifiably claim that it would cut down on the number of deaths from the disease. There were, of course, instances in the 1700s where, as a result of this operation, an individual would actually come down with the disease. Whenever this happened, those who were suspicious of inoculation immediately seized upon such incidences to condemn the whole procedure.[39] In truth, vaccination was more generally accepted by the 1840s. But, prior to this, it was rejected for a variety of reasons, in particular because the idea of preventing a disease from taking place was just too alien for the public mind to accept. While the presence of disease in the historic past seemed to most to be both natural and inevitable, the existence of pain was not so readily accepted. There was, in fact, in the pre-industrial period an almost constant search for new remedies, that is for items that might either ease pain or produce a cure. In this day and age, both physicians and the public-at-large were quick to respond to almost any drug that promised a measure of relief. In time, the hopes of previous generations in this regard would be realized. But that did not happen until the 19th and 20th centuries, when modern medical science came up with both vaccination and chemotherapy. Once it did, society was well on the way towards conquering the great endemic and epidemic diseases.[40] However, before these new techniques were developed, European society was exclusively dependent upon extremely crude drugs, the vast majority of which were of doubtful value. Europe's reliance on these highly suspicious drugs was according to one 18th-century observer, William Rowley, really a form of madness.[41] Biologically, they were of little use, but psychologically they seemed to satisfy this age's craving for at least some kind of protection against the great deadly and disabling diseases. The number of drugs that were being used grew continually over time. By the late 19th century, just prior to the advent of modern microbiology and modern chemotherapy, the lexicon of prescribed drugs had climbed to some 2,743 separate items. Only a few of these supposed drugs, such as quinine and opium, have survived pharmaceutically. The largest number of them, conscientiously listed in the

19th century as capable of healing, such as olive oil, mustard and liquorice, are no longer considered clinically useful.[42]

The overwhelming majority of the so-called drugs used in the past years were of plant or vegetable origin. Most apothecaries, or drug stores, were stocked with a wide variety of what would now be described as medicinal herbs, including such items as sage, ginger, and, in time, digitalis. After plants, the second most important group of drugs, used in the pre-industrial period, were derived from metals, primarily mercury, arsenic and antimony. Nearly all of these products were surrounded by some kind of mystique. Very ordinary and commonplace plants and metals somehow, someway took on an almost magical character in this period. For, this was an age that was obviously eager for any kind of protection that it could get its hands on.[43] Given this somewhat panicky attitude, people kept ascribing to plants and metals curative powers that they simply did not possess. Often recommended by physicians and almost always accepted by the masses, most of these remedies were advertised as either pain-killing analgesics or infallible cures for one disease or another. Beyond the drugs derived from plants and metals, there were, of course, other ways of curing diseases that were generally accepted. The most trusted medical treatment of the times was bleeding. The practice of bleeding was based on the time-honored medical idea that diseases invaded the body from the outside and needed to be relieved. Once bad humors entered the system, they literally had to be let out, and bleeding was then considered to be one of the best ways of accomplishing this. Even the noted Veronese physician Fracastoro, one of the most progressive medical thinkers of the 16th century, was convinced that bleeding was imperative if syphilis was to have any chance of being cured.[44] Purging was practiced for the same reason, in order to dispel the poisons that were obviously building up inside the body.[45] Beyond these practices, the air was, of course, also suspected of harboring corrupt matter that might enter the body and do some harm. Because this was thought to be true in a previous age, perfumes and fumigants were constantly being used, all in a desperate attempt to purify the air of its death-dealing stenches.[46]

As might be expected, all sorts of remedies were prescribed against plague. Purifying the air and keeping it free from harmful smells was, according to the London College of Physicians, of primary importance. Obviously accepting the miasmatic interpretation on the origins of disease, the College strongly suggested at one point fumigating by plunging hot stones into a solution of vinegar and rosemary. At the same time, they also recommended perfuming with a mixture of garlic, cloves, sage and a herb known as wood of sorrel. Both procedures, they assured the public, would clear the air of any dangerous miasmas. Yet another of the cures that the College advocated for plague consisted of making a hole in the top of an egg, emptying its content and filling the empty space with saffron. They recommended saffron, which is actually derived from the crocus plant, because it was considered by a large number of physicians to possess some extraordinary powers. Once made, the concoction was first pulverized, then mixed with mustard and finally drunk with ale.[47] During the 16th century, at least, this concoction was thought to be a rather sure cure for plague. Portions of this particular prescription also appeared in Thomas Vicary's famous antidote for plague published in 1586. In it, he advised the English public to: "Take . . . English saffron the weight of a half-penny, and a farthing worth of Graines, a quart of long Peppers, a penny weight of Dace and stale Ale, stampe your heart and pound your saffron, and mingle them together, and then drink it."[48] The use of herbal medicines was also an important part of the equally well-known recipe which was published just prior to the London epidemic of 1603 under the title of Kings Medicine for the Plague. It included a prescription guaranteeing that "this will (by God's helpe) preserve you [from plague] for the space of a whole year." This remedy consisted of sage, rue, which is an evergreen shrub, elderleaves, bramble leaves, ginger, woodworm, wine and vinegar, judiciously mixed together and drunk every morning after fasting the night before.[49]

Not only were vegetable remedies tried over and over again during this era, so also were a variety of cures prepared from metals. During the epidemic in southern France in the early 1720s, the French government spent large sums of money purchasing compounds that were widely used to aid the victims of bubonic plague. In the remedy that was most popularly prescribed, the key ingredients were first of all saltpeter, now better known as potassium nitrate, and then secondly antimony. Antimony, like nearly all metals, is potentially very poisonous. In spite of this fact, this particular metallic substance, which is very similar to arsenic in its affects upon the body, was continually used to promote vomiting in those who were ill with the disease. Vomiting was at this time just as respected a medical procedure as were bleeding and purging. And like the other two techniques, it was seen as a vital means of dispelling bad humors from the body. The most common plague recipe of the early 1720s which was then being pushed by the French government advised those who were preparing it to "Take saltpeter . . . crush it, place it in a German crucible, place the crucible in a furnace. . . . When the saltpeter is melted, add coarsely ground charcoal . . . [then] Cool in a glass stand." Once this was done, the recipe went on to suggest: "Take four pounds of Hungarian antimony -- break into small pieces, . . . add one pound of the prepared liquor of nitrate [saltpeter], . . . and one half gallon of rain water, boil for two hours on the fire."[50] After this was done, the powder, left over from the process, was cooled and the decoction was then given to the patient in some kind of liquid in order to promote vomiting. The most unfortunate part of this treatment was that the vomiting tended to remove large quantities of life-giving potassium from the victim's body, thus endangering his life even further. This age could not, of course, have possibly known anything about this rather intricate biochemical process. What this case does point up is the fact that the use of drugs in the historic past was in the main highly experimental; some of those experiments worked, most did not.

No drug in the history of medicine prior to the 19th century was considered more effective against syphilis than mercury. For almost 400 years, most physicians in Europe would have unhesitantly agreed with John Andree that: "Mercury . . . is . . . known by all skilful practioners of the healing art to be the only medicine which will cure the Venereal Disease."[51] Exactly how mercury cured syphilis was a mystery to most medical men, a point that Andree readily admitted when he said: "The method of which mercury arrests this disease is not yet known."[52] Other physicians suggested the use of mercury and antimony together, but on its own or in combination the value of mercury was rarely doubted in an age when effective cures were relatively scarce to begin with.[53] Mercury was first used as a cure for malignant syphilis and its accompanying skin pustules around the year 1500. Prior to that, however, mercury did have a fairly long history, one that dated back to the first Christian contacts with the Arabs. Mercury had been used by Arab doctors to treat a wide range of skin disorders. It was normally prepared by them as a salve, the mercury customarily being mixed with saliva or lard before it was applied in order to cushion its more corrosive qualities.[54] Its potency thus reduced, mercury was apparently capable of absorbing a significant amount of bacteria, in turn reducing the irritation on the outer surface of the skin. Skin disorders such as scabies were apparently so common during the High Middle Ages that European society quickly latched on to this Arab practice. Centuries later, when malignant syphilis struck, mercurial ointments were immediately used in an attempt to reduce some of the ugly, external symptoms of the disease.[55]

By the middle of the 16th century, mercury was being widely used against syphilis in one of three ways, either as a plaster judiciously applied to the skin, or as an inhalant, or finally, and most dangerously, in pill form.[56] After the use of mercury, the symptoms of syphilis normally disappeared, meaning, as far as this age was concerned, that the disease had somehow been healed. But, then, these symptoms would have disappeared in any event, what with the disease now entering its latent or tertiary stage. Without adequate knowledge of how syphilis naturally proceeded, mercury was continually praised over the course of centuries for producing an almost miraculous cure. Even the great Fracastoro, upon analyzing all the other remedies that had been suggested for syphilis, wound up declaring: "But most people do better by dissolving everything in quicksilver."[57] The excessive use of mercury, which can quickly reach toxic levels within the body, did lead to individual cases of poisoning. This began to occur with greater frequency as mercury was increasingly prescribed for internal use in pill, powder or liquid form. Taken in ever-expanding amounts during the 17th century, mercury treatments often produced profuse salivation. In such instances, patients were often seen foaming at the mouth for periods of up to six weeks after they were treated. This highly experimental technique, which was known to the medical profession as fluxing, was considered by many to be a life-saving procedure. For them, fluxing fell naturally into the same medical category as bleeding, purging and vomiting. It was simply viewed by many doctors as yet another important way of casting corrupt material out from the body.[58] However, by the 18th century, fluxing was increasingly falling into disfavor, primarily because of its excessive use. The French observer Astruc complained bitterly at this time that fluxing "always weakens and destroys the tone of the stomach, and prevents its faculties, which bring on violent vomiting, violent purging, dysentery, spitting of blood, fainting, swoonings and sometimes death itself."[59] While the overuse of mercury was being condemned in some quarters, mercury itself continued to be prescribed right down to the early part of the 20th century as medicine's best hope for curing syphilis.[60]

Mercury was not the only cure for syphilis which at one time or another had a great deal of support. For a while in the 16th century, it had been rivalled by yet another drug, guaiacum, a remedy which the Spanish had introduced to Europe during the decade of the 1510s. The Spanish had first come into contact with guaiacum on the island of Santa Domingo, where the Indian population had been using it as a standard cure for mild cases of syphilis. According to the Spanish physician, Nicholas Manardes, it was discovered in Haiti by "A Spanyarde that did suffer great paines of the Poxe, whiche he had by the companie of an Indian woman, . . . one of the Phisitions of that countrie, gave unto hym the water of guaiacum, wherewith not onely his greevous paines were taken awaie that he did suffer: but [he] healed verie well of the evill."[61] In a society that was obviously desperate for remedies, guaiacum was soon being hailed by those who advocated its use as the universal panacea for syphilis. Von Hütten, who suffered rather intensely from this disease, was one of guaiacum's leading supporters. Praising the drug's effects he wrote: "If we ought to Give thanks to God for Good and Evil, how much are we bound for his gift of Guajacum; yea, how much doth the joy and Gladness for his Bounty to us, surpass the Pains and Sorrows of our past Sickness."[62] Not only were laymen singling this new drug out for praise, so also were numbers of those in the medical profession, including the great Paré who called it "the number one cure" for syphilis.[63]

Guaiacum was itself of vegetable origin, a drug that was distilled from an evergreen tree that grew wild throughout the Caribbean area. When the Spanish penetrated the West Indies they came across medicine men who were capable of preparing a decoction of guaiacum. The recipes that they used evidently went back for generations. Their method was promptly transferred to Europe where, according to Hütten, the whole process could be accomplished in three rather easy steps. Wood from the tree was first cut and then pounded into a powder. A single pound of the powder was next taken and kept soaking in eight pounds of water overnight. On the second day, the mixture was heated, just short of boiling and allowed to cool. The resulting foam was immediately skimmed from the vat and eventually used as a kind of drying powder for syphilitic eruptions. The remaining liquid or decoction was then drunk by the patient with the expectation that it would relieve the symptoms. Hütten was so sure that guaiacum would cure the disease that he insisted that it was the only medicine that was needed for syphilis. In his writings he went even further scornfully attacking the medical profession for not accepting guaiacum more thoroughly and for literally experimenting with hundreds of other supposed cures for the disease. Experimentation was going on. A confusing array of other cures, all hailed as timely remedies for syphilis, were introduced during the first half of the 16th century. All sorts of decoctions, variously produced from china root, actually an ordinary climbing shrub, sasparilla, a rather common central American bush, and sassafras, originally derived from the North American laurel tree, were each in turn heralded as a sure cure for this disease. In time, nearly every one of them fell into disuse, including guaiacum. After an initial vogue, each was replaced by what later generations of Europeans thought was the only true cure for syphilis, mercury.[64]

While syphilis was heavily medicated many other diseases such as smallpox, typhus and tuberculosis were not. Smallpox was considered by most, of course, to be a natural disease, one that did not need any attention, especially when it struck in its milder form. It has been estimated that during the time when Voltaire was alive that over 80 percent of all Frenchmen had the disease at one stage of another in their lives. In the 18th century when this was happening, the standard treatment for smallpox, when medical attention was called for, consisted of either administering cordials, really just pain-killing alcoholic beverages, or else prescribing purging and bloodletting.[65] Beyond these measures, little else was done. However, at about the same point in time, inoculation was gaining favor, at least, in some quarters. The "buying of smallpox" was increasingly being practiced, largely at the urgings of the medical profession which knew very well that a mild case of the disease could infer lasting immunity.[66] Typhus was still another disease that traditionally received little or no active treatment, although at times digitalis was used in an attempt to control the disease's often prostrating fever. Digitalis, which was widely used for a variety of ailments prior to the 19th century was a herbal medicine, one that derived from a wild European plant known as the foxglove. For generations, this drug was used experimentally first as a purgative, thereafter as an ointment and then finally as an expectorant. Initially discovered in the 16th century, digitalis was used rather unsuccessfully in the treatment of typhus. It was only around 1800 and after much experimenting, that it was, at last, discovered to have chemical properties capable of controlling the human heart muscle.[67]

The discovery of America added considerably to the number of drugs that were circulating within European society. Included among this veritable flood of new remedies was yet another product which was widely acclaimed, quinine. Quinine first became popular in the decade of the 1630s. It owed its notoriety to the fact that the Countess of Chincha, the wife of the Viceroy to Peru, had been miraculously cured of a rather serious fever after taking a powder derived from a certain tree. The tree in question soon became known as the Cinchona tree. By the middle of the 17th century, the bark of this tree was steadily imported into Europe, where it was quickly being processed into quinine.[68] It was initially used against a wide variety of febrile disorders, including typhus, malaria and influenza. Like many other drugs, it was viewed, at least at the beginning, as being almost magical, literally capable of producing extraordinary results. The well-known London physician, Sydenham, recorded how the Jesuits' bark, as it was more generally known, had originally been seen by him as an exciting new cure. Commenting briefly, but to the point, he declared: "Jesuits' bark has been famous in London for the cure of intermittent fevers for upwards of five and twenty and that rightly."[69] In time, however, the medical profession began to lose faith in quinine, especially when it discovered that even large quantities of the drug were not arresting some fevers.[70] Even more alarmingly, the amount of quinine that was being given was not being regulated very closely, with the result that a number of people were being poisoned.[71] Just like other drugs, quinine was proving to be dangerous when it was not used with restraint. Highly praised to begin with, its overuse coupled with the fact that it failed to stop the return of many fevers led to its declining reputation towards the end of the 17th century.

In spite of numerous disappointments with a wide range of potential cures, the medical profession was constantly on the lookout for new ways of treating disease. Given this hope, it is not surprising to discover that two of Europe's most widespread diseases in the 19th century, cholera and tuberculosis, were treated by a wide variety of both old as well as new remedies. Early on in the century the favorite technique of some for dealing with cholera remained the old idea of bleeding. Because the microorganism involved here, <u>cholera vibrio</u>, attacked the intestinal wall, thus preventing the absorption of nutrients, diarrhea inevitably ensued whenever cholera struck. The result of the diarrhea in up to 50 percent of all cases was dehydration and subsequent death. Not knowing this, of course, the medical profession only encouraged the loss of more liquids by promoting bleeding. Most physicians, on the other hand, who employed the technique honestly believed that they were aiding the patient in line with the time-honored assumption that by bleeding they were actually helping corrupt matter to escape from the body. What bleeding did, in actuality, of course, was to accelerate the process of dehydration, thereby quickening the arrival of death. The practice of purging also contributed to this dangerous process of dehydration in certain individuals. The purgative that was used most often by this time was a preparation known a calomel, a drug that was essentially a form of mercury. When calomel, actually mercurous choloride, was used it immediately deprived the patient of badly needed body fluids, thus once again hastening the chances of dehydration.[72] Meanwhile, during the cholera epidemic of 1831, Russian doctors were making use of some entirely new techniques. In that year, the Imperial Government began to back the use of a new substance, a metallic drug by the name of bismuth. Bismuth of nitrate, used in salt form, was conceptually a rather radical departure from anything that the medical profession had ever used before in cases of cholera.[73] The great novelty that was involved in bismuth was that this drug was being administered not to encourage diarrhea, but more importantly to check it. Bismuth did not prove to be all that effective. However, it growing acceptance did represent a significant philosophical breakthrough. For it demonstrated that some medical men were now beginning to realize that in cases of cholera the loss of fluids should somehow be stopped. The very same notion lay behind the use of yet another salt, an acetate of lead, which was increasingly being prescribed at this time to check the vomiting that so often accompanied an attack of cholera.[74]

Throughout the progressive waves of cholera that struck Europe in the 19th century, opium was used with increasing frequency.[75] Opium was not, of course, considered to be a cure. But the pain-killing morphine that it contained did aid the victims of cholera, many of whom experienced a great deal of excruciating pain. Morphine helped by quickly diminishing the pain that they felt, by relieving anxiety and by bringing on sleep. Opium never saved any lives, but it did make the last hours of some terminally ill with cholera at least, in part, more bearable. Beyond the rising utilization of opium, doctors continued to make use of other potential cures. In parts of France, for instance, a cereal made from mustard was commonly employed as a plaster, but without much apparent effect.[76] In England, an older remedy, fumigants, this time based on chlorine, were sometimes tried, but again without any apparent beneficial results.[77] Meanwhile, some Russian doctors tried injecting a solution of water and vinegar into the blood stream of certain patients hoping thereby to arrest the loss of liquids.[78] Diluted acid baths were also employed in some places in Europe in a desperate attempt to restore circulation, which often collapsed in the victims of cholera in the outer portions of the body due to the excessive dehydration that was taking place.[79] Very few of these highly experimental techniques ever succeeded. As a result, the medical profession was thrown back, especially in the 1830s, and 1840s, on some of its older practices, including bleeding, purging and vomiting. One Scottish physician, representing the thinking of many, vigorously defended the need for purging in cases of cholera. Pointing to the way that he had done it in India, he explained: "I commence with 1 1/2 ounces of caster oil, and continue giving one ounce every twenty minutes, until the bowels freely open by it. The patient is kept in this position by force, and not allowed until the operation of the medicine, the slightest motion."[80] Most physicians during the earlier epidemics of cholera would probably not have agreed with the use of force, but they would have argued in favor of the therapy that was being employed here.

Tuberculosis went untreated during much of the 19th century primarily because it was thought to be an incurable disease. Even as late as the 1840s, the standard medical text on consumption, written by George Gregory, openly admitted that the medical profession was completely baffled when it came to this disease. Speaking of the situation that was then existing, Gregory wrote: "I must record the failure of every plan which human ingenuity has hitherto devised for the effective cure of consumption. It is indeed melancholy to reflect how little this disease occurring, as it does, in the prime of life . . . is under the control of medicine."[81] Tuberculosis was considered to be so incurable during these decades that victims of the disease were not even admitted to hospitals. Not only were consumptives regarded as hopelessly ill, there was according to Gregory little likelihood that a cure would ever be found for the disease. Obviously in a state of despair, he went on to comment that: "The uniform experience of mankind in all ages, on this point, suggests a doubt whether any material improvement in the mode of treating consumption can be anticipated, or any important change effected in the mortality occassioned by it."[82] The pessimism that was so often expressed about tuberculosis did not prevent some of the more daring physicians practicing at the time from trying to come up with a cure. Not too surprisingly, most of the remedies that they evolved during the 19th and early 20th centuries tended to be of an experimental nature. A prime example here was the work being done by the French physician Antoine Portal. During the early stages of his career, Portal devoted himself almost exclusively to the study of post-mortems, all in an attempt to learn more about the disease's pathological course in the body. Generally a cautious man, Portal became so discouraged by his inability to come up with any truly positive findings that later on, towards the end of his career, he turned to the experimental use of digitalis in a desperate attempt to find some kind of cure for the disease.[83]

During the 19th century, the search for a drug that would ultimately cure tuberculosis was a disappointing one. At one juncture, sulfur was considered as a good possibility and so, somewhat later on, were gold salts.[84] These experiments were so unrewarding that after 1850 medical men began to desert the idea that there was a possible chemical solution for tuberculosis. Some of the more enterprising minds of the time now began to look in a different direction. Most of the panaceas that were being put forward in the second half of the century involved the idea of building up the strength and endurance of those who had come down with the disease. It was during these decades, for example, that the modern science of nutrition was first born. It developed in the hands of those physicians who firmly believed that tuberculosis could be cured by means of a healthier diet. Many others became convinced that tuberculosis could be overcome if the patient was given the right combination of rest and exercise. To this end, mild forms of exercise, including walking and horseback riding, were increasingly prescribed as part of an overall therapeutic program that was specifically designed to bring about the recovery of consumptives.[85] Along the same lines, but closer to the turn of the 20th century, fresh-air therapy, which was known as hyperaeration, enjoyed considerable popular vogue. This particular treatment consisted of exposing a patient to the benefits of fresh air all day long, especially during the spring, summer and fall months of the year.[86] Even though the medical profession as a whole was becoming progressively more optimistic about finding a cure for tuberculosis, really tangible results tended to elude most doctors. Cures were being produced but at a very slow pace. The disappointment that many still felt around 1900 produced a new reaction, one that once more began to favor the use of drugs. All of a sudden, almost anything that might conceivably help was, in fact, being prescribed. While there were a large number of remedies that were being offered, one medical tract chose to focus in on what it regarded as the three best alternatives. It suggested that those who were ill with the disease or those who wanted to prevent it might look, in particular, to: "The preparation of cod-liver oil [which] has a world-wide reputation . . . . Iron is [also] frequently prescribed . . : . In children who are in any way anemic, the saccharated carbonate of iron is most beneficial . . . . Arsenic is recommended as a general tonic, Fowler's solution being one of the most convenient forms."[87] Actually, the public was being offered a rather confusing array of potential remedies, all of which only served to prove that as of the early 1900s, European society still did not have a truly effective means of preventing or curing this disease.

The failure of medical science prior to the 1910s to come up with any kind of workable chemical formulas against the great deadly and disabling diseases contrasts rather remarkably with what was about to take place for an entirely new age involving the use of drugs was just about to begin. It started, according to many historians, with the discovery of Salvarsan in 1912. Ever since that one breakthrough, modern science has been able to develop a continuing array of drugs, the vast majority of which have been capable of both checking and curing a large number of fairly serious diseases. The first of these so-called wonder drugs was Salvarsan, a compound that was originally synthesized in the laboratories of the well-known German bacteriologist, Paul Ehrlich. Also known as Arsphenamine, Salvarsan was essentially an arsenic compound that was specifically developed by Ehrlich as a cure for syphilis. Ehrlich's major preoccupation as he worked on Salvarsan was to come up with a compound that was capable of killing the spirochaete without the compound doing a great deal of damage to the human tissue surrounding the infection. His "magic-bullet," as he called it, was it is true, based on a metal that was notoriously poisonous. Still, he has been able to subdue it enough to make it a workable tool inside the human body.[88] His compound was tried repeatedly and found to be clinically effective against syphilis. However, given the fact that the highly deceptive third stage of this disease was still not totally identified in the 1910s, there is today some question as to just how far into the body Salvarsan could reach. That question was, of course, not really considered at the time. Instead, Salvarsan was almost universally acclaimed by the medical profession as a significant advance over mercury. Moreover, it proved its value on numerous occasions. For example, in one famous case, Salvarsan was given to more than 6,000 British troops during World War I who were known to be suffering from syphilis. The drug seems to have cured the vast majority of them without any indications of any harmful side effects. The same was not the case for a tiny minority that took Salvarsan, somewhat less than one percent. As it turned out that group was significantly affected. All of them did begin to suffer from headaches, delirium and vomiting, all characteristic signs that are normally associated with arsenic poisoning.[89] In spite of some drawbacks then, Salvarsan continued to be used on a regular basis and with its introduction the modern age of chemotherapy is often said to have begun. The use of chemicals, either of a herbal or metallic origin, to destroy harmful substances that had invaded the body had been one of the long-standing dreams of the medical profession in the historic past. Those hopes have, of course, only been truly realized in modern times. Starting with the early production of aspirin and continuing up to the more recent discovery of antibiotics, modern chemistry has finally produced the kind of remedies and cures that previous generations of Europeans had sought but never found. The development of acetylsalicylic acid, or aspirin, in the 1890s was a kind of a prelude to this new, pain-killing age. A mild analgesic that temporarily reduces body temperature, pain and the swelling that normally accompanies an infection, aspirin was used almost universally during the flu epidemic that struck Europe in 1918 and 1919. Even though that particular epidemic did take hundreds of thousands of lives, many more who had the disease managed to recover from it. For most of them, aspirin went a long way towards relieving the persistent pains in the head, back and limbs that seemed to go along with each and every case of the disease.[90] Not too unexpectedly, old practices also lingered on mixing in with some of the newer ones. For one thing, laxatives, in actuality the time-honored idea of purging, were continually being prescribed, along with aspirin in 1918 and 1919. The two together were, more or less, the standard way of treating flu at that time.[91] The period just prior to 1914 was one of the most remarkable in the long history of medicine. For not only was modern microbiology born in this period, so also was modern chemotherapy. Entirely new insights into the possible harmful effects of certain drugs were also being made. Increasingly, for example, the medical profession came to distrust a wide variety of older metallic substances. As this new attitude gained ground, a whole series of once highly respected drugs, including mercury, were systematically abandoned. This critical feeling towards the remedies that had been used so often in the past also affected some herbal medicines, many of which were now being jettisoned as clinically useless.[92]

Most of the diseases that at one time or another had dominated the European past would begin to disappear during the first half of the 20th century. Almost all of them would be vanquished by the coming of modern chemotherapy. Plague, of course, was long gone from the European scene. It had disappeared during the 18th century, never to return. But elsewhere in the world particularly in Africa and Asia, the war against plague was steadily being won. By the middle of the 20th century, the rats who carried this disease from one African or Asian port to another were progressively being eliminated by Warafin. Warafin was an anticoagulant that the World Health Organization used effectively for decades to control rat populations, and thus plague, in the less-developed areas of the globe. The fleas, which for centuries were involved in the transmission of bubonic plague from animals to man, have likewise fallen victim to modern chemistry. Here, a number of insecticides, including Dicophone, which is better known as DDT have proven to be extraordinarily effective. Unlike plague, typhus was still present in Europe during the early part of the 20th century. But like plague, it too was transmitted by means of a vector, in this instance body lice. For a number of key decades, before it fell into disfavor, DDT was extremely effective in controlling the lice that are commonly associated with the spread of typhus.[93] Beyond the obvious control of rodents and vectors that the development of certain vital chemicals provided, modern antibiotics have also been employed against a whole array of illnesses. Over and over again, they have proved their value, especially against the great bacterial and rickettsial disorders. Streptomycin, which was first developed by the American scientist Selman A. Waksman in the 1940s, is now used all around the globe to treat the victims of tuberculosis. So also is tetracyclin, yet another member of the antibiotic family. It has proved capable of killing not only the bacteria that cause plague and cholera, but also the rickettsia that are directly responsible for typhus.[94]

Once modern medicine began to arm itself with these new drugs and chemical substances, one disease after another began to disappear from the European scene. One of the very first of the new wonder drugs to be developed early on in the 20th century was penicillin. Penicillin was a typical antibiotic in that it was physically capable of puncturing the cell wall of certain bacteria, thus killing them almost immediately. Among the numerous forms of penicillin was a product known as Penicillin G in aluminum monsterate or PAM. This form of penicillin was used extensively to control what had been one of Europe's greatest scourges, syphilis.[95] This particular antibiotic turned out to be so useful in the treatment of syphilis that it quickly replaced Salvarsan as the major remedy for this highly elusive disease. By the 1940s antibiotics were also being employed in the fight against tuberculosis. This was definitely the case with streptomycin, which was initially tested against the tubercular bacillus. As soon as it was learned that it could destroy a bacterium, researchers realized almost instantaneously that they had, indeed, come up with a wonder drug. Shortly after this breakthrough in the middle of the 1940s, the discovery of yet another potent antibiotic, IHN, more specifically isonecotine acid, raised medical hopes even higher that tuberculosis might be completely eliminated.[96] This, of course, did not happen, but by the middle of the 20th century, virtually all of the great infectious diseases from the European past were either gone, in decline or under control.[97] The ability of certain chemical products, in particular the antibiotics, to maintain that record may well depend on whether the microorganisms involved here ultimately prove strong enough to develop any real resistance to these highly effective chemical agents.

The birth of modern chemotherapy was practically-speaking the beginning of a new age, while philosophically it marked the end of an older one. For more than half a millennium, the medical profession in Europe had unhesitantly believed in the value of drugs. Its faith had been so great that it kept ascribing to quite simple and quite ordinary plants and metals powers which they did not intrinsically possess. For centuries then Europe was unquestionably a drug-oriented society. In the words of one 18th-century critic of the medical profession, William Rowley, the thinking of most physicians was dominated by an ever-maddening desire for one drug after another. At one point towards the turn of the 19th century, he complained bitterly that most doctors were in turn, "Quick-silver mad, Digitalis mad, Arsenic mad, Sugar of lead mad," and so on.[98] Perhaps the helplessness that most doctors felt in the face of so many deadly and disabling diseases accounts for their well-documented belief in the ability of certain drugs to treat and to heal. That faith was finally vindicated in the 20th century. From a certain angle of vision then, Europe is now what it was in the past, a drug-orientated society. Only now instead of placebos, it has drugs that are truly effective against the great infectious diseases. From Ehrlich to Waksman, the originators of modern chemotherapy have undoubtedly ushered into existence a new and much more pragmatic age in the history of medicine. But in doing so, they also fulfilled what was for centuries in the medical profession a long sought after goal.

Most of the drugs that were used in the past were almost inevitably hailed, at least at the start, as sure cures. The great discoveries of the 1940s, in particular the antibiotics, were also proclaimed as wonder drugs, only this time with more scientific validity. Modern chemotherapy has, of course, led to the control of a large number of diseases. But, at one and the same time, it has not produced their total eradication. So while antibiotics have proven to be the most useful drugs that the medical profession has ever had at its disposal, they have not simultaneously eliminated whole diseases. This is because these drugs are not all-powerful. Warning about the limits that characterize all antibiotics in 1965, the Canadian Dr. C.J. Wherrett advised his colleagues that: "Somehow we must convince the entire public that victory [over disease] is not to be taken for granted, that is equivalent to abandoning a fire because the flames have died down and ignoring the fact that embers are still aglow underneath."[99] Wherrett's cautious attitude here rests on the proven ability of certain microorganisms to mutate to the point where they are biologically capable of resisting the action of certain antibiotics. In the world beyond human perception, new strains of bacilli are developing all of the time, many of them strong enough to resist antibiotics that were, a decade or so before, highly effective against them.[100] Only the future will tell whether modern chemotherapy has produced a truly long-lasting or only a temporary type of defense against most of the great bacterial and rickettsial disorders from the past.

Most of the glaring misconceptions about disease that were held in the European past vanished during the latter part of the 19th and early part of 20th centuries. For as soon as it became clear that microorganisms were actually responsible for disease, the medical profession at long last had the key insight that it needed to come up with the chemical cures that have been such an integral part of 20th-century medicine. For an extended period, of course, medical men had been looking outside of the body for the cause of disease. The classic explanation for disease that was handed down from one century to another was that it was caused by foul or putrid air that had somehow invaded the body. In line with this belief, it seemed only logical to previous generations of medical men that the poison that had entered the body should be expelled. Boils, pustules and other swellings emerging on the surface of the skin were regarded, according to this theory, as natural attempts by the body to heal itself by expelling these poisonous humors. The drugs that were produced in the European past, whether they were based on plants or metals were primarily designed to aid and abet the process. Drugs were useful, it was thought, in so far as they helped the body to do its own work, either by encouraging fluxing, vomiting, bleeding or purging. There was then a cause and effect relationship between the way that doctors thought of the origin of disease and the kind of drugs they sought. All of that came to an end, needless to say, with the advent of microbiology. For what microbiology actually did was to teach Europeans to think about the origin of disease in a new and entirely different way.

CHAPTER 8

MEDICAL OPINION

The first part of preservation is, to purifie and purge the ayre from all evill vapours, sentes, stench, corruption, putrification, and evill qualitie. For which cause, it is necessary to make good fumes in our houses, of sweet and wholesome wood.

--Thomas Lodge, A Treatise of the Plague (London, 1603), p. 4.

The overall history of medical opinion between the 14th and 20th centuries may be divided into two ages, an earlier one dominated by hard and fast philosophical assumptions and a later age characterized by a more scientific attitude. Prior to the 19th century, medical opinion in Europe was influenced by a powerful set of assumptions that were, somewhat ironically, a mixture of both Christian ideals and Graeco-Roman suppositions. The intellectual outcome of this rather peculiar blend of religious and secular thinking was a set of ideas about the origin of the great deadly and disabling diseases that lived on for centuries up to the early part of the 1800s. Because these assumptions, centering for the most part on the divine, planetary and miasmatic explanations for the presence of disease, carried with them the weight of dogma, they tended to dominate the thinking of the medical profession generation after generation. New ideas, of which there were many, were advanced to challenge these prevailing assumptions. But, generally-speaking, they were ignored right down until the end of the 18th century largely because they did not carry with them either the stamp of theological or philosophical authority. In the highly conservative age that tended to predate the European Enlightenment, a close study of human anatomy and pathology was played down in favor of more traditional explanations for the presence of disease. Even the pioneering work of Fracastoro in the 16th century and Kircher in the 17th century, which insisted, albeit without a great deal of actual evidence, that microscopic agents were the real cause of disease, was essentially rejected because that work ran counter to more well-established ideas. In comparison, the 19th century in the history of medicine marks a significant break with the past, for it was during that century that modern medicine really began. It was during this period of time that nearly all of the ideas that are now currently associated with modern medicine were born, including what was increasingly being learned about physiology, pathology, vaccination and microbiology. Indeed, the sheer magnitude of the reception that Koch's discoveries received in the 1880s and 1890s is in itself a kind of testimony to a profession that was progressively breaking away from the thinking that had dominated the past.[1]

A number of the great deadly and disabling diseases struck Europe in the late 15th and early 16th centuries at the very moment when that society was in the midst of a gigantic religious revival. The unprecedented misery being caused by the reoccurrence of bubonic plague and the sudden and almost simultaneous arrival of typhus, syphilis and influenza, undoubtedly reenforced the popular belief that disease was of divine origin. The Bible, for example, was replete with stories that diseases were constantly being sent by God as a form of divine punishment for the sins of man.[2] The rise of Protestantism, at this time, with its tremendous emphasis upon the Bible, obviously encouraged the already common belief that disease was fundamentally a form of divine wrath. Around 1500 many theologians and a large body of physicians certainly believed, for example, the widely-accepted notion that syphilis was "a plague sent down from Heaven."[3] Deep into the 17th century, this argument could be heard repeatedly whenever and wherever bubonic plague happened to strike.[4] In the rather memorable words of one English Bishop, mankind had brought the plague onto itself by: "Our impassion towards our Brethren miserably wasted with war and famine . . . , our heavy oppression of our Brethren at home . . . . Our cheap and irreverent regard to God's Holy Ordinances, of his Words, Sacraments, Sabbaths and Ministers, our wantonnesse and toyishness of understanding, in corrupting the simplicity of our Christian Faith."[5] What lay behind the idea that disease was a form of divine punishment was, of course, the even more fatalistic assumption that the suffering which was brought on by disease could not possibly be avoided. That feeling of hopelessness and despair lingered on in Europe for an extended period, not finally being overcome until the latter part of the 19th century.[6]

The arrival of one infectious disease after another at the dawn of the Modern era also coincided with an equally strong belief in astrology. This trend was so powerful that by the early part of the 17th century, the minds of most medical men had become rather thoroughly saturated with astrological assumptions.[7] What was the case then was also true of an earlier period. Like most of his contemporaries in the 1600s, the Spanish physician de Villalobos believed that disease was the direct result first of sin and then, thereafter, of divine displeasure. God's pique, he argued at the time when syphilis was first being introduced into Europe, was more than justified and was visibly manifesting itself through the actions of certain planets.[8] In the context of the times, Mars and Saturn were primarily responsible for bringing on all sorts of diseases. Just how they did it was explained in 1665 by the English observer John Gadby, who commented that: "All Astrologers affirm, That all popular diseases are irritated by Mars and Saturn . . . and indeed the skilful . . . may readily read these dismal effects in their Natures. Mars is a planet fiery hot and dry Cholerick; and therefore Author of all Pestilential diseases: Saturn is a Planet, Earthy, cold and dry and Author of all tedious and durable infirmities."[9] Both the divine and celestial explanations for the presence of disease had their psychological impact, for they tended to carry the minds of most observers away from a more natural interpretation for disease.[10] In so doing, they made the origin of disease seem so far away that it was generally assumed by the many that these ailments would never be brought under human control.

Over the course of time, these extra-terrestial explanations for disease became entwined with some more down to earth beliefs about the origins of disease. This particular synthesis was the direct result of the revival of Graeco-Roman learning which was taking place during the period of the Renaissance and which tended to accentuate all over again the earlier teachings of Hippocrates and Galen. The work of these two classical thinkers had done much to advance the most celebrated of all medical explanations for the presence of disease, the miasmatic interpretation.[11] The miasmatic view was predicated on the notion that disease entered the body by means of foul and corrupt air currents. Exactly why the air was periodically contaminated in this way was unclear to both Hippocrates and Galen. However, later on during the Middle Ages it was increasingly assumed that God was responsible for these occurrences and that the actual presence of these poisonous substances in the air was somehow linked to the movement of the planets. Moreover, according to this theory, the putrid matter that caused disease hung invisibly in the air. And because it was invisible its coming was exceedingly difficult to predict. Even the great Fracastoro, philosophically, at least, the founder of modern microbiology, was personally convinced in the 1530s that when it came to syphilis "the source and seat of the evil was in the air itself."[12] This belief was so strong that for centuries almost no one escaped its intellectual grasp. Whenever and wherever either an old disease or a new disorder showed up, the medical profession invariably explained its coming in miasmatic terms. Rather typically, in 1568, the Scottish physician Skeyne, writing about the reappearance of plague, explained to his readers that: "Ane pest is the corruption or infectioum of the Air, or ane venemous qualytie and maist hurtfull Wapour thairof."[13]

Century and century, this ingrained assumption about the origins of disease went unchallenged even as one new disease succeeded another. In the 1780s, for example, the normally factually-minded Haygarth could declare without any fear of rebuttal whatsoever, that: "the natural smallpox appears to be communicated thro' the air."[14] Even as late as the 1840s, the presence of cholera in Scotland was explained away to the satisfaction of most by the long-accepted belief that the "disease is induced by some deleterious vapour or gas. "[15] It can be truly argued that no idea in the history of medicine lasted so long or was accepted by so many in such an unquestioning way as the miasmatic explanation for the presence of disease.

Over the course of centuries, the miasmatic point of view was generally-speaking a static concept. However, every so often this basic assumption was embellished by certain thinkers, many of whom were strongly influenced by their own personal experience with one or another of the great infectious diseases. Like most great theories, the miasmatic point of view had to be adjusted now and then to accommodate new insights. Among others, William Clowes, after watching the spread of syphilis became convinced that the disease, while admittedly starting in the air, was also being communicated by means of touch.[16] Based on what he had observed, Clowes concluded that syphilis was a highly contagious disease, one that was more than capable of being passed from one person to another. As it turned out, the doctrine of contagion, now gaining more and more adherents was rather easily incorporated into the miasmatic interpretation of the origin of disease. In fact, the two ideas proved to be unusually compatible, just as long as one accepted the notion that the disease was first contracted through the air. From there, it logically followed that once a person had become infected in this manner, the disease could obviously be conveyed to others as a result of physical contact.[17] While these exercises were taking place, speculation continued over the actual origin of corrupt air. For not everyone was satisfied that these air currents were, in fact, predetermined by planetary motion. Among the skeptics was the English student of influenza John Caius.

Caius became progressively convinced that the putrid air that caused disease was actually stored in the ground, only to be released every so often by an earthquake.[18] Much later than this in the 1720s, the French observer Astruc denied that this was true. He insisted in the case of plague that the real source of the morbid matter that caused the disease was infected bodies. It was decaying cadavers, he argued, which were actually reinfecting the air for the most part.[19] All of this speculation, and there was a fair amount of it, never got past the most basic and fundamental assumption of the times, that the air was primarily responsible for the presence of so much disease. This belief lived on into the latter part of the 19th century, still persisting even in the face of mounting evidence that disease was, in fact, caused by tiny microscopic agents that attacked the body.[20]

During the era when medical thinking was dominated by the miasmatic theory, it was widely assumed that once the morbid matter from the air entered the system it would adversely affect the body's various humors. This, in turn, would produce what the profession was fond of describing as a "melancholy and phlegmatic state."[21] One of the considerations that kept disturbing the advocates of the miasmatic theory, however, was the fact that the vast majority of those who inhaled "infected air," even during an epidemic, never got sick. According to the English apologist Lobb, this apparent contradiction did not necessarily disprove the miasmatic theory, for, as Lobb pointed out, at least in the case of plague: "The Danger of being infected with the Plague very much depends on the Quality of the infected Matter emitted into the Air, and the Nearness of Persons to receive it."[22] Over the course of numerous generations, the miasmatic point of view was continually saved by a series of mental adjustments just like the one that Lobb was able to make in the early part of the 18th century. Not only was this myth rarely challenged, it was constantly being popularized and thus reenforced. Even the great Shakespeare helped to keep the idea alive, speaking to his audiences at one point of "a Planetary Plague, when Jove Will o'er some high vic'd City, hang his poison in the sick Air."[23] Meanwhile, according to some observers, man was not totally helpless even if he was being subjected to these rather dangerous air flows. In the words of William Kemp, there were ways of safeguarding oneself. Writing in the 1660s, he pointed out that: "For as the air is corrected by smells, so is it also by fumes of which there are a multitude prescribed."[24] Not only were scented smells and fumes of all types employed against the deadly odors that hung on in the air, so also was burning. For burning was seen as yet another way of keeping the air pure and fresh.[25]

The miasmatic theory regarding the origin of disease directly influenced the type of medical treatments that were being employed in the period before the Industrial Revolution. It was generally believed, for example, that once the so-called "morbific matter" entered a person's system from the air, the body would try to regain its formerly healthy state by throwing off the poisonous substance or substances that had invaded it. Such things as fevers and abcesses along with vomiting and purging were seen as purely natural attempts on the part of the body to push out this putrid matter. The job of the physician according to the logic of the times, was to aid and if possible to accelerate these obviously life-giving processes. This attitude was so universally accepted in the 17th century that in treating cases of typhus, it was suggested that: "The Fever sometimes requires Vomiting, Purging and Bleeding -- especially in the beginning . . . , [to help] Nature endeavouring to expell the Morbifick matter."[26] Even the far-sighted English physician Sydenham, who is now regarded as one of the precursors of modern medicine, argued strongly at this time in favor of the need "to restore the health of the patient by the elimination of morbific matter." This was necessary, he went on, because diseases "arise partly from the particles of the atmosphere, [and] partly from the different fermentations and putrefactions of the humours."[27] When this happened, it was necessary for the physician, in Sydenham's view, to step in and to produce a cure. This could best be done by releasing the poison, for as he argued in the treatment of those with "smallpox, now just coming out . . . it will be servicable not only to bleed, but likewise to give a vomit."[28] This way of approaching disease inevitably filtered down to the local level. One study that was done on rural France in the 1780s and 1790s proved rather conclusively that in this part of the continent phlebotomy, or bleeding, was the most commonly practiced medical treatment of the day. It was closely followed by the administration of emetics, which were normally prescribed in order to induce vomiting.[29] And even as late as the first cholera epidemics of the 19th century, emetics and purgatives were still being given as the standard cure for this particular disease.[30]

Rather curiously, "the Morbifick matter" that was commonly thought to be invading the body was never seen as something that was actually alive. Whatever the substance was that was corrupting the human body, it was generally considered to be inorganic.[31] Only a few thinkers prior to the 19th century, working speculatively and without any sort of microscopic evidence, were imaginative enough to advance the idea that something organic might actually be saturating the air. One of these more enterprising thinkers was the Veronese physician Fracastoro, who lived in the early part of the 16th century. Fascinated by the idea of contagion, Fracastoro began to argue that syphilis was passed through the air by tiny, invisible objects which he rather graphically described as seminaria. The word seminaria as he used it might be historically translated as seeds, more modernly as germs. Focusing primarily on syphilis, Fracastoro argued that: "Contagion is a precisely similar putrefaction which passes from one thing to another: its seminaria [germs] have great activity, they are made up of a strong and vicious combination, and they have not only a material but also a spiritual antipathy to the animal organism."[32] Fracastoro obviously believed that these invisible substances were living organisms, a concept which later on would become the basic assumption underlying all of modern bacteriology and virology.

The notion that disease might possibly be caused by chemical substances too minute for the naked eye to see was kept alive from one century to another by other thinkers as well.[33] Among them was the German Jesuit Athanasius Kircher, who in the 1650s actually predicted the eventual coming of microbiology. Rather cleverly, Kircher combined the prevailing miasmatic theory with his own belief that the air was inhabitated by tiny infectious organisms. Kircher picturesquely referred to these organisms as "animata effuvia," indicating that he believed that they were living substances. He speculated that at the start these small creatures were lifeless, but he went on to say "under the influence of ambient heat and in proportion to the degree of infectious decomposition, [they] produce an offspring of innumerable imperceptible worms, so that the more [of these] corpuscles [that] are present in the effuvia, . . . [the more] they may be considered no longer as evidence of life but as actual living effuvia."[34] The germ theory, which had first been enunciated by Fracastoro, had now been restated by Kircher in a way that was not all that far removed from reality. As it turned out, however, the idea that they were putting forward at this time was just one of a number of competing explanations, one that quickly lost out to much more dominant theories. The idea that tiny microorganisms were, in fact, responsible for most disease did have its advocates into the 18th and 19th centuries. But the notion was always played down in favor of the prevailing assumption that the most immediate cause of disease was foul and putrid air. There was, of course, growing proof that these tiny organisms did exist. The new microscopes being developed by the Dutch were proving that some bacteria did exist, but their connection with disease was not firmly and finally established until the latter part of the 19th century.[35]

Towards the end of the 18th century, belief in the germ theory was at a very low ebb. Still, the medical profession had to face the all-too-evident fact that the vast majority of those who were caught in an epidemic sweep and were supposedly breathing in infected air, never came down with the disease in question. A large number of physicians had noted this phenomenon in the past and commented upon it with great curiosity. The failure of infected air to disable the many was, when it was considered, a rather glaring inconsistency in the miasmatic theory, one that was cleverly explained away during the 1700s by the emerging doctrine of predisposition. Increasingly, through this century, it was argued by some that corrupt air only penetrated the body of those who were already predisposed to pick up that particular disease.[36] The idea that some people were predisposed toward a disease was used most often to explain the rather disturbing growth of tuberculosis that was taking place in the general population. These unfortunates were, according Robert Morton, who wrote on this topic in the 1720s, bound to get consumption because they possessed a natural predilection for it. Expanding his belief, he went on to say that: "An Original Consumption is that, which arises purely from a Morbid Disposition of the Blood, or Animal Spirits, which reside in the System of Nerves or Fibers."[37] By the early part of the 19th century, the idea of predisposition which had originally been formulated to save the miasmatic theory from an inconsistency, had itself become a much more sophisticated doctrine. More importantly by the 1830s, as Dr. Henry Gaulter explained, the idea of predisposition had grown to encompass the belief that predisposition, in addition to being natural in some, could also be acquired by others. Gaulter defined this process, more exactly, saying: "Acquired predisposition includes whatever impairs the general health, especially by injuring the digestive organs, previous disease, habitual intemperance, excessive labor, imperfect nutrition, with other physical evils."[38]

Throughout the long period when the miasmatic point of view held sway, it managed to coexist very nicely with the idea of contagion. At first glance, that coming together would not appear to have been all that inevitable, especially if one considers that these two theories really claimed that disease came from entirely different sources. Actually, the potential differences between these two assumptions were rather easily reconciled. The idea that an infection could be passed from one individual to another was first highly publicized in the case of plague. Later on, it also seemed to be true of syphilis. And once syphilis was recognized as essentially a venereal disease, it was virtually impossible for most physicians to deny the conclusion of the Spanish observer de Isla that: "The Serpentine Disease is an epidemical contagious disease."[39] The doctrine of contagion was as of the early 1600s so ingrained that it could no longer be ignored. But once it was accepted, it was almost immediately married to the already prevailing assumption that the air was the source of all illness. This synthesis was extremely easy to bring about. All it required was that medical men accept the basic notion that corrupt air was the ultimate source of disease. From there on in, it was easy enough to argue that those who were infected in this way, to start with, could then pass the disease on to others by means of touch.[40] The period of medical thinking that emphasized the miasmatic point of view was, without question, a conservative one. During this age when basic assumptions counted for a great deal, the miasmatic view was ingeniously preserved, century after century, with only slight variations. Few, if any, ever really challenged this elaborate scheme for explaining the widespread presence of so many different diseases. What irregularities did emerge were usually explained away by some recently developed bit of logic. In the context of the times, most physicians, even if they had heard of the germ theory, would have remained skeptical about it. After all, they had been trained to think of disease as coming from an entirely different source.

The rise of modern medical science in the latter part of the 19th century not only depended on the development of new techniques, but perhaps even more importantly on the elimination of certain older ways of thinking. With most of the medical profession prior to 1800 essentially tied to a conservative way of doing things, only a few in the historic past were venturesome enough to turn to innovation. During the course of the 17th century, two medical thinkers stand out as part of this tiny minority. The first of them was the Englishman Sydenham. Evidently a skeptic by nature, Sydenham came to distrust a number of medical practices that were widely accepted in his own time. Always interested in finding new ways to treat the all too common fevers of his day, Sydenham used quinine experimentally. He also favored the use of cold applications instead of heat as the best means of controlling a rising fever. Some of his experiments, in particular the excessive use of mercury to treat those who had syphilis, plainly went too far. Still, given the fact that most physicians at this particular point in time did not fully understand the physiological consequences of what they were doing, his work in this area must be viewed as a search for a new cure.[41] Just as open minded in this regard was Sydenham's famous contemporary, the Dutch professor of medicine, Sylvius de le Boë. Sylvius was himself an early student of post-mortems. As a result of his anatomical studies, he became convinced that acid and alkaline were naturally balanced substances in the human circulatory system. His discovery was, to say the least, a rather novel insight into the chemical workings of the human body. But, that discovery was not popularly accepted in his own day, largely because the age was almost completely ignorant of even the most elementary facts concerning the body's chemistry.[42]

Whatever knowledge the medical profession had about the workings of the human body in the early part of the 18th century, and it was really very little, was gained from inorganic studies. Most of the body's basic functions, and in particular the organic and chemical changes that were produced by the various diseases that attacked it, were still very much of a mystery. The obviously enlightening science of physiology was, for example, still a hundred years away from full development. With so little knowledge available to medical men, the field was wide open to all kinds of speculation. A few facts could quite often give birth to some very elaborate philosophical assumptions, and they did. Some of the theories that were being developed in the 18th century concerning syphilis were highly characteristic of the baffling mixture of truth and error that surrounded most diseases. The well-known Italian physician Baglivi, for example, writing in the 1710s, was personally convinced that syphilis was caused by a kind of venereal ferment, which the body fitfully tried to expel by means of its own glandular system. He based his belief on his own observation that the disease's eruptions on the skin tended to approximate the major glands known to be in the body.[43] Later on in the same century, the noted Scottish surgeon Hunter helped to publicize the idea that gonorrhea and syphilis were the same disease. He simply concluded that the dripping associated with gonorrhea and the initial stage of syphilis were just slightly different forms of the same basic disease. As it turned out, his thinking on this point was accepted almost universally and was not actually corrected for another fifty years.[44] In a day and age when accurate assessments about the nature of certain diseases mixed freely with all kinds of misconceptions and misinformation, an enlightened few turned out to be amazingly correct in their conclusions. One of them was the Italian autopsist Georgio Morgagni. Working on cadavers, Morgagni came to the conclusion that syphilis was, indeed, a generalized disease, one that was capable of affecting different parts of the body. Unfortunately, his basic insight into the actual pathological course of syphilis inside of the body was essentially lost for the next one hundred years because no one picked it up and perpetuated it.[45] For in this age of hard and fast medical opinions, new knowledge like that being advanced by Morgagni was often set aside in favor of more comforting older views.

Whatever new knowledge about disease came into existence before the 19th century, its growth and development was dependent upon an experimental sense. At a time when the Enlightenment was just beginning and customary ways of thinking were still strong, no experimental technique caused more controversy than the one that first surrounded inoculation and then vaccination. Inoculation was a folk tradition that was practiced in certain parts of the Middle East long before it was introduced into Europe during the early part of the 18th century.[46] As soon as the operation was brought back to Europe, it was greeted with both skepticism and scorn. Large numbers of people simply would not believe that it was possible to combat a disease with a disease, the whole idea being, quite obviously, too novel for them.[47] It was often noted by those who were in favor of variolation that deaths from smallpox inevitably declined whenever inoculation was introduced. While this was true statistically, this particular bit of information did not convince the majority who were already predisposed to reject the process.[48] The practice of inoculation which was usually feared and distrusted by the public-at-large, was followed towards the end of the 18th century by Jenner's now famous experiment with the use of cowpox. His development, shortly after this, of a workable vaccine was wholeheartedly accepted by a number of his devoted followers, but most of those who heard about it were, more than anything, opposed to it. It was not until the 1850s and 1860s that public acceptance of vaccination really started to grow.[49]   Growing popular approval of vaccination after 1850 was not an isolated incident, for it came just at that moment when both doctors and laymen alike were becoming more tolerant of some of the newer medical techniques which were then being introduced.   The rigid conservatism of the past, which had repeatedly downgraded the idea that disease could be prevented was now giving way to a more promising age, one in which all levels of society were more hopeful about overcoming disease.

The 19th century was in many ways the most remarkable in the long history of European medicine, for many of the misconceptions that had held back the birth of modern medical science were dissolving during these crucial decades.   The workings of the human body, which had previously been shrouded in mystery, were now being revealed thanks to the advent of modern physiology.[50] More importantly, once the regular processes of the body came to be understood better in the first half of the century, the way was finally opened for the development of pathology as a legitimate area of scientific inquiry.[51] Moreover, around the middle of the 19th century, the first definite links between certain well-identified bacteria and some of the more common diseases were finally being established, at least in the minds of a few scientists. Gradually, in the period after the 1850s, the medical profession did come to accept the increasingly tantalizing idea that bacteria were, indeed, the cause of most illnesses. The bacteria that were now being implicated in the spread of disease were not an entirely new phenomena. Some of them had literally been known for generations, but very few thinkers historically had ever ascribed to them any sort of real toxicity. Now, it was becoming abundantly clear from the work of Koch and others, that these tiny microorganisms were responsible for most of the deadly and disabling diseases that had haunted Europe for so long. To have asked the medical profession to revolutionize its thinking on this score almost overnight was, of course, asking a great deal.[52] But, rather remarkably, the bulk of those who were practicing medicine in the latter part of the 19th century did accept the new evidence in an exceedingly short period of time. Once the microscopic explanation for disease came into its own, the miasmatic point of view simply dissolved. This older conception about the origin of disease, which had been part of medical thinking for more than a millennium simply evaporated in the face of this newly acquired evidence.

Before the modern science of pathology could emerge more fully, one other philosophical impediment to modern medical thinking had to be cleared away. The stunning triumph of modern physiology and pathology during the 19th century was not only a victory for closer observation, it was, as has already been noted, an entirely new way of thinking about the physical origins of disease. One older idea, however, concerning the way in which disease was transmitted would have to be resurrected in order for modern medical thinking to proceed on a a a more empirical course. Rather ironically during the early part of the 19th century, the age-old concept of contagion had suddenly fallen into disfavor. For centuries up to this point: "Contagion before the germ theory . . . [had been] visualized as the direct passage of some physical influence from a sick person to a susceptible victim by contact or through the atmosphere."[53] In spite of ancient lineage, the concept of contagion was consistently being challenged by a growing number of medical thinkers during the early 1800s. Doubt concerning the validity of this notion was spreading within the medical profession. It was growing largely because most physicians had seen the vast majority of individuals that they knew escape disease even though they were in close physical contact with those who were ill. There were just too many exceptions to the idea that a disease should easily and automatically spread from one person to another. Totally unaware of the existence of immunity, the idea of contagion was, momentarily at least, being discarded by a large percentage of those in the medical profession. The coming of microbiology a few decades later would prove, of course, that contagion actually did exist. The concept of contagion was reestablished then decades later, but on an entirely new basis. For this new age was beginning to understand that contagion existed, but only because tiny microorganisms were being passed either by air, water or food from one victim of a disease to another.[54]

The revolutionary changes in medical thinking that characterized the second half of the 19th century were dramatically accelerated by the newly founded science of bacteriology. There were literally dozens of scientists who were involved in this pioneering area, but three names stand out from the rest for their truly unique contributions, they were Villemin, Pasteur and Koch. Villemin, who was one of those who was committed to the idea of contagion, demonstrated conclusively through a series of experiments in 1865 that tuberculosis could be passed from one laboratory rabbit to another.[55] Villemin's highly ingenious experiments in this area tended to increase the suspicion among certain medical men that microscopic agents must be responsible for the spread of this disease. Shortly after this, Louis Pasteur, who was a chemist by training, mustered rather conclusive evidence that bacteria were at work in the fermentation process that led up to the production of wine. Fascinated by the potential of these microorganisms, Pasteur, ably assisted by several others, went on to demonstrate that both anthrax in sheep and cholera in chickens were caused by bacteria. While a series of animal disorders were being linked to the existence of several well-known bacteria, it was Koch who was finally credited with establishing an unassailable connection between bacteria and a variety of human disorders. After years of study, Koch discovered in 1882 the microorganisms responsible for tuberculosis in humans and then followed up that obviously sensational find by uncovering the tiny organism that was the cause of cholera.[56] Koch's work represented a turning point in the history of medicine. For with him, the evidence in favor of the idea that disease was caused by certain microscopic agents had become so overwhelming that it could, in fact, no longer be ignored.

The first tell-tale signs that medical science was beginning to take on a more scientific character date back to the 1830s and 1840s. The growing sophistication of medical thought, both then and in the decades that followed produced an ever-expanding volume of highly accurate knowledge concerning the great infectious diseases in Europe. All sorts of new insights were being produced not only about tuberculosis, but also in regard to syphilis, cholera and influenza. However, it was the truly remarkable discoveries concerning tuberculosis which really signalled to the times the fact that medical science was at long last on its way towards unravelling the mystery that had once surrounded the origin of disease. Prior to this in the 1830s, the French physician Philippe Ricord, working among syphilitics in Paris, had been able to prove for the first time that gonorrhea and syphilis were actually separate and distinct diseases. He did this by injecting "pus" from certain gonorrhea patients into a number of volunteers. Since syphilis did not develop in the controlled group, he accurately concluded that the two disorders must be entirely different diseases. From here, Ricord went on to examine syphilis even more closely, logically dividing the disease into three separate stages. As a result of his research, Ricord was among the very first to see that syphilis had deep-seated consequences, an impact that had gone unrecognized up to this particular point in time.[57] Beyond the rather amazing insights that he produced, Ricord typified that new breed of medical men who were now coming to the forefront in the profession, for he was personally quite dissatisfied unless he could plumb a disease experimentally for more and more knowledge about its true pathological course.

When cholera struck Europe initially in the early 1830s, it was, of course, a mysterious ailment. But, increasingly it, too, was subjected to the investigative powers of a profession that was progressively gaining in epistemological maturity.[58] In many ways, cholera was among the most difficult diseases that the medical profession had to handle. It proved to be extraordinarily difficult to understand because it required that medical men change their way of thinking. What they had to do was to accept the seemingly far-fetched notion that cholera was actually transmitted by water and not by air.[59] The key figure in promoting this radical new interpretation was the English physician John Snow. Characteristically thorough, Snow examined the impact of cholera on "no fewer than 300,000 people of both sexes, of every age and occupation, and of every rank and station." Using the statistics that he had amassed, Snow discovered that "one group being supplied with water containing the sewage of London" was, indeed, far more susceptible to cholera than those who were drawing their supply from a cleaner source.[60] From this and earlier studies that he had done, Snow concluded that cholera was transmitted by water, especially that which had been contaminated by what he euphemistically described as "cholera evacuations."[61] It was not unusual in this age of steadily advancing scientific perceptions, for one insight to lead directly to another. In this particular case, not only did Snow uncover the real manner in which cholera was spread, he also argued, rather perceptively, that the disease's impact most probably varied with the amount of contaminated matter that was taken in.[62] While Snow was rather positive in reporting his findings, others were not so ready to accept them. The consequence of all of this, as the well-known German physician Max von Pettenkofer was to note, was that his conclusions quickly became a matter for "scientific disputation."[63]

Even before Snow had put forth his somewhat controversial discoveries, medical science was already investigating both cholera's etiology and its pathology much more rigorously. Two Russian scientists, P. R. Gorianinov and N. N. Malakhov, had, in fact, expressed the belief in the 1830s that cholera was caused by "microscopic agents belonging to the animal kingdoms." Unfortunately, their findings were almost immediately attacked by the Moscow medical establishment as "contrary to our view of the natural world."[64] In spite of opposition, a handful of medical thinkers did continue to keep alive what in time came to be known as the germ theory. These more imaginative types would, of course, eventually feed the more fertile minds of Pacini and Koch, both of whom came up with the idea that bacteria were the cause of cholera.[65] One of the most unheralded areas of 19th-century medicine was autopsy. Even though this field did not receive a great deal of publicity, some truly momentous discoveries were made as a result of post-mortems. By the 1850s, for instance, pathological studies that had been done on cadavers had definitely established that cholera was an enteric disorder, one that systematically attacked, according to German and French pathologists, "the mucous membrane of the small intestine."[66]

Not everyone, of course, was convinced of these new findings. There were still plenty of skeptics around. Even as late as 1886, the validity of Koch's discovery of the Vibrio cholerae was being questioned by some physicians who simply did not believe that cholera was caused by water-borne bacteria. At one point the English doctor George Buchanan even chastised Koch over cholera in a major British publication declaring that "it would seem that Dr. Koch arrived too hastily at his affirmative conclusion [about cholera]."[67] Among Koch's most formidable detractors was his fellow German Max von Pettenkofer. In the 1880s, Pettenkofer was just as famous as Koch, having won an outstanding reputation for his advocacy of public health measures to prevent the spread of infectious disease. An uncompromising opponent of the microscopic theory of disease, Pettenkofer and a group of his students purposely swallowed water that was literally teeming with cholera bacteria. None of them suffered any ill effects whatsoever, an act that momentarily, at least, discouraged acceptance of Koch's findings.[68] However, it was not really long before the bacterial cause of cholera was so firmly established that the concept won almost universal acceptance. Medical science, as of the 1880s, had obviously mastered the mystery behind cholera; the next disease to fall was to be tuberculosis.

The eventual conquest of tuberculosis was likewise dependent upon the overthrow of certain long-established medical myths. Once these misconceptions were cleared away, the medical profession could finally begin to view tuberculosis much more realistically. The first philosophical obstacle that medical science had to overcome in the case of tuberculosis was the mistaken assumption that this disease was, in the words of the great Bayle, "nearly always incurable and fatal."[69] This obviously fatalistic assumption, which was so prominent in the years before 1850, kept discouraging and demoralizing that tiny minority that honestly believed that the disease was curable. The major reason why tuberculosis was viewed so hopelessly was because the disease was usually diagnosed for the first time in its later, terminal stages. Encouraged by this time-honored belief about tuberculosis, as late as the 1870s, medical men were still looking for evidence to prove its hereditary character. Among those who adherred to the doctrine that certain individuals and families were predisposed to the disease was the English physician C. Thomas Williams who argued: "One of the most striking proofs of the hereditary character of phthisis is the presence of tubercles, often demonstrated in the lungs of a foetus or a young infant of consumptive parents; another is to be found in instances where a consumptive and a healthy person marry and the children become consumptive."[70] As long as the medical profession was tied to the idea that some were literally foredoomed to this disease by poor constitutions, very few doctors were ever willing to look for other possible explanations for the presence of tuberculosis.

There were, of course, other misconceptions about tuberculosis which were just as widely held during the 19th century. Among them was the lingering notion, first expounded in the early part of the century, that tuberculosis was not a communicable disease. In the 1870s, by way of illustration, the standard English medical text written by August Flint and William H. Welch still maintained that: "The doctrine of the contagiousness of . . . [tuberculosis] has now as hitherto its advocates, but the general belief of the profession is in its non-communicability."[71] This highly erroneous assumption was quickly dispelled in 1882 as a direct result of Koch's discovery of the Mycobacterium tuberculosis. For that particular organism proved to be extraordinarily contagious.[72] Koch's approach to the study of bacteria had been strongly influenced by the work of Villemin two decades earlier. The iconoclastic Villemin had evidently never really subscribed to the myths that continued to surround tuberculosis in the 1860s. Far more daring than most, Villemin, who worked primarily with rabbits, became personally convinced that tuberculosis was caused by a single agent which was, indeed, highly contagious.[73] Villemin knew that he was advancing ideas that represented a departure from previous thinking. He was quite conscious, as he said, that his "facts and interpretations [would] be opposed by those with different views."[74] Villemin's ideas had a powerful impact upon Koch. When Koch announced, for example, his discovery of the bacteria that were responsible for tuberculosis, he started out his now famous article by referring directly to Villemin's earlier contention that tuberculosis was a contagious disease.[75] Rather remarkably, one highly imaginative experiment by Villemin had, in fact, paved the way for Koch's monumental discoveries of the early 1880s that had, in turn, produced an entirely different way of thinking about how this disease came into existence.

Koch's surprising discovery literally revolutionized medical thinking for decades to come. From that moment on, tuberculosis would be viewed as not only a treatable disease, but as a curable one. Even before this, however, a number of hospitals and some physicians were already working from the premise that consumptives could be cured. One of the very first hospitals in all of Europe to take in and treat those already suffering from tuberculosis was the Brompton Hospital in London. As early as 1848, that hospital was able to report that up to 25 percent of its tuberculosis patients had their symptoms relieved, and yet another six percent had seen their condition almost totally arrested.[76] While pioneering work of this kind was going on at the Brompton Hospital, a small group of physicians was equally active in the area of treatment and cure. Among them were two noted Swiss doctors, Conrad Meyer-Ahrens and Alexander Spengler. Meyer-Ahrens was in the 1840s an extremely vocal advocate of the idea that scrofula, here defined as tuberculosis among the physically weak, could be cured by a judicious combination of sunlight, fresh air, bathing and appropriate diet.[77] This belief was picked up and propagated almost instantaneously by yet another Swiss physician, Spengler. Spengler began his career as a country doctor. Very early on in his practice, he could not help but notice that fresh mountain air in the Alps was somehow capable of having a therapeutic affect on those suffering from tuberculosis. Soon after this, he established a health spa at Davos in the Swiss Alps. That institution became the model for hundreds of other sanitaria which in the course of time would come to dot the European countryside. All of them went up, of course, in the full expectation that tuberculosis could and would now be cured.[78]

Koch's discovery of the bacteria that were involved in the spread of tuberculosis encouraged him to go one step further and try to develop a vaccine that would prevent the disease in the first place.[79] For a while, Koch believed that he had come up with a product that would save Europe from tuberculosis in the same way that Jenner's discovery had liberated the continent from the scourge of smallpox. In 1890, before an International Congress of Physicians which had assembled in Berlin, he announced somewhat rashly, as it turned out, that he had produced "a means . . . of bringing the process of tuberculosis infection in laboratory animals to a standstill."[80] Koch's unexpected announcement was naturally greeted by the whole medical profession, for his work in this area was generally viewed as the prelude to the future development of a vaccine that would be equally capable of checking the growth of tuberculosis in humans. Koch's new product, which became known as tuberculin, was used experimentally throughout the 1890s, but it proved to be incapable of stopping the spread of the disease.[81] In spite of this obvious disappointment, tuberculin did become an extraordinarily useful diagnostic tool in the hands of the medical profession, for it did prove capable of determining whether or not an individual had built up some kind of immunity to tuberculosis or not. So, while tuberculin never became the vaccine that the medical profession had hoped it would be, it did eventually serve as a generally reliable means of detecting the disease's presence inside of European society.[82]

In the course of four relatively short decades, that is from the 1880s to the 1920s, modern medical science, had begun to amass a fair amount of information about tuberculosis. As early as the 1890s, the majority of medical men in Europe, for instance, knew that tuberculosis could and did vary its impact from one person to another and that "all are not at all times equally susceptible."[83] This fundamental medical insight, which had often been noted in the historical past in relation to other diseases, was at this particular time just beginning to make an impression. Among those who were struck by this fact was the German-born biologist Bruno Lange. Lange, and a number of his contemporaries, were, of course, just starting to see in the capacity of some to resist the onslaught of tuberculosis the very modern concept of immunity.[84] Koch's obviously pivotal discovery of the <u>Mycobacterium</u> <u>tuberculosis</u> also gave to the medical profession a real understanding of exactly how bacteria operated inside of the body. More especially, the profession learned that bacteria have a tendency to cluster and multiply, particularly in the type of tissue that could provide them with a highly favorable kind of environment.[85] Each decade brought new discoveries. By the 1910s, rather sophisticated microscopic studies, using staining techniques originally pioneered by Koch, had, for example, successfully separated the two major forms of tubercular bacilli, the human and the bovine.[86] Other studies, based on microscopic evidence, were by the early 1900s not only exploring the untapped concept of immunity, they were actually establishing the way in which leucocytes attacked and destroyed certain kinds of microorganisms.[87] By the 1920s, microbiology had already come of age. As it matured, it began to reveal a world that the medical profession prior to 1882 could not possibly have imagined because it was tied to an entirely different way of thinking about natural phenomena.

In the decades after World War I, the medical profession was in a much better position to deal with the problems caused by tuberculosis. This improved position was a consequence of the fact that it was now armed with two new techniques for combatting tuberculosis, the first of which involved surgery, the second a vaccine. The new surgical approach of the time focused on the practice of introducing air into the pleural membranes that directly surround the lungs. The pressure that subsequently built up had the affect of collapsing one infected lung. This technique literally shut down that lung and gave it an opportunity to heal. This type of operation which became known as artificial pneumothorax, or AP, was used successfully throughout this period saving thousands of lives.[88] In the meantime, Koch had died without ever realizing his personal dream of creating a vaccine that would be capable of subduing tuberculosis. Nevertheless, the idea that he had first advanced with tuberculin in the 1890s did live on. That idea finally reached fruition in the 1920s as a result of the efforts of two French scientists, Calmette and Guerin. Together they developed a vaccine which was more popularly known as BCG. BCG did not turn out to be as powerful a vaccine as the one that Jenner had perfected a century earlier. It was never as effective largely because the work of Calmette and Guerin was beset with problems. In the main, they found it extremely difficult to attenuate the tubercular bacilli that they were dealing with to the point where they could inject them into humans. It was only after prolonged effort, that they finally came up with a vaccine that they could administer to humans. Even though the product lacked the miraculous qualities associated with Jenner's discovery, the medical profession still had a partially effective vaccine in BCG. It turned to be particularly effective in the treatment of the very young. In 1932, the prestigious Pasteur Institute in Paris officially sanctioned the use of BCG, a move that obviously made it more acceptable to the popular mind. In its statement, the Institute confirmed "the fact that vaccination in infancy definitely reduces the spontaneous effect of virulent tuberculosis in infants in the first and second years of life. This response," the Institute's report went on to say "may be compared to those who are not vaccinated and are often subject to the deterioration and even death from the bacteria."[89] Given the increasing use of BCG and the more effective means of controlling tuberculosis that were now available, it was difficult for most observers to believe that just 50 years before, this tuberculosis had been generally regarded as an incurable disease.

The discoveries being made about tuberculosis were at this time being matched by research that was going on elsewhere on other diseases. In terms of its psychological impact, one of the most far-reaching discoveries of the early 20th century was Ehrlich's development of Salvarsan. Salvarsan, it will be recalled was an arsenic compound that was widely used around World War I to treat those who were suffering from syphilis. But just as important as the drug historically was the concept that inspired its development. For Ehrlich had really inaugurated the age of chemotherapy by advancing the notion that if bacteria could be attacked and destroyed in the body naturally, they could also be undermined by means of chemical substances introduced from the outside.[90] Ehrlich's unique insight really became the working assumption behind the development of all new drugs in the 20th century. Ehrlich's belief, which was partially proven in the case of Salvarsan, ultimately led to the discovery of streptomycin in the 1940s. At least, the philosophical concept was there. For in his research what Waksman was trying to do was to find a substance that would break down and destroy the human strain of Mycobacterium tuberculosis. He succeeded in doing this after years of exhaustive testing, finally establishing to his own satisfaction that the bacteria that caused tuberculosis were, indeed, "particularly sensitive to streptomycin."[91]

During the first half of the 20th century, other medical discoveries of an equally dramatic nature were also being made. The microorganism that was responsible for typhus was discovered in the late 1910s, while, shortly after this, in the early 1930s the first viruses were being uncovered and linked to influenza. The discovery, in 1933, of Type A influenza and then Type B, just prior to World War II, inexorably carried medical science deeper and deeper into the world of microbiology.[92] More and more highly specialized studies in the field of microbiology were steadily being produced. Thanks to them, medical researchers by the 1940s were beginning to understand that the antigens that grow on the outer membranes of bacterial, rickettsial and viral cells were, in fact, the specific agents responsible for disease.[93] This kind of information gave to modern medicine a unique opportunity to fight back against these diseases, for, modern science could now develop vaccines that were specifically designed to destroy these highly toxic antigens. The amount of knowledge accumulating in the field of medicine since the time of Koch's great discoveries exists in striking contrast to the past. The changes that this expanding body of knowledge produced represents a revolution that has few parallels in human history. Of even greater significance was the fact that most of this knowledge had immediate practical application. If medical science has come close to subduing the great deadly and disabling diseases from the European past, it is primarily a consequence of the great turnabout in medical thinking that happened in the last half of the 19th century.

If the word science can be defined intellectually as a willingness to go beyond existing presuppositions and to venture into entirely new areas of thought, then the medical profession existed in a pre-scientific state prior to the 1880s. Before this key decade, most medical thinkers were, in the main, permanently committed to a set of well-defined philosophical assumptions about disease that tended to impede the development of a more scientific attitude of mind. For centuries, before the age of microbiology, the thinking of medical men was constantly preoccupied with ideas that involved either the divine, the planetary or the miasmatic interpretation of the origin of disease. Only a few daring thinkers were ever able to break away from these prevailing patterns of thought. Those men, including such famous men as Fracastoro, Kircher, Sydenham and Morgagni, are usually heralded as the precursors of modern medical thought, and they were. But, what is often forgotten is that these men and others who were like them, rarely found their new ideas accepted in their own times. Their beliefs were simply too novel for their peers to accept. As a result, they were downplayed largely because centuries of ingrained thinking had convinced the medical profession that certain long cherished philosophical assumptions about disease were, in fact, true.

By the beginning of the 19th century, much of that traditional thinking had, of course, been incorporated into the prevailing miasmatic explanation for the cause of disease. Most of the ideas that had dominated medical thinking for centuries suddenly vanished in the following decades with the coming of a more scientifically-oriented type of medical inquiry. They disappeared in favor of a more modern way of looking at disease, one that was pioneered by Pasteur, Villemin, Koch and Ehrlich. What made this new age possible, of course, was that these men had based their findings on microscopic studies. When they did, they helped to create a feeling within the medical profession in favor of more microbiological explanations. Historically-speaking, two moods have gripped the medical profession in Europe, one was rather conservative, the other more tolerant of novelty. These two separate and distinct eras were dominated by entirely different attitudes and explanations. The few who challenged the prevailing thought patterns of the earlier period here can not be taken as representative of the past. For they were, indeed, the few and not the many. Their ideas would have to wait until the beginning of a more scientific era before they could be appreciated. Recognition of their achievements came late because the overall history of medical thought in Europe was radically divided into two eras, each with its own unique way of looking at the natural world.

CHAPTER 9

PUBLIC HEALTH MEASURES

> With the increasing mortality [from plague] the [Privy] council urged that while the plague was no doubt God's punishment for wickedness good care . . . in making orders would work great benefit. Especially did it stress the value of pest-houses: all the great cities of Christendom had them.
>
> --Charles F. Mullett, The Bubonic Plague and England (Lexington, 1956), p. 91.

Many of the newer attitudes about disease that were now emerging in the last half of the 19th century dramatically influenced government policy. For as of then, governments were actively supporting programs that would help to eradicate disease. Prior to this period the primary aim of most governmental activity in the field of public health had been to isolate those who were seriously ill from those who were still obviously healthy. The favorite method that governments had for doing this was to quarantine the victims of diseases, for the most part in separate buildings, which in the case of plague were popularly known as either pest-houses or lazarettos. This long-established practice began to fade around 1800, for with the coming of a new and more modern means of vaccinating the public, the idea of isolation began to give way to a belief in prevention. Preventing disease from occurring was also the motive behind the major public health campaigns of the 19th century that aimed at improving sanitation and cleaning up the water supply. The 19th century also witnessed the rise of numerous organizations wholly dedicated to the idea of combating disease. In England, early on in the century, these included local boards of health, while sometime later, in Germany, they encompassed national organizations committed to the complete elimination of tuberculosis.[1] All of these attempts at promoting public health were inevitably influenced by prevailing intellectual attitudes. Early efforts in the field of public health, especially those that emphasized the notion of quarantine, were actually inspired, of course, by the rather fatalistic assumption that disease was incurable. Those who thought in these terms kept insisting that the best way to promote public health was to remove those patients who were sick from those who still had their health. But, as thinking about disease changed and as "symptomatic . . . treatment" began to give way to "causal treatment" in the 19th century, truly energetic programs that favored not only public health but the actual conquest of disease were introduced.[2]

The idea of quarantining the victims of disease grew out of Europe's discouraging experience first with plague and then with syphilis. The tragedy produced by the coming of the Black Death convinced both public authorities and the medical profession that while this disease was being moved about by air currents, it was also being communicated by means of physical contact. This was not, in actuality how bubonic plague was transmitted. Nevertheless, this age, which was increasingly fearful of contagion, did tend to agree with the definition of the German physician A. Orthmann, who argued, rather persuasively in his own time: "what we call contagion is a poisonous sprout, which emerges from the body of a sick person. It is easy enough therefore to generate a similar illness in others by means of some form of touch."[3] During the pandemic of plague that struck Europe in the late 1340s, those who were suffering from this disease in the cities of Germany were normally forbidden to handle or sell either food or beverages for fear of further contamination.[4] Very similar attitudes were expressed during the outbreak of malignant syphilis that took place in the 1490s. In England, meanwhile, it was reliably reported that syphilis "was [being] communicated and constantly communicated from the infected to the healthy by the employment of the clothes, vessels, baths, etc., used by those already suffering from it."[5] Fear of contamination also led to the expulsion of large numbers of syphilitics from the urban areas of Europe at this time. But, just as in the case of the plague, it was soon discovered that pushing syphilitics out onto the highways was simply another way of spreading the disease.[6]

The periodic return of plague to a number of leading sea ports on the Mediterranean coast after the 1350s, convinced many local authorities that they should act more decisively. In these cities, quarantine soon began to take on an institutional character, what with the building of pest-houses and lazarettos for the complete isolation of those who were already ill, or, for that matter, even suspected of having the disease. Marseilles erected its first quarantine station in 1383, while the two chief Adriatic ports of Dubrovnik and Venice already had lazarettos by the early part of the 15th century.[7] Those who were unfortunate enough to be confined in these special institutions were usually incarcerated for some forty days, a period of time, which in this highly religious age, was thought to be equivalent to the forty-day ordeal that marked Christ's temptation in the wilderness.[8] By the dawn of the Modern era, most of the principal commercial centers in Europe had their own lazarettos. In the larger pest-houses, a full staff of both physicians and nurses were normally in residence. Still, it was extremely difficult to find individuals who were willing to work in these disease-ridden institutions. Indeed, the story has been told of one Milanese official, who, upon visiting a pest-house "went into a dead faint for the stinking smells that came forth from all those bodies and little rooms."[9] While most pest-houses and lazarettos were evidently dreadful places, they were generally considered to be necessary, not only for quarantining the victims of plague, but also for the confinement of known syphilitics.

City governments regularly took on the responsibility for isolating those who were sick. Public authorities in the urban areas of Germany often confined syphilitics to small hospitals, including those persons who were only suspected of having the disease.[10] Beyond this, in the major commercial center of Augsburg in southern Germany, members of the rich and powerful Fugger banking family, stepped in with their own funds. They built a special hospital exclusively for syphilitics, which became known, rather appropriately as the Poxhouse.[11] In other places on the European continent, where hospitals did not exist, town councils often passed laws that confined those who were seriously ill with syphilis to their own homes, while in Aberdeen in Scotland, syphilitics were legally forbidden to hold conversations with "fleshers, backers [and] brewers . . . for the safety of the town."[12] Once syphilis grew tamer in the 1550s and no longer seemed to represent the menace that it had in the past, the isolation of known syphilitics, so rigorously enforced prior to this, was no longer deemed necessary. But authorities did continue to believe that it was their moral duty to protect the public against those who came down with bubonic plague.[13] In England, gatherings of all types were normally banned whenever an epidemic occurred. In Venice, which had already established a board of health as early as 1486, teams of medical officials moved from one house to another during an epidemic, disinfecting as best they could all of the clothing and goods that they could find. Their techniques were not all that effective. But this one effort was characteristic of Venice, which really led all of Europe in the development of public health facilities that deliberately aimed at the containment of disease.

During most epidemics of plague, fear of those who had the disease was often matched by a fear of those who had died from it. As far as most public authorities were concerned, the mounting number of dead during an epidemic were just as great a threat to health largely because their rotting corpses were, they believed, filling the air with putrid and, thereby, poisonous substances. In the midst of the great epidemic of pneumonic plague that struck Venice in 1348, the Doge and the Great Council appointed a special panel to study the growing menace being posed by the presence of so many corpses. The panel quickly recommended that the dead be carried by boat to an isolated island, where they were to be buried at a depth of at least five feet.[14] The idea of burying bodies deep in the ground soon became a very important sanitary measure. If they were placed too close to the surface, it was thought at the time, the accompanying putrefication would measurably increase the amount of infection that was saturating the air. This point was made, rather forcefully, by the Privy Council in London in 1625, when it ordered that: "the Graves be digged so deep as that those bodies which lie next to the surface of the earth be interned and covered three feet deep at the least, the contrast whereof being generally observed . . . , cannot choose but be of a great occasion of increase of the Infection, by corrupting the Air in great measure."[15] Apparently then, isolating the dead during an epidemic was to some public health officials in the pre-industrial period just as vital a step as quarantining the living.

While some governments were resorting to a variety of imaginative methods to protect their population from infectious diseases, most eventually became dependent on pest-houses or lazarettos. In time, these institutions, as the chief defenders of public health, grew to become rather sophisticated edifices. In 1607, Paris erected a new lazaretto that soon became the envy of other cities. It was strategically located outside of the city's limits so as to reduce the chances of contamination. The building itself was designed like a fortress, with tall outer walls isolating the principal part of the lazaretto from any and all contact with the general public. Staffed by doctors and nursing sisters, those who attended the sick lived, judiciously, apart from them in a separate building.[16] Lazarettos being built elsewhere were also increasingly elaborate institutions. In Italy, where public health measures seemed to be ahead of the rest of Europe, lazarettos were usually used to confine the sick, while pest-houses were set aside for those who were convalescing. In both instances, however, the principal aim was just as much to protect the public as it was to help the sick and dying.[17] By the 18th century, lazarettos were taking on a new function. They were progressively being used to quarantine those travelling aboard ships that were suspected of carrying plague. Now catering to the well-to-do, many of the new lazarettos began to take on the appearance of a regular hotel. The Englishman John Hunter, who toured most of the major lazarettos in Europe in the late 18th century, found them replete with well-kept rooms, taverns, chapels and wine-cellars, all of the comforts that were needed in this day and age to make quarantine somewhat more bearable.[18]

Beyond the building of lazarettos and the declaring of quarantines, the pre-industrial period had very few ways of responding to an epidemic. The only other method that was used with any kind of regularity was to employ the army at certain critical moments to encircle and isolate areas that were highly infected. This obviously drastic step was taken, for example, in Spain in 1640 when army units were deployed to surround infected towns and prevent the further exodus of those who were already sick with plague. This calculated move was not a military exercise but a rather determined bid to create a sanitary cordon that would protect neighboring areas from the disease.[19] Spanish officials, in charge of southern Italy, took a very similar step in the early 1690s. They constructed a cordon that was 45 miles wide and which included some 360 small military posts in order to isolate three towns in the area of Bari that were being racked by an attack of bubonic plague.[20] The most conspicuous use of military force against the expansion of a disease came in the form of the Austrian military frontier that criss-crossed the Balkans. The militarized border here was also a well-thought-out sanitary corridor established against Turkey, the country where recurrent epidemics of plague were thought to originate. Permanently patrolled by some 4,000 troops, the border was regularly dotted with check-points and quarantine stations. Anyone suspected of carrying the disease or any cargo that seemed suspicious could be and often were quarantined for up to 84 days. Using these precautions, the government of 18th-century Austria believed that it was safeguarding its principal population centers not only from plague but from other potentially dangerous infectious diseases as well.[21] While the use of the military was by no means universal, later on Russian and Spanish officials asked for and received military aid to surround infected pockets where cholera had broken out during the initial attack of that disease in the early 1830s.[22]

Prior to the 19th century, public health facilities were relatively rare and those that did exist were largely confined to some of the wealthier urban areas in Europe. Progress was being made in the cities, but on a limited scale. Hospitals, by way of illustration, were growing in numbers and becoming much more sophisticated institutions. By the last two decades of the 18th century, many of them were even adding well-stocked pharmacies with trained interns capable of dispensing the drugs that they held.[23] The majority of hospitals at this time were not general hospitals, but instead highly specialized institutions catering to special groups such as ex-soldiers, the poor and those in need of immediate maternity care.[24] The standard of nursing in these hospitals was apparently very high, with most nursing nuns completely devoted to their profession. Their efforts, however, before the age of modern medicine had dawned were evidently confined to considerations like cleanliness and consolation.[25] While most hospitals before the Industrial Revolution were rather small, a few were truly gigantic. The great charity hospital in Paris, the Hôtel-Dieu was, in reality, a general hospital that could take in up to 4,000 patients during the 18th century. Unfortunately, this hospital was often overcrowded. Even worse it tended to shove together patients of different ages and different sexes, all suffering from a variety of ailments.[26] Apart from institutions like the Hôtel-Dieu, which often collected the poor rather than actually helping them, the masses were, generally-speaking, excluded from medical attention prior to the 19th century. For the most part, they had to depend on superstitious cures, some of which included the use of drugs and some not.[27]

This prolonged period of neglect came to an end just after 1800 with the introduction of a whole series of public health campaigns that were designed to promote vaccination. These programs were the very first health measures in Europe actively to include mass elements. One hundred years later around 1900, vaccination was, of course, a universally accepted medical practice, but for several decades before this there was widespread popular resistance to vaccination. Inoculation, which was practiced in parts of Europe prior to Jenner's famous experiment with cowpox, was not a good precedent for reassuring the public. It is true that the practice of inoculation had some powerful champions both in the medical profession and from among the ruling elite, including, for example, Catherine the Great of Russia.[28] In addition to this kind of support, variolation with smallpox pus was on its own an extremely successful medical technique. Given all of these considerations, the operation should have convinced the majority in the 18th century that it was a worthwhile endeavor. But, just the opposite occurred; the majority of the population remained unconvinced, even frightened by the idea. Thomas Dimsdale tried to allay some of these fears, arguing at one point in the 1760s that: "Experience . . . and instances of so many thousands succeeding by this method without any considerable bad effects from it, either immediate or remote, are irresistible arguments for its support and justification, and the best proof of its utility and safety."[29] Dimsdale was in this passage praising the new and more effective Suttonian method of administering smallpox vaccine to those who had not previously come down with the disease. This new technique cleverly avoided the older method which featured a deep incision and which often caused a secondary infection. What it did was to infiltrate the pus into the blood stream by a series of small punctures or scratches.[30] In spite of this improved method, variolation remained an extremely rare operation through much of the 18th century.

In 1796, Jenner, as has already been pointed out, came up with an entirely new method for protecting individuals against smallpox. In May of that year, he inoculated an eight-year old boy with cowpox. Part of Jenner's now famous experiment required that he revaccinate the boy in question with variola vaccine. Writing about what happened, Jenner reported: "In order to ascertain whether the boy, after feeling so slight an infection of the system from the cowpox virus, was secure from the contagion of smallpox, he was inoculated with variolous matter taken from a pustule. Several slight punctures and incisions were made . . . and the matter was carefully inserted, but no disease followed."[31] Jenner followed up this experiment with others. The results were so promising that he became immediately convinced that he had, indeed, found the perfect defense against smallpox. After some initial resistance, Jenner's new method for protecting against this disease was increasingly accepted by both medical men and those in the upper reaches of society.[32] But, mass elements held back. As a result, vaccination did not really become widespread until the 1840s.[33] Here and there, lower class elements were literally shocked into accepting the new procedure. Just such a situation developed in Palermo on the island of Sicily in 1801. One year earlier, an epidemic of smallpox had swept through the city taking some 8,000 lives. The toll had been so great that thousands of survivors began clamoring for vaccinations in 1801. All together, more than 10,000 of the city's inhabitants were vaccinated, most of them accompanied through line by their parish priests.[34] Mass vaccinations also took place in other cities. When this happened, it was usually the result of propaganda by one or another of Jenner's growing army of admirers within the medical profession.[35]

During the opening decades of the 19th century, both variolation and vaccination were practiced simultaneously throughout Europe. Without a doubt, hundreds of thousands and even millions were protected from the scourge of smallpox by one or the other of these operations.[36] But, the majority were not. They stubbornly resisted often pointing to the small number of those who died after either variolation or vaccination as proof that these procedures were unsafe. In Paris, where public authorities were diligently trying to advance the practice of vaccination, popular reaction was skeptical indeed. Doctors reported, for example, that many artisans and ordinary workers were of the opinion that "smallpox is a natural disease and one ought to have had it."[37] Beyond this obvious impediment, public resistance in the French capital was often amplified by the slip-shod way in which vaccinations were performed. In 1818, the

French Ministry of the Interior received a report on this matter. It pointed out: "Lower-class children are too carelessly vaccinated, too carelessly observed thereafter and too carelessly followed up until the vaccination has been completely effective."[38] Those who were poorly vaccinated should have been revaccinated, but they evidently were not. Many of those who were inadequately vaccinated came down with the disease over the course of time, for smallpox was still rampant in many parts of Paris. To those who were already doubtful about vaccination, this only proved that this new procedure could not possibly protect the population against the ravages of smallpox.

All over Europe then, those public authorities that were interested in pushing vaccination had to convince a generally reluctant public. In Italy, in the province of Bologna, the local sanitation commission had to struggle for more than two decades in order to win over a hesitant population. Government proclamations in the 1810s warned mothers that vaccination was the only known way of protecting their infants against the dangers of smallpox. Nevertheless, it was not until the 1830s that this propaganda had any kind of telling effect. By then, the commission was openly guaranteeing the safety of the operation and was assuring the public that vaccination now had the full backing of all doctors and surgeons in the province.[39] Meanwhile, in England, popular resistance to vaccination was soon being led by an Anti-Vaccination League. As late as the 1870s, the League was regularly publishing testimonials that attacked the idea of vaccination. In one of its monthly bulletins, a League spokesman, a P. A. Taylor, proclaimed: "That after learning of the evidence upon which faith in vaccination was based much to his surprise he was led gradually to the conviction that the cherished system of vaccination was a mere dillusion - a baseless superstition; that it afforded no protection from smallpox."[40] Public skepticism about the value and worth of vaccination obviously continued deep into the 19th century. Much of that distrust was a legacy from the past, but some of it, at least, was a consequence of the fact that vaccination was still a very imperfect procedure.

In spite of popular resistance, local governments, seeing an advantage in vaccination, were constantly trying to persuade the public of its value. In St. Petersburg, the vaccine was normally provided free of charge from an early date. Moreover, the local dispensing clinic bragged that it had vaccinated some 34,617 children between 1801 and 1817 without a single death taking place.[41] This assertion was more than likely an exaggeration, since children did die from the operation in other parts of Europe. The percentage here was exceedingly low, probably somewhere in the neighborhood of one percent or less. Public health officials could have pointed, if they had wanted to, to statistical charts showing that overall death rates from smallpox were, in fact, rapidly plummeting with the rise in the number of those being vaccinated,[42] for statistics were definitely on the side of those who favored the further extension of this public health procedure. In spite of this, the public was often less concerned with statistics than with the dangers that sometimes surrounded the practice of vaccination. Those who supported the idea of vaccination kept praising the procedure even though during much of the 19th century vaccinations, for one reason or another, were often poorly administered. As late as 1883, in the English city of Leicester, of 4,819 newly born children, only 1,732 were successfully vaccinated the first time around. The rest, to the obvious distress of their parents, had to be vaccinated again, sometimes up to three or four times before the child was adequately protected.[43] These failures tended to diminish public confidence in a process that would eventually work and work well.

During the century, physicians were rarely sure that the operation would be a success. Moreover, some of them lived in dread of the vaccine actually going bad and killing the child that they were trying to aid. One 19th-century physician who had some setbacks with the vaccine openly confessed that "the cowpox has proved a severe disease. In three or four cases out of five hundred, the patient has been in considerable danger, and one child actually died." Evidently fearful of the vaccine, this physician went on to declare that he "should not be disposed to introduce this disease."[44] The death of children from the injection of cowpox vaccine was, in part, caused by the practice of arm-to-arm vaccinations. Here, the so-called lymph formed a common pool which was in turn used over and over again for one operation after another. Many physicians did not at first recognize just how unsanitary a procedure this actually was. Beyond this, there was an extended period of time during which there was no such thing as pure, uncontaminated lymph. This along with the septic lancets that were often used for cutting undoubtedly contributed to the all-too-frequent secondary infections that mass elements kept complaining regularly went along with vaccination.[45] Later on, towards the end of the 19th century, the well-known English physician, S. Monckton Copeman, who spent a great deal of time researching the consequences of vaccination, admitted that the vaccine that was then in common use was extremely difficult to keep free of contamination.[46] Copeman's avowed aim was to produce both a pure and stable vaccine, one that could be kept free of bacterial contamination. Eventually, he came up with the idea of storing individual doses of calf lymph in glycerine. And this, coupled with the almost complete abandonment of the highly dangerous arm-to-arm method, led by 1900 to the production of a much safer vaccine.[47] With the development of a purer vaccine, the opposition to vaccination which had lingered on for so long now began to fade almost completely.

By the early part of the 20th century, the idea of vaccination had become universally accepted as the best means available to medical science for preventing disease. After this, vaccines were progressively developed in the inter-war period against a number of deadly and disabling diseases including plague, typhus and tuberculosis. However, none of them proved to be anywhere near as efficient as the vaccine against smallpox.[48] Powerful claims were originally made for BCG, the substance that was developed in France in the late 1920s by Calmette and Guerin. Unquestionably BCG did provide millions of infants with at least a measure of protection against tuberculosis.[49] But, by the 1940s, it was abundantly clear to most observers that BCG would never provide the same degree of protection as that which was gained by cowpox vaccine. Summing up what the profession now realized, the principal discoverer of antibiotics

Selman Waksman wrote: "BCG vaccination never succeeds in completely preventing the development of tuberculosis, the degree of immunity produced by BCG being at best no greater than that produced by a natural infection which results in a positive reaction to tuberculin."[50] The discovery in the middle of the 1940s of antibiotics that were capable of destroying both bacteria and rickettsia immediately diverted public attention, at least momentarily, away from vaccines and in the direction of chemotherapy. Nonetheless, vaccination remained an integral part of many public health campaigns, in particular those that followed World War II and were directed against the spread of such viral disorders as smallpox and influenza. Looking back over time, Jenner's momentous experiment had indeed worked a kind of psychological miracle. It was, without a doubt, the first truly successful public health measure in European history, one which had turned public opinion towards the idea of preventing disease instead of accepting it.

Public hygiene, like nearly every other important public health measure, was a product of the 19th century. Once it was recognized, for example, that both typhus and cholera tended to develop in the midst of squalor, governments hurriedly began clean-up campaigns, particularly in the sprawling cities. Increasingly, of course, the periodic outbreaks of typhus were now being closely linked to the presence of contaminated sewage.[51] This fact about typhus was becoming more and more evident at least to some. During the epidemic of typhus in Silesia in the late 1840s, a commission had been set up to investigate the causes of this disease. Rudolf Virchow actually rose to prominence in Germany as a member of this investigative team. Ardently supporting the cause of public hygiene, Virchow condemned the filth which he said carried typhus and which was allowed to exist in the poorer districts of Silesia.[52] Meanwhile, in England, the coming of cholera, which time after time struck the poorer areas of London and other cities, likewise encouraged a growing movement in favor of much cleaner conditions. Led by Southward Smith and Edwin Chadwick, those who favored more stringent public health procedures in England would also insist on the removal of stagnant sewage as their very first priority. In line with this goal, men like Smith and Chadwick actively pushed for the development of a modern system of sewage. When that happened the poor were effectively removed from their own waste products, probably for the first time historically.[53] Both public hygiene and improved sanitation then went a long way towards helping to conquer typhus and cholera.

During the last half of the 19th century, European society began to organize a series of local, national and international bodies, all dedicated to combating the spread of infectious diseases. The rise of a growing number of organizations specifically brought into existence in order to encourage public health did have an historical precedent, for the existence of local boards of health can be traced back directly to the Italian city-states of the 14th century. Originally created as provisional bodies to meet a particular crisis, like the coming of plague, these organizations soon took on a permanent character. Many of them acquired their own bureaucracies, one that was usually topped off by a powerful directing committee and lesser officials. Beyond these key individuals, community leaders were often co-opted onto these organizations to hold the very important position of "protector and officer of health, with power and authority . . . to carry out any provision relevant and useful for preserving this place clean and free of any infectious plague."[54] By the 16th century, boards of health and health officials were common in most Italian cities. But elsewhere in Europe, organized efforts to control disease were apparently rare. Apart from such centers as Lyons and Brussels, most of the more important European cities were totally unprepared for the coming of disease on a massive scale.[55] As of 1580, Paris, also one of the conspicuous exceptions, did have a Provost of Sanitation, whose function it was to uncover all cases of plague in the city limits and to transport the sick to local hospitals.[56] On the other hand, while most cities in Europe failed to come up with a board of health, many were by 1800 steadily appointing chief medical officers, whose job it was to advise the town council on ways of preventing the outbreak of plague and other dangerous diseases.[57]

As the 18th century progressed, national and imperial governments all over Europe began to pay increasing attention to the diseases that were draining off large parts of their populations. The dominant economic theory of the age, mercantilism, placed a great deal of importance on the idea of a productive and expanding population. The German mercantilist philosopher Christian Wolff even went beyond this in 1721, arguing that the power of the state was crucially dependent upon a healthy population, itself experiencing an ever-rising standard of living. In order to achieve this, he argued, the spread of contagious diseases would have to be contained and the health of the German nation improved by means of state intervention. The idea of a "healthy life" was now viewed in mercantilist thought as one of the prime responsibilities of government.[58] The idea of medicine directly serving the interests of the state led in France to the creation of the Royal Society of Medicine in 1778. The function of the Society was to study sanitary conditions, determine the presence of endemic disease and investigate the therapeutic advantages of mineral water and other known remedies.[59] This new type of thinking also went on to encourage the rather novel idea of establishing a corps of medical police. This concept was first advanced by Wolfgang Rau in 1764, a German from the city of Ulm. Insisting that every monarch needed both fit and healthful subjects in peace and war, Rau argued that the state must, as a matter of policy, care for the health of its subjects. He also contended that medical police should be used whenever necessary in order to achieve this goal.[60] Medical police never did formally come into existence, but the elaborate public health measures of the 19th century certainly did represent a triumph for this type of thinking.

The sudden and all-too-perplexing outbreak of cholera in the early 1830s found most European countries inadequately prepared to handle the coming of disease on a more massive scale. In the midst of this particular crisis, urban governments quickly began to form cholera committees, all desperately trying to cope with the accumulating problems that were associated with the presence of this disease. The Moscow

Cholera Council was characteristic of what was primarily an urban effort against the disease. Members of this council made a determined bid to inspect as many houses as possible, to enforce sanitary regulations and to isolate suspected cases from those portions of the population that were still healthy.[61] Cholera commissions performing very similar functions sprang to life elsewhere, most notably in Rotterdam in 1866 and Hamburg in 1892, again in response to major epidemics that were then occurring in these port cities.[62] The majority of these commissions, while they lasted, were rather poorly organized, although a few were models of efficiency. In the French provincial town of Quimper, in Brittany, for example, things went smoothly. Here, the town council fought the coming of cholera in 1832 with a sanitary commission that was superbly organized. This town of 10,000 people was administratively divided into six sanitary districts, each headed by a commissioner. Each commissioner was given wide-ranging powers to inspect and quarantine, along with a budget for the purchase of drugs.[63] These often momentary responses beginning in the 1830s to what was obviously a dire situation were actually just the beginning. In ensuing decades, these commissions served as a guide for more permanent public health organizations, which in the decade of the 1850s steadily became an integral part of government efforts to encourage public hygiene. To a significant degree, the rise of various boards of health was a response to the emerging public demand for greater protection against infectious diseases. Typically, at Exeter, in southwest England in 1831, "resolutions were passed at a public meeting . . . to raise a subscription for providing . . . for . . . the poor, and for purposes tending to preserve the health of the City."[64] It was also suggested at this time in Exeter that it would "be advisable that eight additional apothecaries be engaged to attend the sick, should the Cholera make its appearance in this city."[65] In the majority of cases, these preparations, whether they were well planned or purely makeshift, failed to stop cholera, which just swept through all of the cordons that were put up against it.[66] Nevertheless, the unexpected return of cholera in the late 1840s, did inspire the passage of legislation that led directly to the creation in 1853-1854 of a General Board of Health for England, which in turn supervised a series of local boards. Each local board had the power to appoint an officer of health, normally a practicing physician who had the authority to impose health and sanitary standards.[67] This breakthrough which originally came in England was followed shortly after by parallel developments on the Continent, for by the middle of the 19th century, both governments and the medical profession were now equally prepared to fight the impact of disease instead of just submitting to it. These normally local, and sometimes voluntary, efforts to stem disease were progressively complemented as the century wore on by the foundation of national and international organizations fully dedicated to the control and even eradication of disease.

In 1895, the Germans founded just such an agency. It became known as the German Central Committee for the Control of Tuberculosis, and it was established as a purely voluntary agency. By the following year, the committee had managed to enlist widespread support from within the medical profession. Showing real initiative, the leaders of the committee also decided to go outside medical circles and win as much public backing as possible for their cause. University lecturers, government ministers and army generals were all energetically recruited for the committee. With representation drawn from all parts of German society, the committee carefully planned a series of fund-raising campaigns. Fear of tuberculosis, along with the public's desire to see the work of this committee succeed brought in rather large donations. By 1900, the committee had become so successful that it was supervising a network of no less than 33 public clinics and 16 private sanitaria, while simultaneously planning the creation of 38 more hospitals for those suffering from tuberculosis. Financial aid from the committee flowed to all institutions in German participating in the campaign to combat this very deadly disease.[68] Other national organizations soon followed from the German example, one of them being founded in Russia a short while after this.[69] The steady emergence of local and national institutions dedicated to the conquest of cholera and tuberculosis next inspired the foundation of international bodies that were also committed to the protection of the public's health. This development began with the First International Sanitary Conference which was held in

1851. That particular congress may be rightly regarded as the precursor of today's World Health Organization.

The First International Sanitary Conference that met in Paris in 1851 was primarily called into session as the result of spreading public fears occasioned by the return of cholera. All together, 11 European states and Turkey were officially represented at the proceedings of the congress. One of the bolder delegates to the congress, Anthony Perrier, from Britain, openly condemned older practices which he said had failed to stop the return of cholera. At the plenary session of the congress, Perrier caustically denounced those who persisted in "the routine path of practices that were outmoded, useless, . . . and harmful to public health."[70] Medical thinking, in general, was definitely becoming more daring in the 1850s, to the point where older and more well-established views were now being seriously challenged. This dramatic turnabout in medical thinking encouraged the Austrian physician G. M. Menis, at the congress, to condemn the long-accepted practice of isolating and quarantining the victims of disease. Such measures, he declared, in the case of cholera, "far from opposing the ravages of the disease, only made it more frightening and fatal."[71] The conference disbanded without actually reaching a consensus on a single point. Nevertheless, an extremely important precedent favoring the idea of international cooperation had been set. Ten other international conferences followed in the period from 1859 to 1903, many of them characterized by rancor over etiology and policy. But finally, after years of effort, a series of European governments in cooperation with the United States and Brazil, formally created in 1907 a permanent supra-national agency known as the International Office of Public Hygiene. Based in Paris, this international body soon began to grow, adding its own secretariat headed by a Director and a Secretary-General.

In the period before 1914, the International Office of Public Hygiene took on a number of pressing problems, focusing its organizational efforts on the control of certain infectious diseases and the need to eliminate water pollution.[72] The League of Nations, born just after World War I, soon absorbed the work of this agency in conformity with the League's Covenant which charged it with the responsibility to "endeavor to take steps in matters of international concern for the prevention and control of disease."[73] Hereafter, the League's Health Committee accepted the daunting task of checking the further expansion of disease. Its work, at least to begin with, was largely investigative. But it was of great importance. For its well-documented studies and reports on the prevalence of disease and the use of drugs were among the first international attempts to bring to light information on these two pressing public health problems. The Health Committee also strongly encouraged the use of statistics in nearly all of the reports that it received from its member states. By thoughtfully blending this type of information, the committee was able to piece together an increasingly revealing picture of the incidences of various diseases in Europe.[74] Beyond this, statistical studies done, for example, in Bulgaria, at the direct urging of the committee, proved that congenital syphilis existed in certain well-defined rural areas in that country. Once these facts, previously unknown, were brought to public attention, health authorities in Bulgaria felt compelled to treat the disease with Salvarsan and other generally accepted remedies.[75]

Beyond the detection of disease, the Health Committee of the League dealt with a wide variety of other public health problems, including the constantly expanding use of opium. This social problem had arisen right after World War I, a direct result of the all-too-frequent administration of morphine on the battlefields of Europe between 1914 and 1918. The Health Committee and the various states that were members of the League were both involved because together they were responsible for enforcing the International Opium Convention of 1912. That agreement made it mandatory for physicians and druggists to report the sale of opium and any of its derivatives above a certain specified quantity.[76] In addition to its many functions, the mere existence of the Health Committee was bound to have an influence on its member states. For instance, when the new nations of Poland and Hungary were created in the wake of the Russian and Austrian empires, both took decisive steps to introduce new public health schemes, the results of which they were required to report to the committee. Poland quickly created a National Department of Sanitation, while Hungary immediately made the registration of all infectious diseases compulsory for all physicians.[77] This kind of moral pressure was obviously operating in older countries as well. In Italy, the Ministry of the Interior was deliberately reorganized to include a Department of Public Sanitation with its own corps of inspectors and agents.[78] The Health Committee of the League also fought for the introduction of vaccination programs, especially against those diseases where vaccination was still somewhat of a novelty. Here, the committee championed the idea of vaccinating against typhus, a disease which by 1939, thanks to public efforts, was on the verge of actually being extinguished in Europe.[79] All of these myriad activities were subsequently taken up and expanded after the Second World War by the World Health Organization, the latest of those international agencies that were especially dedicated to advancing the cause of public health.

While the periodic pandemics of cholera that took place in the 19th century certainly provoked local, national and international organizations to act, it was, in fact, the growing public outcry against tuberculosis that led to the ultimate triumph of the idea of promoting public health. This happened because the eventual decline of cholera after the 1860s and the gradual eradication of smallpox left public attention rather firmly focused on the advance of tuberculosis. In an age of expanding literacy and concern, programs specifically designed to stop tuberculosis won more and more popular backing. One hundred years before this, the pioneering work of Antoine Lavosier, the great French scientist, who was also a leading advocate of public health, barely had an impact at all on public opinion.[80] A century later, both greater personal hygiene and joint efforts to prevent disease had become the concern of the many. This growing awareness was aided by the fact that medical knowledge was now rapidly spreading through the whole of society. Physicians often spearheaded the drive to educate the public more fully than ever before. In the major French city of

Lyons, local doctors were instrumental in creating an Office of Public Relief, a Dispensary and a Council of Public Health. This last named agency was particularly effective since it intriguingly involved neighborhood committees in its work.[81] As the 19th century progressed, the physical well-being of all members and levels of society suddenly became a pressing concern. Because of this, the focus of most organized activity was increasingly on tuberculosis, since it was the most widespread and debilitating disease that then existed inside of European society.

The day was now gone when tuberculosis patients had been totally isolated, as they had been in Spain and Italy, by royal decree, or expressly forbidden to enter a hospital, which was the practice in England right up to the middle of the 19th century.[82] By the 1880s and 1890s, a much more solicitous attitude towards the victims of this dreaded disease was obviously replacing the ostracism of the past. Beginning in the 1890s, clinics, dispensaries and sanitaria all began to dot the continent, each of them built in the growing belief that tuberculosis could be cured. The first wholly public facility that was established to aid those suffering from this disease was founded in Edinburg by Robert Philip in 1887. Hundreds of others soon followed.[83] The first German clinic entirely devoted to the care of tuberculosis patients was opened in 1890 in Halle, a city that already had a long history of progressive thinking in the area of public health.[84] In time, sanitaria became the classic means of caring for those who had tuberculosis. By 1900, most of them had become rather sophisticated institutions, capable of saving lives. The one that was built just outside of Vienna prior to World War I was a marvel for its time, with numerous buildings devoted to therapy and a helpful daily regimen based upon improved nutrition and exercise.[85] Many of these institutions were by then steadily discharging patients who were either much improved or completely cured. All of this convinced Philip that there was a lesson to be learned in the way that European society was treating tuberculosis that could be extended to all other infectious diseases, for, as he said, the study of tuberculosis is "luminous with principles that give just proportion to the disease, and inspire fresh efforts toward the realization of the ideals of health."[86]

By the early 1900s, the prevention of disease was being progressively tied by Philip and other medical thinkers to individual efforts to lead a healthier type of existence. Most physicians by the 1920s were coming to realize that on their own, individuals were perfectly capable of protecting themselves against the onset of tuberculosis. The ideas of greater cleanliness and hygiene were constantly being stressed for children through public campaigns. This was done because they were the ones who were most susceptible to the bacteria that caused tuberculosis.[87] The potential impact that diet could have was also being thoroughly explored at this time by a medical profession that was much more willing to consider each and every possibility. Philip was also a leader in this field too, primarily because he was convinced that there was an intimate connection between poor nutrition and the victory of tuberculosis over certain individuals.[88] Among those who agreed with him was the English physician Edward Squire, who in 1893 expressed the medical profession's evolving belief that tuberculosis could be systematically overcome. Reflecting this new attitude towards the disease, Squire pointed out: "That consumption depends largely upon conditions which are preventible, is becoming universally recognized by the medical profession; and it is believed that a collection of the hygienic rules in which preventive measures must be based will be found useful."[89] Squire's formula for remedying tuberculosis included a judicious blend of rest, the stabilization of body temperature, exercise to promote circulation, and a much more nutritious diet. Healthy growth was vital if one was going to ward off tuberculosis, Squire argued. And a healthy constitution was dependent, he insisted, on the intake of meat, "the great flesh-forming food, and sustainer of energy."[90] While he emphasized the importance of protein, Squire also insisted on a well-balanced diet, one that likewise included fats and vegetables.[91]

Prior to the beginning of the 19th century, the vast majority of Europeans never actually came in contact with either a pest-house or a hospital. For these institutions, along with whatever attempts were made to improve sanitation, were almost exclusively confined to the cities.[92] These largely urban facilities really existed at a time when a full 85 to 90 percent of the European population was on the land and could not take advantage of them.[93] Beyond this form of deprivation, regional studies have proven that the overall number of doctors in society was very small and that they were very thinly distributed through the countryside.[94] Moreover, most physicians in this era were from the upper reaches of society and their services were, in actuality, rarely available to the mass of Europeans before the year 1800. According to one of the leading experts in this area, the American historian George Rosen: "In Germany, many physicians were in the service of the numerous princes, while in England and France they were associated with the world of wealth and fashion."[95] The only contact that most artisans and peasants ever had with the world of medicine before the Industrial Revolution was through an apothecary.[96] In reality, it was not until the start of the 19th century that the masses were finally brought within the care of the medical profession. These contacts were initially encouraged by programs devoted to vaccination and then, thereafter, by the rise of clinics, dispensaries and general hospitals. It was, of course, the dominant diseases of the century, smallpox, cholera and tuberculosis, that stimulated most of these new endeavors. All three of them really encouraged the creation of public health programs during the century. And in sociological terms, public health in this day and age meant improving the opportunities for mass elements to resist the onset of these particular diseases.

The growth of public health facilities on a truly massive scale coincided exactly with the changing intellectual attitudes towards disease that were now taking place. The passive acceptance of disease that had once so characterized majority feeling was progressively giving way to a new spirit, one that was confidently predicting the defeat of the great deadly and disabling diseases.[97] Many physicians, like those attending the various International Sanitary Conferences of the 19th century vehemently disagreed with one another over questions concerning policy, treatment and etiology.   But these conflicts were in themselves an indication of a pressing desire by many to find the right way to overcome infectious disease. The staidness of medical thought prior to the 1800s contrasts all the more then with this new kind of intellectual vitality which was just about to give birth to the age of microbiology. This new and more modern attitude also inspired the growth of public health facilities. Europe's modern 20th-century medical establishment which can now deliver so much more care actually owes its origins to 19th century developments, especially in the area of public health. For it was during this century that the medical profession gave up the older public health idea that the victims of disease should be shunned and isolated. Countering that belief, it came up with the much more modern notion that the purpose of public health was to involve the medical profession in the prevention, treatment and cure of disease.

CHAPTER 10

DEMOGRAPHIC AND
SOCIOLOGICAL CONSEQUENCES

> **From the beginning of agriculture and urbanization till well into the present century infectious disease was the major overall cause of human mortality and the most important stabilizer of population. Now the whole pattern of human ecology has . . . changed.**
>
> **--MacFarlane Burnet and David O. White, <u>Natural History of Infectious Disease</u> (Cambridge, 1972), p. 1.**

Prior to the coming of the Industrial Revolution, Europe was a very impoverished society. Average life-expectancy in early Modern times was quite low. Just exactly how long most Europeans lived in this obviously dangerous age is still not known, but it was probably in the neighborhood of 30 years.[1] It has, for example, been definitely established that in the 1690s males living in the German city of Breslau only survived on average until they were 27. While in England and Wales, at the same time, life-expectancy for males was only slightly higher at 32.[2] While most Europeans could not expect to live statistically past 30, this figure is in itself somewhat misleading primarily because it is only an average.[3] As this information suggests, the heaviest toll of the times fell, in actuality, upon the young, in particular the very young. In certain parts of northern France, by way of illustration, one out of every four infants was dead by the age of two, while in some rural areas of Normandy only 58 percent of the population ever reached the age of 15.[4] These fearsome tolls were the direct consequence of war, famine, and, most of all, disease. The key role that disease played in holding down population growth in the pre-industrial period was pinpointed a few years ago by two contemporary demographers, Thomas McKeown and R. G. Brown, who argued, rather persuasively that : "The relatively high death rates in all countries in the . . . past, are chiefly attributable to a higher incidence of infectious diseases."[5] It is now generally accepted by nearly all historians and demographers that the ubiquitous presence of bacterial, rickettsial and viral disorders of all kinds unquestionably dampened down population growth in Europe right up to the beginning of the 19th century, with the young being most affected. Less is known about the precise sociological impact of these diseases, although the popular impression is that poorer elements, primarily artisans, workers and peasants, did suffer disproportionally from the great deadly and disabling diseases of the past. They seemed to die from them more often and at a considerably younger age.

The Industrial Revolution immediately raised up the European standard of living. The most dramatic breakthrough of all featured an important rise in the level of nutrition. These advances were soon reflected in the fact that between 1800 and 1900 life-expectancy in Europe jumped from less than 30 years to more than 50.[6] Before this, Europe had been suffering from "a crisis of subsistence," to use the famous phrase coined by the contemporary French social historian Pierre Goubert.[7] For not only was Europe generally impoverished before the Industrial Revolution, it was at the same time an obviously disease-ridden society. Within this essentially impoverished society, disease helped to limit population growth in Europe from the 14th to the 18th centuries to a mere 20 percent each century. By contrast, between 1800 and 1900, the population of Europe was to more than double.[8] Just like previous centuries, the 19th century was to have its characteristic diseases, but demonstrably they were having a much less pronounced influence upon the rise of population. What has just been said strongly suggests that the demographic impact of any disease must be carefully weighed against the conditions that exist in the larger society in which it is occurring. While Europe was still essentially impoverished and the masses were suffering from a low level of nutrition, disease was much more disastrous, for it did shorten life considerably. While it is true that diseases were still commonplace during the 19th century, it was also the case that their potential impact on population growth was checked by both rising rates of nutrition and expanding levels of immunity. Diseases may have been just as prevalent from pre-industrial to industrial times, but death from them was progressively being delayed until later on in life. The fact that diseases were now affecting individuals at a different stage in life was first revealed in the 19th century by declining rates of infant mortality. Improved diet, in particular the steady addition of protein and vitamins, was undoubtedly a critical factor here, giving the general population an opportunity to ward off disease, a chance that they had not been given in previous centuries. This, along with the progressive acceptance of both vaccination and sanitation, was bound to push down death-rates and push up life expectancy during this crucial century of industrial expansion.[9]

In the historic period that stretched from the 1340s to the 1770s, the population of Europe, then, was continually being kept in check by the coming of a series of catastrophic diseases.[10] During this extended era, there were murderous visits from syphilis, typhus and influenza, but none of these disorders ever matched the ferocity of plague, which by itself probably drained off something in the neighborhood of 50 million lives. Half of all of those who died from plague were claimed during the Black Death of the period of 1347-1351, the greatest population disaster that Europe was to suffer between the fall of the Roman Empire and World War II.[11] Unlike later epidemics of plague that largely affected urban areas, the Black Death reduced population levels both in the cities and in the countryside. Urban life was quickly paralyzed by an attack of plague. The prosperous Italian city of Siena was hit just this way in 1348. Almost instantly, the disease carried off half the city's population, killing some 25,000 people within a few months. A large number of civil servants were among those who died, bringing the normal functioning of the city's government to an abrupt halt. For months, the city seemed to be overwhelmed, but even with a reduced population it soon began to make a rather surprising recovery. In time, the economy began to revive, but at a less efficient level since all kinds of special skills had been lost to the city's now dislocated economy. As it was, tax revenues were down and so also was business from the surrounding rural areas since cultivation had likewise declined. Still, the greatest loss was not economic, but actually social. Too many talented people had died in Siena in 1348 for the city to make a truly complete recovery.[12]

The Black Death of 1347-1351 also deprived numerous villages of their population. In the rural areas of Europe, population recovery was even more difficult than in the cities. In the rural parts of Hainaut, in what is present-day Belgium, for example, a large number of villages were almost completely depopulated. Worst still, some of them were hit by recurring epidemics of plague in succeeding years, keeping their populations continuously low. The number of live-births in these villages fell dramatically, in several instances to a mere quarter of what they had been prior to the arrival of plague.[13] The village records for Albi in the Massif Central certainly reveal this particular pattern. In 1343, Albi's registers included the names of some 2,699 individuals. Fifteen years later, in the wake of the Black Death, the total number of those still registered had slipped to just 1,357. Moreover, the names of a number of families were by then completely absent from the records, indicating, of course, that whole families had perished in the midst of this obvious demographic crisis. The names of many new families also appeared on the role in 1358 with some regularity, suggesting that a great deal of migration from one locale to another had taken place since 1343.[14] That particular development could be seen all over again in eastern France, where the cities of the region began to recover their previous population levels rather quickly largely as a result of migration from rural areas. One of the district's principal cities,

Colmar, was actually receiving a continuous flow of immigrants, in the main peasants who were systematically deserting the villages within a 10 to 15 mile radius of the city.[15] These shifts guaranteed a restoration of population for many cities but severely crippled the economy of many villages, which were totally unable to make up their population losses. The cities, by contrast, were quite successful in attracting newcomers primarily because they were still centers of wealth that could well afford to pay a high price for the incoming labor from the rural areas that their economies now needed so badly.[16]

After the pandemic of 1347-1351, plague began to take on a more localized character, for the most part concentrating its periodic attacks on the cities of Europe.[17] Over the course of the next 300 years, urban areas were constantly being drained of their population. The all-too-frequent return of plague to certain key port cities, along with the seemingly permanent presence of other horrifying diseases such as syphilis and typhus, often gave the cities a very unsavory reputation. That negative attitude towards urban life was summed up at the end of the pre-industrial period by Rousseau who scoffingly proclaimed that: "The cities were the abyss of the human species."[18] The cities, always apparently rife with one disease or another, did continue periodically to suffer a catastrophic loss of population during this era. In the late 1400s, for instance, Hamburg lost 50 percent of its population in a singe attack of plague, while Lübeck, to the north, simultaneously lost a quarter of its citizens.[19] Much later than this in 1648, the Spanish city of Oriheula lost 5,000 of its residents, all of whom passed away in just a few short weeks. This turned out to be an economic disaster for this particular market town since the figure represented up to one half of its total population.[20] Large cities were obviously not spared. London, in 1665, lost nearly 100,000 people within a few months during the great epidemic of that year.[21] In spite of these unprecedented losses, the cities of Europe usually regained pre-plague levels of population within an extremely short period of time. The opening up of new employment opportunities, especially for the unskilled, turned out to be an extraordinary inducement, one that encouraged a massive flow of rural poor into the cities.

The total number of deaths from plague was normally so great in the cities down through three centuries that the experience seemed to awe and overwhelm most observers.   As a result, few contemporaries remembered very much beyond the fact that hundreds and thousands had died seemingly in an instant.   This is why the municipal records for the French provincial city of Rouen are so striking.   For here, a carefully detailed record was kept of most of those who died from plague in the city's six districts between September, 1668 and January, 1669. Most of the victims were dutifully classified both by sex and age, providing us with a truly unusual historical record of exactly who suffered the most from this very deadly disease.   The records, in this instance, are still somewhat incomplete in the sense that the survey covered only 82 percent of those who actually died. Of the total number who died and for whom information is actually known, 42 percent were adult males, while 28 percent were adult females.   Only 13 percent of those who passed away were children. Information about the other seven percent could not be confirmed.[22]   If these figures are a reflection of previous attacks of plague and there is some reason to believe that they are, then one of the principal demographic consequences of this disease was bound to be a rather disastrous effect upon fertility, for most of the adults who died, given the low level of life expectancy at this time, would have been either in their twenties or thirties. It is a well-established fact that the number of children born after a visit of plague normally dropped somewhat precipitously. This happened in Hainaut and in countless other places, an outcome that could be expected considering that so much adult mortality had taken place so recently.

The ability of cities to recover rapidly from high rates of adult mortality was poignantly demonstrated in the case of the English city of Norwich after 1579. An epidemic of plague had hit the city in the late 1570s. It swept away a third of the city's population. In spite of this, the number of baptisms in Norwich was soon soaring. There was also a sudden increase in the number of marriages in the city in the early part of the 1580s. These somewhat unexpected changes in the wake of what had been a demographic disaster were most likely due here, as in other instances, to a rush of immigrants from the countryside. Most of them were evidently eager to enter the city and to take up positions in the work force that had been recently vacated by those who died.[23] Villages, by contrast, were not as fortunate. When plague struck Stoke-in-Teignhead in southern Devon in 1546-1547 or Saint-Christophe-des-Bois in the area of the Loire in 1686, the restoration of population was much more difficult to achieve.[24] In Stoke-in-Teignhead, the death-rate from plague rose six times over what it normally had been for this particular village.[25] The loss of heads of households spelled an immediate decline in fertility that was, practically-speaking, impossible for the village to make up. So, in spite of the fact that the cities of Europe were periodically wracked by horrendous adult mortality whenever and wherever plague struck, they ironically recovered much more quickly than did the villages of the time. Small hamlets were, it is known, hit by plague much less frequently than cities after the period of the Black Death, but they apparently suffered much more lasting economic and demographic consequences.

While plague was unquestionably the greatest of the catastrophic diseases that managed to penetrate Europe prior to the Industrial Revolution, there are several others that also struck suddenly and arbitrarily, often taking away tens of thousands of lives. The most important of these diseases were typhus, syphilis and influenza, which like plague also took a significant toll of the adult portion of the population. Typhus, which had historically been linked to war, tended to kill off large numbers of soldiers either on the battlefield or in their very unsanitary base-camps. Those who died in these epidemics were principally young males in their twenties, many just approaching marital age.[26] This inference about typhus was definitely confirmed during the 19th century when more detailed studies revealed that typhus was primarily a disease of young males in their late teens and early twenties.[27] Syphilis likewise produced a demographic crisis, but, on the surface at least, only in the 1490s and for a few decades thereafter while it was operating as a truly fatal disorder. Because syphilis was often transmitted by means of sexual intercourse, it too retained an adult character, since everyone "knew by this time that it was generally acquired by venery."[28] Influenza also seems to have operated in the historic past against the adult population. This particular age group evidently took the brunt of the disease, for example, in 1770 when flu struck at parts of Normandy, in this instance killing off tens of thousands.[29] While overwhelming evidence does not as yet exist regarding the age distribution of those who died during catastrophic attacks of epidemic disease before the year 1800, preliminary evidence does suggest, perhaps a bit mysteriously, that adults were the ones that died most often.

If, in actuality, mortality from epidemic disease in the pre-industrial period did have a distinctive adult character, then two conspicuous features of the long-range demographic pattern in Europe before 1800 can be more readily explained. For the loss of so many young and medium-aged adults, numbering over time in the tens of millions must have meant a precipitous decline in the total of those available for marriage. This, in turn, must have led to a decline in fertility. In the cities, this fact was usually masked by immigration which automatically elevated the number of marriages and births. However, in the countryside, where the vast majority of the population lived, these human losses often proved to be irreversible. Mortality among marriageable adults due to disease, along with the mortality among children, which was often evidently the result of organic failure, together undoubtedly account for the extremely slow rise in population that Europe experienced between the 14th and 18th centuries.[30] Beyond this, mortality figures before the Industrial Revolution have also shown a remarkably sharp tendency to fluctuate. Whereas, in modern times, the total number of deaths in any one area changes very little from one year or decade to another. By contrast, in the pre-Industrial era, they often lacked stability, being strongly affected by very high death-rates from epidemics occurring in a very short period of time.[31] While infant mortality appears to have remained constant then over long periods, fluctuating levels of adult mortality, periodically elevated by a wide variety of infectious diseases, probably accounts for the often precipitous rise and then decline in the crude death-rate that took place in so many areas of Europe. With the coming of industrialization, the arbitrary character of these figures would start to fade away and overall death-rates begin to even out. To a significant extent, this smoothing out was due to the influence of two new and highly potent killers, smallpox and tuberculosis. While they dominated in the 18th and 19th centuries, both of these disorders took life in a steady as opposed to spectacular way.

The growth of the European population was, then, consistently kept down between the 14th and 17th centuries by an extraordinary amount of adult mortality that was directly related to the presence of infectious disease. This was coupled with the frequent death of infants, most of which was apparently caused by organic failure. To a large degree, poor diet accounts for this situation. For malnutrition, especially the lack of certain key nutrients probably explains why there was such a conspicuous lack of immunity to disease in the adult population. In all probability, poor nutrition was also the reason why so many vital organs failed to develop in so many children, leading, of course, to premature death. By the 18th century a new factor had entered the picture, for by then catastrophic diseases were no longer assailing the European continent as before. With the general passing of epidemic disease, overall adult mortality did begin to decline. But the death-rate among children, which had always been especially high, did continue at its previous level. High-rates of infant mortality in the 17th and 18th centuries were clearly traceable to a variety of causes, chief among them being smallpox. Smallpox occasionally operated epidemically, but most of the time, it functioned as an endemic disease subtly killing off eight to ten percent of its youthful victims. In England, which may be taken here as an example, profound demographic changes were beginning to take place in these decades. Those changes were to be representative of what was soon to happen in the rest of Europe. The number of children being born in England after 1740 was definitely on the rise, while the number of adults dying each year was very much on the decline.[32] These rather dynamic demographic shifts, following immediately upon the disappearance of the great catastrophic diseases in Europe, should have propelled population figures upwards. But, the gains were not as spectacular as one might have expected. The perplexing rise, soon after this, of so many deadly childhood diseases, including whooping cough, diphtheria, measles and, even more dramatically, smallpox, knawed away at these gains. The population of Europe was still being kept in check only this time by diseases that seemed to be singling out the young.

The demographic statistics that have been collected for the period from 1750 to 1850 are, in actuality, somewhat imprecise, with the cause of death in far too many instances determined in the most cursory way imaginable. This disturbing reality has led McKeown and R. G. Record to argue, quite cogently, that "the data [for this and earlier periods] (on mortality and natality) are so treacherous that they can be interpreted to fit any hypothesis."[33] While their observation, which was made in the mid-1960s is still essentially correct, it is, nonetheless, accurate to point out that smallpox was an increasingly deadly disease during the 18th century and that "the pattern of smallpox in the cities became more and more a disease of infants and young children."[34] Death-rates from smallpox among the young kept soaring alarmingly during the 1700s. When smallpox did strike, it usually claimed anywhere between eight and 33 percent of those infected. Throughout the German-speaking areas of Europe, smallpox kept operating epidemically, consistently killing off a third of the young affected. By contrast, it would take only ten percent of those that it made ill when it functioned endemically.[35] Very similar rates for both epidemics and endemics were being reported from England throughout these years as malignant smallpox steadily gained sway.[36] Inevitably, it was the extremely young who died, especially those under the age of three.[37] Closely-kept records in France for the early part of the 19th century underlined the commonly held view that those who were most likely to die were those in the age group from one to four. At the very same time, those who were most likely to escape the reach of this disease were those who were eight to 15 years of age. Their good fortune was probably the result of the fact that they had already acquired some degree of immunity thanks to an earlier exposure to the disease.[38]

The presence of so many infectious diseases in the past, constantly reducing either the adult or infantile populations, naturally limited family size. The loss of one or the other marriage partner to plague, typhus, or tuberculosis, not only reduced the size of a given family, it very often, operated, for a while as least, as a check on further fertility. This occurred because it usually took a while for the survivor to find another marriage partner. Beyond this, the perpetuation of infant mortality due to organic failure and disease also meant that only a specific number of those individuals who were born actually attained adulthood. The figure here for pre-industrial times was somewhere in the neighborhood of 60 percent. All of these pressures, which were largely the consequence of the fact that Europe was historically an impoverished and undernourished society kept normal family size to about four persons. French Intendants, working in rural areas during the reign of Louis XIV, regularly interpreted a hearth to be a household of just over four persons.[39] A century later, a national commission established in 1776, under the jurisdiction of the Council of State in France, to investigate the demographic impact of infectious diseases, discovered that the average poor family in the country had four children, of whom characteristically only two survived to adulthood.[40] At about the same time in Worcestershire, in west central England, an area, by the way, that was notorious for typhus, parish records show that average family size rarely exceeded more than four persons.[41] In 1800, just prior to the birth of the Industrial Revolution, the population of Europe was estimated to be some 189 million people, just about double what it had been in the early 1340s. What increase there had been came very slowly over the course of nearly 500 years. The gains that were made were only partial largely because they were taking place inside a society that was conspicuously disease-ridden and where infections had systematically killed off first large numbers of adults and then later on children.

The rising standard of living that Europe was to experience in the 19th century did not bring the presence of infectious diseases to an immediate end. In spite of the introduction of public hygiene and a great improvement in the level of nutrition, disease sometimes seemed just as rampant as it had been in the pre-industrial period. Tuberculosis, a tame disorder in previous generations, was now apparently gaining in virulence and steadily spreading to the point where it was virtually saturating all of the continent. Typhus, tuberculosis, cholera and influenza, which hit mainly at the adult population, along with numerous infantile disorders did continue to exist, taking millions of lives. Yet none of these afflictions really acted as a check upon population in the same way that diseases had in the past. For during the 19th century, the population went zooming up, more than doubling in a century that also saw life-expectancy rise rather amazingly from 28 to 50 years. Given these facts, it can only be assumed that the general population was so much stronger biologically that it was better able to withstand the continued presence of infectious diseases. All of this suggests even more strongly, of course, that the impact of disease can only be understood against the background of events that are occurring in the larger society in which those diseases are operating. In the 19th century, it is fairly obvious that improved diet and a rising standard of living were together steadily reducing the influence of disease. During these decades, declining infant mortality was undoubtedly the key factor spurring the growth of population in Europe. Alongside this development, the pattern of adult mortality likewise underwent a change, being progressively delayed until later on in life. These two considerations, taken together, unquestionably account in general terms for just why the European population was growing so rapidly. The final conquest of endemic and epidemic diseases during the 20th century only accelerated this process, forcing European society for the very first time to think of ways to control the growth of population, a function once performed by the great deadly and disabling diseases.

In the history of Europe, tuberculosis first began to gain ground in England where, as one of the more subtle of the infectious diseases, its influence for long periods of time was all-too-easy to underestimate. Nonetheless, by the early 1700s, it was taking one out of every five lives in Great Britain.[42] By the early 1800s, that ratio had risen to one in every three and half.[43] After reaching a peak in the first few decades of the 19th century in England, it waned in that part of Europe only to become shortly after this the most universal disease of all on the Continent. More than half of the European population probably suffered from this debilitating disease during the century, with one in every three adults by the 1880s actually succumbing to it.[44] Tuberculosis, a long, lingering and obviously disheartening disease, was normally first acquired in childhood. The medical profession understood this clearly by the end of the 19th century, even though the disease itself did not usually prove terminal until sometime during the adult years.[45] After lying in the system often for years, it was repeatedly noticed that the most common variety of tuberculosis, "consumption develops most rapidly between the ages of 18 and 25."[46] It is true that one out of every three terminal cases of tuberculosis did evidently occur between the ages of 18 and 25. But the vast majority of those dying from this disease did so often after a prolonged illness, with slightly more than 50 percent of the fatalities from this disease taking place after the victim had passed the age of 30.[47] Such widespread mortality, taking up to three million adult lives every year in Europe around 1900, might conceivably have stymied population gains during this time. But it did not primarily because the majority of those dying did so after the child-rearing ages had already gone by.

By the time of World War I, tuberculosis was a declining disease in Europe. In the more highly industrialized countries where levels of nutrition and the standard of living had advanced the most, deaths from tuberculosis were falling to the point where only ten percent of the population was dying from this disorder. In Belgium, the rate was even lower being down to 8 percent. Meanwhile in countries such as Ireland and Hungary, which were still overwhelmingly agricultural and where living standards were considerably lower, deaths from tuberculosis were as of then three to four times higher.[48] Tuberculosis in the 19th century was the most spectacular killer that Europe had known since the great disasters that were associated with plague. But the crisis of subsistence that had amplified the impact of diseases upon society in the pre-industrial period was now definitely coming to an end. As a result, the influence of tuberculosis was not being felt so intensely, probably because tuberculosis was a lingering disease, which unlike plague and smallpox did not kill instantly. This meant that many of the victims of this disease had already founded families before they actually passed away from it. Adult mortality from disease, from all the evidence, was now taking place later on in life. The growing sturdiness of the European population up to World War I and the enhanced ability of nearly all levels of society to either cast off an infection or delay its terminal stages helps to explain why tuberculosis did not stifle population growth the way that other diseases had in the past.

Even though Europe as a whole was growing healthier and better able to forestall the consequences of disease, the continent was still struck by two major epidemic diseases between 1830 and 1919. The two were cholera and influenza. The very first invasion of cholera, which came in the early 1830s, was by itself a rather chilling reminder of the epidemics that had harassed Europe so often in the pre-industrial period. Cholera was not, however, a disease that affected the entire length and breath of the European continent. For, in actuality, it was a disorder that hit hardest at two eastern countries, Poland and Russia. Death tolls in these two parts of eastern Europe were noticeably higher both in the 1830s and thereafter than they were in the more economically advanced states of western Europe. The number of those killed by Asiatic cholera was ten times greater in the eastern part of Europe, for example, than in the more industrialized states of Britain and France.[49] In eastern Europe, the more impoverished and undernourished rural areas of these countries were to suffer the most, with death-rates in the cities of St. Petersburg and Moscow relatively low for a country that was literally blanketed by the disease.[50] Evidence that has been accumulating in the field of historical epidemiology suggests that epidemics spread most rapidly among those who were least able biologically to defend themselves. That conclusion was substantiated by developments in rural Russia in the 19th century. The agricultural portions of Russia had one of the lowest standards of living in all of Europe after the 1850s, with the result that they continued to be the geographical homeland of cholera for the next five decades.[51]

Like tuberculosis, cholera was primarily a disease of young adults. The medical profession during cholera's century-long stay in Europe was constantly surprised by statistical evidence that showed that children rarely died from this disease. In Marseilles, where truly extensive records of those fatally afflicted with this disease were kept in 1849, the age group that proved to be the most susceptible to cholera were adults between the ages of 20 and 50. Within that special group those who were between 30 and 40 turned out to be the most susceptible of all. These statistics, backed by the impressions gathered by a large number of medical observers, suggest that when it struck, cholera should have immediately reduced rates of fertility. But significantly like tuberculosis, this disease also failed to disturb the overall growth of the European population. The vast majority of those dying from cholera in the example of Marseilles, some 75 percent of the disease's victims, were, in point of fact, over the age of 30, a little bit beyond the age when families were normally formed.[52] Because this was the case, fertility was not dramatically undermined by the coming of cholera. Even more importantly here, cholera, while it was often viewed as a frightening disease, was really not all that prevalent. It probably never killed more than 10 million people during the 19th century. While this figure seems high to begin with, it was not great enough to dampen down the overall population gains of the pre-World War I era in Europe.

Along with cholera, influenza was also a disease that took on an epidemic form. When it did during the course of the 19th century, it also regularly attacked adults. Prior to 1889, while influenza was still a relatively mild disorder, the young were by contrast the ones who were most likely to be infected. In the period from 1847 to 1889, influenza was a disease that caused widespread morbidity, but it was so tame that it was only fatal on rare occasions. Newly born infants and those who were up to five years of age were the ones who normally contracted this disease. Still, they were usually able to throw it off in a matter of a few days.[53] When influenza apparently mutated in the late 1880s and underwent a gigantic metamorphosis, it simultaneously became an adult disorder. In the city of Dublin at this time, it was now being reliably reported that the disease "spared the lives of children of tender years, but killed large numbers of adults."[54] Throughout the two great pandemics of the early 1890s and the late 1910s, influenza continually took a high percentage of adult lives. An extraordinary proportion of those dying in London and Paris in 1918-1919 were adults between the ages of 20 and 45. The toll was largely concentrated in this age group, a somewhat surprising result considering that a very high percentage of the men from these two cities were already serving in the armed forces.[55] As disturbing as the continued onslaught of tuberculosis and the periodic appearances of cholera and influenza were in this period, they never had the same telling effect that diseases had previously had. Diseases before the coming of the Industrial Revolution had obviously disturbed population trends in a way that was not true of the 19th century.

Other diseases, ones that were less well publicized than tuberculosis, cholera and influenza also operated against the adult population during most of the 19th century. Typhus was in this category, living on past the Napoleonic Wars mainly as an endemic disorder. Local studies, tracing the presence of this disease in certain families over long periods, have definitely shown that death from typhus was most likely to occur among young adults between the ages of 15 and 25.[56] Syphilis, meanwhile, continued to be a disease which also normally afflicted young adults. Records that were kept in Paris in the 1830s show an amazing consistency here. The overwhelming bulk of those admitted to the city's Venereal Hospital were, not too surprisingly, between the ages of 20 and 30.[57] Victims of syphilis rarely died after coming in contact with the bacteria that caused the disease. Death, when it did come from this disorder, usually took place later on in life. Syphilis was evidently a very subterranean disease during the later part of the 19th century, killing more than was officially imagined, but probably not until they reached their forties or fifties. Neither the deaths that were sporadically caused by typhus nor those that were a result of syphilis ever really pulled down population figures. They were, for the most part, marginal diseases. But functioning alongside tuberculosis, cholera and influenza, they did contribute in their own way to the high rate of adult mortality that characterized the 19th century. In spite of this, the cumulative effect of all of these adult disorders was simply not enough to match the demographic effects of disease during an earlier and more impoverished era.

The relative balance that Europe achieved between births and deaths prior to the great population explosion of the 19th and 20th centuries had been maintained for centuries by poverty, malnutrition and disease.[58] The massive poverty of this era was largely featured by a poor diet that was so lacking in nutrition that the masses were effectively left with inadequate levels of immunity to combat disease. Moreover, it is probably true that during this period as one historian has put it, rather frankly, that disease actually "anticipate[d] deaths that would have occurred [anyway] in the near future."[59] In this more desperate age, both high rates of infant mortality, probably attributable to organic failure, and adult mortality, mostly caused by infectious disease, obviously limited both fertility and any really significant increase in population. Given the very low rate of life expectancy, at best around 27 years, during these centuries, it is relatively safe to assume that a high percentage of deaths came just before the actual age when marriage might have taken place. The frequency of premature deaths undoubtedly restricted the formation of new families as well as limiting the size of those families where one or another of the parties had died. Disease, which persistently undermined population growth prior to 1800, operated in an entirely different social and economic environment in the period after this.[60] To begin with, infant mortality declined, the direct result of better nutrition, higher levels of immunity and the growing acceptance of vaccination. Adult mortality, always elevated in the past in relation to overall population figures, continued for several generations at its previous rate, but it was now being postponed until somewhat later on in life, all of which made family formation and the successful rearing of children much easier in the 19th century than it had been in a previous period when death had commonly occurred on average so much earlier in life.

It is a well-established fact that between the 14th and 20th centuries hundreds of millions of Europeans died from infectious diseases. What is far less clear to historians who are working on disease patterns is just exactly what social classes were most affected by the coming of one or another of these deadly diseases. A precise sociological explanation of disease has been extremely difficult to construct largely because most observers in the past were so overawed by the consequences of disease that the best they could do was to count the number who had died. Only a few ever bothered to trace the social origins of those legions of people who had passed away. The vast majority of chroniclers, historically, are silent on this vitally important sociological consideration. Only during the 19th century did trained observers begin to establish an irrefutable link between poverty and disease on a truly regular basis. Social reformers, like the German Rudolf Virchow, pioneered the use of statistics as the best means possible for unmasking the social consequences of diseases. Writing in 1849, Virchow declared: "Medical statistics will be our standard of measurement: we will weigh life for life and see where the dead lie thicker, among the workers or among the privileged."[61] In the decades after the 1840s the connection between poverty and disease was made even more firmly by a number of social activists. This insight came at the end of an era. For the progressive elimination of poverty in European society in the century after this helped immensely to reduce the impact of certain diseases.[62] Disease was now on the wane, but for centuries prior to this, disease had, of course, lingered on. While a great deal more evidence needs to be assembled, the growing impression among those who have studied the issue is that during the long reign of these deadly and disabling diseases in Europe, the greatest toll was among those who were less well off.[63]

Prior to the Industrial Revolution, mass elements did suffer disproportionately from the presence of infectious diseases. There was, however, one conspicuous exception to this overall generalization. Whenever an extremely virulent disease came crashing into Europe both those at the top and the bottom of society seemed to suffer equally. This was especially true during the period of the Black Death, the initial invasion of syphilis and influenza and at that very critical moment in the 18th century when variola minor began to give way to the extreme form of smallpox. However, a high proportion of the time after the 1350s, plague acted undemocratically, principally killing off the malnourished and the underprivileged. By contrast, the Black Death was much more democratic, evidently taking lives from all levels of European society. According to the literature of the times, elite elements were badly decimated with both knights and kings affected by this all-consuming disease which "let no man stande."[64] The Church was also seriously hurt, losing a high percentage of its manpower.[65] In the archdiocese of York, for example, a full 44 percent of the clergy was killed off during plague's epidemic sweep through northern England.[66] Sometimes, middle-class elements took even greater losses. An examination, for instance, of the town records of Perpignan in southern France revealed that 64 percent of the scribes and lawyers, who formerly worked in the city, were killed off by an attack of plague in 1348.[67] Such extraordinary losses of life, not always but quite often matched elsewhere in Europe, tell the story of a disease operating against a society that was, in the main, biologically helpless against it. It was little wonder in these circumstances, then, that sonnets composed at the time spoke moralistically of God's wrath against the rich.[68]

The impression that has been created over time is that few social classes were spared the misery of the Black Death. Attempting to counter this general conclusion, some specialists have insisted that plague even in the 1340s did have a destructive social character, being primarily a proletarian disease. Partial evidence in favor of this minority view has been uncovered, for it is known that in certain German cities upper class elements died from plague only half as often proportionally as did mass elements. This discovery, along with others, has led some to conclude that plague practiced a "selective type of mortality that favored those who were comfortably situated."[69] While the precise sociological consequences of the Great Pandemic of 1347-1351 have not, as of yet, been fully investigated, plague definitely did take a more severe toll of the poor in the centuries that were to follow. Epidemics in the long era leading up to the 1700s did, on occasion, cause panic among the rich and well-to-do, who sometimes fled the cities of Europe when the news first broke that a major disease had invaded.[70] The better-off, heading for their country homes, characteristically deserted Paris during the epidemic of plague that punished that city in 1665.[71] This practice was not exclusively confined to the pre-industrial period; aristocratic and business elements fled the city of Paris in 1832, when for the first time in generations an epidemic of gigantic proportions, in this instance cholera, swept through Europe. All levels of Parisian society were frightened by the advent of cholera, but, then, it was obviously much easier for the rich to evacuate the city.[72]

While well-to-do elements often had the opportunity to desert the cities during such a crisis, enough stayed on during endemic periods and less severe epidemics to prove that after 1351 plague was a disease that typically singled out the poor and downtrodden. The sudden appearance of bubonic plague in the 14th century in the Cambria region of France doomed many of the poorer elements in the area to an early death. For nearly a century after its first attack, the disease travelled from one place to another in Cambria, the greatest number of deaths occurring among those who were either in moderate circumstances or actually impoverished.[73] Meanwhile a very similar pattern was taking place in Scotland.[74] When plague struck Paris in 1523, as it did with some regularity, the French lawyer Nicholas Versosis poignantly described the disease's impact upon the lower orders in the city. He explained that "death was principally directed towards the poor so that a very few of the Paris porters and wage-earners who had lived there in large numbers before the misfortune, were left."[75] A few decades later, the Venetian Ambassador to England noted a very similar situation developing in the city of London. Commenting in the 1550s, he pointed out: "They have some plague in England well nigh every year . . . . The Cases for the most part occur amongst the lower classes, as if their dissolute mode of life impaired their constitutions."[76] One physician, searching about in his mind to explain this particular dichotomy finally concluded that "the air about the poor patients is more infectious than about the rich."[77]

The pre-industrial cities of Europe were normally populated by a large class of beggars and paupers, often existing in a very sickly state. In the middle of the 14th century, the thriving Italian economic center of Florence was thought to have, at least, 17,000 of these unfortunates.[78] These downtrodden elements could be found in most cities right into the early part of the industrial era. These poorly nourished groups were also the ones who were most likely to be attacked by one or another of the great infectious diseases. In the German cities of Hamburg and Nuremberg, it is known that their ranks were constantly being decimated by plague. But, again, these two cities never really suffered any sort of permanent loss of population largely because they were perpetually receiving a stream of new immigrants from the surrounding rural areas.[79] Before the coming of the Industrial Revolution, then, a variety of diseases, with plague being the most prominent among them, kept taking away portions of the lower classes in the cities. But these all-too-steady killers never seriously disrupted the urban economy, since they tended to carry away manual laborers and beggars, elements who were rather easily replaced. The historic connection between plague and poverty which could be seen elsewhere was even more firmly established in the cases of Vienna and Moscow. When these two cities were hit by plague in 1679 and 1771 respectively, the disease initially took hold in the poorer districts, spreading out from there to the more well-to-do sections of the cities.[80]

The tendency on the part of a particularly virulent disease that was just entering Europe for the first time to attack all levels of society, so apparent with plague, was demonstrated all over again with the arrival of syphilis. The malignant syphilis of the 1490s and early 1500s quickly infected both those at the top and those at the bottom of society. It was reliably reported at the time that common people were dying, at least in the thousands, from the first effects of this disease. In the very same instant, syphilis was proving to be no respecter of persons, for it was also claiming kings, monks and merchants among its victims.[81] In Italy, for example, Benvenuto Cellini reported, evidently somewhat sarcastically, that: "this kind of illness is very partial to the priests and especially the richest of them."[82] Upper class elements continued to be attacked by syphilis up until the point that they finally devised a way of defending themselves.[83] In time, ideas in favor of virginity and prohibitions against pre-marital sex, like those being advocated by John Calvin and his followers, helped to limit the amount of syphilis that was actually penetrating the upper reaches of society. On the other hand, in the centuries that followed the 1550s, syphilis did become increasingly identified with the lower classes. The Spanish physician Villalobos was convinced at an early date that the disease had the best chance of spreading among those who lived in the poorest of circumstances.[84] In the ensuing centuries, syphilis was normally seen by the larger society as a disease that could principally be found among the poor and promiscuous.

Over the centuries, then, bacterial diseases such as plague and syphilis did become progressively identified with the poor in European society. While this particular connection is fairly easy to establish from documentary evidence, the true sociological impact of such major viral disorders as influenza and smallpox has been much more difficult to determine. Evidently, the much more powerful pathogens operating here consistently attacked all levels of society. The well-to-do, if most of the observations made in the past can be believed, did successfully maintain a fairly high level of immunity over time against certain bacterial diseases. But like the poor, their level of resistance was much lower when it came to an invasion of a viral disorder. As a consequence, all classes seemed to be subject to viral attack, both at those moments when these diseases were growing more virulent and also during more regular outbreaks. The great influenza epidemics of the 16th century made large numbers of people ill, while simultaneously killing many. Even at the time, the disease was popularly known in France as the Trousse-Galant, primarily because so many members of the upper class had come down with the disease that it was almost fashionable to have it.[85] Meanwhile, in England, influenza was appearing in several places, including Oxford where again many "persons of rank became its victims . . . . Professors and students fled in all directions, but death overtook many of them, and this celebrated University was deserted for six weeks."[86] The disease also struck lower down in the social order, with it being reliably reported that: "Of the common sort, there were numberless that perished by it."[87] After these initial deadly epidemics, influenza settled down to become a rather innocuous disease, its sociological character being all but impossible to perceive in the ensuing centuries.

Like influenza, smallpox also steadily attacked both up and down the social order. As this viral infection grew more virulent during the 18th century, most physicians, watching the unrelenting spread of smallpox, would have agreed with the comment that: "this distemper spares neither Age or Sex, Rich or Poor are equally exposed to its influence . . . very few escaped it."[88] But the introduction of vaccination, which caught on first among the rich did mean that this element in society was increasingly escaping the ravages of smallpox. The poor, often left unprotected either because of superstition or neglect, became its principal victims in cities like Glasgow right up until the time when vaccination was, at long last, universally accepted by rich and poor alike.[89] While smallpox seemed to touch everyone during the peak of its virulence in Europe creating truly widespread morbidity, death from this common disease did at times seem to have a rather distinct sociological character. Research on this point done in England and Wales showed very definitely that weaker elements were the ones most likely to perish from the disease.[90] Since those at the bottom of the social order were the ones who were most undernourished, with dangerously low levels of immunity, they seemingly suffered the greatest number of deaths from an attack of smallpox. While this is probably true, the overall picture here is still quite unclear, primarily because those who had first-hand knowledge of smallpox in the historic past, generally-speaking, failed to notice just what social groups were actually being most seriously affected by this viral disorder.

While any final conclusions about the sociological impact of influenza and smallpox must be postponed until the time when even more facts emerge, the distinctive lower-class character of cholera is, from all the evidence, virtually indisputable. By the last half of the 19th century, medical men were growing progressively more conscious of the social impact of certain diseases. Many of them were now beginning to realize as one French doctor noted that "the health of the poor is always precarious, their stature slight and their mortality excessive." By comparison, he went on to point out that "affluence and wealth, that is to say, the circumstances in which those who enjoy them are situated, are indeed the prerequisite for health."[91] During the initial attack of cholera in the early 1830s, it was immediately apparent to many that this disease was discriminating against the poor.[92] Even before the disease struck the city of Exeter in southwestern England in 1832, it was widely assumed by doctors and town officials that the poor would be most affected and special instructions were published "for the information of the poor."[93] With statistics about disease more readily available in the 1830s, it soon came to public notice that cholera was largely sweeping away the indigent in both the urban and rural areas of Europe.[94] The more well-to-do were definitely escaping a disease which was, at least at the start, thought to be so infectious that no one would have the power to resist it once it entered a given area.

Like a growing number of his contemporaries, the English statistician William Farr was becoming extremely conscious of the relationship between poverty and disease. In a government report that he helped to compile in the late 1840s, Farr boldly asserted that "wealth does exert a certain influence on the mortality of cholera and of ordinary causes [of disease]."[95] This theme was picked up a few years after this by John Snow, who accumulated evidence which proved rather decisively that working-class elements were being hit ten times harder by cholera than were those in the upper reaches of London society. Among other things, Snow demonstrated that while only one in every 348 merchants and one in every 265 physicians were being taken ill by cholera, the disease was definitely infecting one in every 35 weavers and one of each 20 fishmongers.[96] In recent years, the French social historian Louis Chevalier has come up with even more convincing proof to show that deaths from cholera did tend to parallel the social and economic inequalities that were an integral part of Parisian society just prior to the 1830s. Personally convinced, as he is, that biology has played a much larger role in history than has previously been imagined, Chevalier studiously compared death-rates first from before and then during the Parisian epidemic of 1832. In 1832, the death-rate for upper-class elements changed only slightly, whereas among poorer elements in the city, particularly wage earners, death-rates from cholera were sometimes accelerated by as much as 500 percent.[97] Throughout the remainder of the 19th century, cholera continued to be associated in the popular mind with squalor. Public health authorities attempting to contain the disease spent much of their time trying to improve sanitary conditions in the poorer sections of the cities of Europe, knowing full well that it was here where cholera usually struck its most deadly blow.

The poverty of the European past still lingered on and characterized some parts of the continent in the later part of the 19th century. When it did, it inevitably meant that some, in actuality, of course, a declining percentage of the overall population, were still destined to "die miserably, [largely] for want of . . . suitable provision."[98] Certain elements, within the working class and peasantry continued to be riddled by infectious disease even as industrialization proceeded.[99] But the impact of disease was less noticeable now because death from disease was being progressively delayed until later on in life. Death, which had previously been associated with all ages, was now being increasingly confined to the fifth and sixth decades of existence. Within this new and evolving context, tuberculosis may be viewed as the characteristic disease of the masses in 19th-century Europe. It did debilitate the young, but those who were infected were usually strong enough physically to ward off its terminal stages for several decades. Again, as in the case of cholera, it was frequently a disease whose greatest onslaught was against those who were less well off economically. As an example here, as early as the 1840s, hospital authorities in London were able to pinpoint the occupations of the overwhelming proportion of their patients with tuberculosis. Most of them turned out to be shopkeepers, clerks, bakers, tailors, and printers, primarily lower-middle class and working-class elements.[100] At first, it was thought that tuberculosis was all but inevitable among those who were forced to work in confined quarters.[101] However, it was soon discovered that the disease was also rapidly spreading to others, many of whom did not work in either stale or unhealthy circumstances.[102]

As tuberculosis evolved, then, as a truly serious disease, it proved to be a social disorder, one that was affecting the broad mass of both men and women in European society. By the 1880s, tuberculosis was so ubiquitous that it was also taking the lives of prosperous elements, but, as it turned out, much less often than it killed those lower down in the social order. At a time when approximately one in every three adults was dying from tuberculosis, this highly infectious disease was in the well-to-do and fashionable Parisian suburb of Fontainebleu taking only one in every five lives. Studies, meticulously carried out over a 40 year period in this exclusive upper middle class area did disclose the presence of tuberculosis, but its death-dealing effect was felt in Fontainebleu only half as frequently as in the general population.[103] Beyond this, physicians working on cases of pulmonary tuberculosis in the 1890s were certainly convinced that this form of the disease was much more ominous among those who were economically impoverished. For the most part, they felt that whatever preventative measures were adopted against consumption should specifically focus on those who had the lowest standard of living.[104] The discovery of tuberculin in the same decade tended to reenforce their impression. For tuberculin could accurately detect the presence of tuberculosis and very soon became just as valuable a tool for social analysis as it was for medical diagnosis. Tuberculin tests conducted around 1900 proved rather conclusively that in the poorer districts of Vienna and Zurich a full 95 percent of the twelve and thirteen year olds reacted positively, meaning that they either had the disease before or were currently suffering from an active case of tuberculosis.[105]

To begin with, tuberculosis was primarily an urban disorder, initially much more rampant among urban elements on the continent. The urban origins of tuberculosis strongly suggest, of course, that the pathogens that were involved here, like so many others, needed numbers in order to survive.[106] This conclusion, confirmed by an ever-expanding volume of facts, did not mean, in turn, that all of the various social groups in Europe's emerging society of the 19th century were equally affected. For the evidence accumulated thus far powerfully supports the general belief that death-rates from tuberculosis were twice as high among working-class elements as they were among those in the business and professional community. And after 1900, those who actually enjoyed a high standard of living were increasingly dying, not from tuberculosis, but from heart disease and cancer. In so doing, they were predicting trends in mortality that would become much more prominent in the second half of the 20th century. After striking the cities, tuberculosis in the late 1800s began to spread out into the rural areas of Europe, eventually extending itself to the peasant population as well. By 1914, in fact, countries that were overwhelmingly agricultural were suffering much higher rates of tuberculosis than were the more highly industrialized nations.[107] What had begun then as a working-class disorder would eventually turn into a disease that would debilitate the peasantry. Either way, tuberculosis was a disease that more often than not took its victims from the lower ranks of society. In this respect, it acted like so many other bacterial diseases had in the historic past. It took the greatest amount of life from those who were the least able to defend themselves biologically.

The poverty of the past was the reservoir within which most disease had originally been bred. That impoverishment inevitably included malnutrition and squalor, both of which had a way of spurring the growth of disease, in particular the great bacterial and rickettsial disorders. Thrown back on their own resources, mass elements, often struggling along at bare subsistence were physically helpless against these diseases. Biochemically, they simply lacked adequate levels of immunity to fight off the invasion of diseases that either wore them out or killed them outright. Weakened to begin with by the stressful conditions in which they lived, artisans, peasants and workers were too often neglected for long centuries by the medical profession, which historically catered to the upper classes. The 19th century, the key century in the history of medicine in so many ways, was also the period in which doctors, along with the remainder of society, began to develop a social conscience. By then, the economic fate of the masses was rapidly becoming a matter of public concern. Increasingly, the medical profession started to support the type of reforms that would finally bring the masses into contact with the great medical changes of the industrial period. Among those who were pushing the profession in this new direction was the German Rudolf Virchow. Advocating the democratization of health and insisting, at the same time that everyone had a right to it, Virchow argued that: "The physicians are natural attorneys of the poor, social problems fall to a large extent within their jurisdiction. Medicine is a social science . . . and must have a voice in government if conditions are to be improved."[108]

Virchow's argument in favor of a more solicitous attitude, first put forward during the middle of the 19th century, did become a reality over the course of the next 100 years. During these decades, physicians progressively led the way, locally, nationally and internationally, in those campaigns that were designed to eradicate infectious disease. Most of the diseases of the past that kept undermining population growth in Europe are now, of course, almost completely gone. A fortunate combination of medical achievements coupled with an ever-rising standard of living in

Europe finally brought a healthier existence to the vast majority. Death, known to all ages in the past, has now been largely confined by these advances to the sixth, seventh and eighth decades of life. Not only have more recent European populations escaped the trauma of early death, the overwhelming proportion of them today are not even conscious of the great deadly and disabling diseases that historically threatened the lives of so many of their ancestors. Without such a living memory, historians can all too easily lose sight of the fact that there was a sociological character to the way that diseases have operated. While this area of historical investigation obviously needs much more intense study, it is still clear from the preliminary evidence that those lower down in the social order were subject to disease more often and earlier on in life. Whenever a new disease struck Europe suddenly and unexpectedly, it normally took a toll from all levels in society. But, over the long-run, those at the top of society, probably because of better nutrition and better living conditions, seem to have lived lives that were, in reality, interrupted less often by infectious disease. In this respect, this tiny minority, functioning at the top of Europe's pre-industrial social order, predicted the freedom from infectious diseases that has, to a significant degree, become the birthright of most present-day Europeans. The poor in Europe's unhappy past were not that lucky, for they were the ones, the evidence is already beginning to show, that were forced by circumstances to take the full brunt of the great deadly and disabling diseases.

CONCLUSION

BIOLOGY AND HISTORY

> **Underprivileged at the start, the working class was even more underprivileged thereafter, and in such a way that the inequality of its economic and social condition was reflected in a definite biological inequality.**
>
> --Louis Chevalier, <u>Laboring Classes and Dangerous Classes in Paris During the First Half of the Nineteenth Century</u>, trans. by Frank Jellinek (New York, 1973), pp. 337-338.

Prior to the 20th century, few Europeans lived what would be considered today to be a healthy existence. Worn down by work, malnutrition and unsanitary living conditions, hundreds of millions of Europeans were pathetically unable to put up any kind of resistance whatsoever to the coming of the great deadly and disabling diseases. Because the majority of Europeans were biologically weakened by those conditions, they were essentially condemned to live out their lives in what was a disease-ridden society. That society was literally saturated with dangerous pathogens which often proved to be far too powerful for the average individual of the times. Different ages, of course, had their own characteristic diseases. In the late Middle Ages and in early Modern times, it was plague. Just prior to the industrial age, the most prevalent disease was smallpox. While in the 19th and 20th centuries, tuberculosis was clearly dominant. Over this extended period, certain diseases obviously rose and then fell in intensity. Their coming and going was, to some extent, dependent upon their virulence, which demonstrably vacillated from one historic period to another. While all the great deadly and disabling diseases between the middle of the 14th and the early 20th centuries had their own individual reigns, what strikes the observer the most about this gloomy era is the constant presence of disease. It existed without any relief at all either for the young or for the adult population. Those who managed to escape one disease were immediately liable to another in a day and age when infectious disease always seemed to be present.

Those living in the last half of the 20th century are now relatively free from the pressures that were imposed by these infectious diseases, for the majority of Europeans do not die today from infectious disease, but from some form of organic failure. If cancer is eventually conquered, this trend will, it is safe to say, become even more pronounced. Considering the fact that one after another of the great infectious diseases have either disappeared or have been vanquished, the time may soon come when pathogenic agents may no longer be a serious threat at all to the European population. If this occurs, infectious diseases of many kinds may simply become just a memory. This has already happened in a number of instances. For most of the diseases that operated before the start of the 20th century are, of course, gone, remembered, in actuality, by only a few. The conquest of the overwhelming majority of infectious diseases over the last century and a half has freed the vast majority of Europeans alive today from one of the most commonplace and sorrowful experiences of the past. Without first-hand knowledge of the diseases that raged so often in previous generations, it is difficult for modern-day audiences to comprehend what life was really like for their forebearers. Year in and year out, they had to face the prospect of living with a debilitating or disabling disease or watch a loved one die, often painfully, from one or another affliction.

With present-day society already beginning to forget the dire effects of tuberculosis and with diseases like typhus and cholera now just vague terms, the frightful impact of diseases on previous generations can really only be brought to light once more by the historian. Studies along these lines are sometimes made difficult largely because the records from the past are incomplete, for prior to the 19th century, deaths in previous generations were often recorded in the most cursory way that one could imagine. Even more troublesome is the fact that they were usually registered, not by physicians, but rather by ordinary, untrained government employees. Beyond these considerations, what complicates the work of the historian in this era is the realization that some of the causes of death, such as deep-seated syphilis, were never even recognized. In spite of these obstacles, which in certain specific cases have prevented the whole story from emerging, the overall pattern of disease in European history has not been particularly difficult to perceive. Fortunately, from the point of view of the working historian, while few doctors ever understood the real cause of disease historically, most of the them were keen enough to observe the symptoms. While a few diseases were symptomatically similar to one another, the overwhelming majority of them produced truly distinctive symptoms, which were often very carefully reported in the past. From a biological point of view, most diseases are unique in the way that they have affected the body. Because this is so, those historians with at least some background in biology, can reasonably expect to be able to determine, if not every specific incidence of a disease, then at least its general development over the course of time. In this respect, biology may be seen as a useful tool for the historian of disease. He obviously needs this kind of knowledge especially if he is going to focus in on symptomatic evidence as his proof of the presence of certain diseases.

Few experiences in European history have been as common as infectious diseases. While the upper reaches of society were presumably able to delay the impact of disease for long periods, the masses were almost never without daily reminders that one or another of the great deadly and disabling diseases was lurking somewhere in their midst. For them a truly healthy existence was at best just a momentary and all-too-fleeting experience. Apart from an occasional bout with influenza, today most Europeans go for years and even decades without experiencing a serious bodily infection. Few in the period prior to the last two generations of Europeans could ever have made such a statement. Why were they so much weaker biologically, so much less able to stave off infectious diseases or delay their terminal consequences until the later decades of life? The answer to a certain extent lies, of necessity, in the life-cycle of those organisms that affected man and in their natural ability to grow stronger and then to weaken. Beyond this, the discovery of modern antibiotics, capable of killing both bacteria and rickettsia, has obviously been of monumental importance. So also has the rising level of nutrition, which all in all has made the average European stronger and better able to ward off diseases thanks largely to higher levels of immunity. In terms of the ability of European society to protect itself from infectious disease, there is, of course, a gigantic difference between then and now. The job of the historian of disease is to help to portray that gigantic difference. And aided by the insights that have been accumulating in the area of biochemistry over the past twenty years, this job is becoming easier to do, for by combining these two fields and by taking what amounts to a new interdisciplinary approach, historians in the future will surely be able to illustrate with even greater accuracy what life was really like for far too many of our more unfortunate predecessors.

NOTES

Part I: The Diseases

[1]Major Greenwood, Epidemiology: Historical and Experimental (Baltimore, 1932), pp. 9-10.

[2]Peter Diosi, "Long Term Changes in the Natural History of Infectious Diseases," Centaurus, Vol. 9 (1964), 288-91.

[3]Norman T.J. Bailey, The Mathematical Theory of Epidemics (New York, 1957), p. 2; and Hans Zinsser, Rats, Lice and History (London, 1935), p. 60.

[4]J.M.W. Bean, "Plague, Population and Economic Decline in England in the Later Middle Ages," Economic History Review, 2nd series, Vol. 15 (1962-63), 424; and S. Mukerjee, "Cholera Phages," in Principles and Practice of Cholera Control, (Geneva, 1970), 39.

[5]Jean-Noël Biraben, Les Hommes et La Peste en France et dans Les Pays Européens et Mediterranéens, 2 vols. (1975-76), Vol. I, Introduction.

[6]J.T.C. Nash, "Evolution in Relation to Disease," Transactions of the Epidemiological Society of London, New series, Vol. XXV (1905-6), 205.

[7]Dieter Wagner, "Wandlungen des Begriffs Epidemie," NTM: Schriftenreihe für Geschichte der Naturwissenschaft, Vol. 9 (1972), 62.

[8]Ian Taylor, "Epidemiology 1866-1966," Public Health, Vol. 82 (1967), 30.

[9]Aidan Cockburn, The Evolution and Eradication of Infectious Diseases (Baltimore, 1963), p. 7.

[10]Rene and Jean Dubos, The White Plague: Tuberculosis, Man and Society (Boston, 1952), p. 70.

[11]MacFarlane Burnet and David O. White, Natural History of Infectious Disease, 4th edition (Cambridge, 1972), pp. 7, 13.

[12]Asa Briggs, "Cholera and Society in the Nineteenth Century," Past and Present, Vol. 19 (1961), 76.

[13]Arthur E. Imhof, "The Hospital in the 18th Century: For Whom?" Journal of Social History, Vol. 10 (1977) 488-89.

[14]Philippe Ariès, Western Attitudes toward Death: From the Middle Ages to the Present, trans. by Patricia M. Ranum (Baltimore, 1974), p. 103.

[15]Iago Galdston, "The Epidemic Constitution in Historic Perspective," Bulletin of the History of Medicine, Vol. 18 (1942), 613; Lloyd G. Stevenson, "New Diseases in the Seventeenth Century," Bulletin of the History of Medicine, Vol. 39 (1965), 1; and R. Preuner, "Epidemien im Wandel der Zeiten," Anglo-German Medical Review, Vol. 5 (1969), 4.

[16]Quoted in Daniel Thomson, "Change in Epidemiology and Preventive Medicine," Proceedings of the Royal Society of Medicine, Vol. 58 (1965), 831.

Chapter 1: Plague

[1]Thomas Vincent, God's Terrible Voice in the City (London, 1667), p. 19.

[2]Arthur B. Faulkner, A Treatise on the Plague (London, 1820), p. 224.

[3]I.F.C. Hecker, The Black Death in the Fourteenth Century, trans. by B.G. Babington (London, 1833), pp. 98, 104-5.

[4]Archibold W. Sloan, "Medical and Social Aspects of the Great Plague of London in 1665," South African Medical Journal, Vol. 47 (1973), 270.

[5]Robert Pollitzer, Plague (Geneva, 1954), p. 11.

[6]A.A. Arata,"The Importance of Small Mammals in Public Health," in Small Mammals: Their Productivity and Population,

(Cambridge, 1975), pp. 351, 353; and M.P. Kozlov, "Sovremennyi Areal Vozhuditelia i Istorii Formirovaniia Prirodnykh Ochagov Chumy na Kavkaze," Zhurnal Mikrobiologii, Epidemiologii i Immunobiologii, Vol. 44 (1967), 10-17.

[7]Frederick F. Cartwright and Michael D. Biddiss, Disease and History (New York, 1972), p. 37.

[8]John D. Comrie, Scottish History of Medicine, 2 vols., 2nd ed. (London, 1932), Vol. I, p. 202.

[9]Paul Ganière, "La Peste Noir et Ses Consequénces Sociologiques," Academie Nationale de Médicine, Bulletin, Vol. 155 (1971), 641; and R.E. Hemphill, "Society, Artists, and the Plague," Bristol Medio-Chirurgical Journal, Vol. 81 (1966), 1.

[10]E. Pifferi and G.B. Scarano, "Le Pestilenze in Perugia nei Secoli XIV e XV," Pagine di Storia della Medicina, Vol. 10 (1966), 53.

[11]Quoted in Herman B. Allyn, "The Black Death: Its Social and Economic Results," Annals of Medical History, Vol. 7 (1935), 231.

[12]Quoted in G.C. Coulton, The Black Death (London, 1930), pp. 12-13.

[13]Quoted in William M. Bowsky, "The Impact of the Black Death upon Sienese Government and Society," Speculum, Vol. 39 (1964), 17.

[14]Quoted in Philip Ziegler, The Black Death (London, 1969), p. 58.

[15]Ziegler, The Black Death, p. 53.

[16]Quoted in Christos S. Bartsocas, "Two Fourteenth Century Greek Descriptions of the Black Death," Journal of the History of Medicine and Allied Sciences, Vol. 21 (1966), 396.

[17]Emil Schultheiss and Louis Tardy, "Short History of Epidemics in Hungary until the Great Cholera Epidemic of 1831," Centaurus, Vol. 11 (1968), 281.

[18]Biraben, Les Hommes et La Peste, Vol. I, p. 85.

[19]William L. Langer, "The Black Death," Scientific American, Vol. 210 (1964), 114, 116.

[20]Quoted in Martin Sprössig, "Die Erfurter Seuchengeschichte und die Moderne Mikrobiologie," Beiträge zur Geschichte der Universität Erfurt, Vol. 11 (1964), 172.

[21]Schultheiss and Tardy, "Short History of Epidemics," 281.

[22]Quoted in Allyn, "The Black Death," 232.

[23]Charles F. Mullett, The Bubonic Plague and England (Lexington, 1956), p. 9.

[24]Quoted in Augustus Jessott, "The Black Death in East Anglia," Twentieth Century, Vol. 16 (1884), 921.

[25]Comrie, Scottish History of Medicine, Vol. I, 293.

[26]Ganière, "La Peste Noir, p. 643.

[27]Pichatty de Croissainte, A Brief Journal of What Passed in the City of Marseilles While it was Afflicted with the Plague in the year 1720, Anonymous trans. (London, 1721), p. 6 (3rd report).

[28]Adam Lonicerus, Ordnung für die Pestilenz (n.p., 1572), p. 29.

[29]Hecker, The Black Death, pp. 96-97, 104-5.

[30]Langer, "The Black Death," 114; and Bailey, The Mathematical Theory of Epidemics, p. 1.

[31]Sloan, "Medical and Social Aspects," 270.

[32]R. Devignat, "Variétés de L'Espèce Pasteurella Pestis: Nouvelle Hypothèse," Bulletin of the World Health Organization, Vol. 4 (1951), 249.

[33]Report of the International Plague Conference Held at Mukden, April, 1911 (Manila, 1912), p. 41.

[34]Nathaniel Hodges, Loimologia: Or, An Historical Account of the Plague in London in 1665, trans. from the Latin (London, 1720), p. 84.

[35]Jean Astruc, Dissertation sur L'Origine des Maladies Épidémiques, et Principalement sur L'Origine de La Peste (Montpellier, 1721), p. 15; and quoted in Walther Kirchner, "The Black Death: New Insights into 18th Century Attitudes toward Bubonic Plague," Clinical Pediatrics, Vol. 7 (1968), 435.

[36]Nicholas Massa, Liber de Pestilentiali (Venice, 1540), pp. 21-22.

[37]Hodges, Loimologia, pp. 139, 151.

[38]J.F.D. Shrewsbury, A History of Bubonic Plague in the British Isles (Cambridge, 1970), pp. 4-6; and L. Fabian Hirst, The Conquest of Plague (Oxford, 1953) pp. 28-30.

[39]Pollitzer, Plague, p. 13.

[40]Ganière, "La Peste Noire," 642; Mullett, The Bubonic Plague, p. 9; and Élisabeth Carpentier, "Famines et Épidémies dans l'Histoire du XIVe Siècle," Annales, Économies, Sociétés, Civilisations, Vol. 17 (1962), 1071.

[41]Arata, "The Importance of Small Mammals," 351.

[42]Shrewsbury, A History of Bubonic Plague, pp. 2-3.

[43]William H. McNeill, Plagues and Peoples (Garden City, 1976), pp. 151-52.

[44]Abrahm S. Benenson (ed.) Control of Communicable Disease in Man, 12th edition (Washington, 1975), p. 227.

[45]W.D. Lawton and M.J. Surgalla, "Immunization against Plague by a Specific Fraction of Pasteurella Pseudotuberculosis," Journal of Infectious Diseases, Vol. 113 (1963), 39.

[46]McNeill, Plagues and Peoples, p. 151.

[47]N.G. Gratz and A.A. Arata, "Problems Associated with the Control of Rodents in Tropical Africa," Bulletin of the World Health Organization, Vol. 52 (1975), 701-4.

[48]Geneviève Prat, "Albi et La Peste Noire," Annals du Midi, Vol. 64 (1952), 17; Gérard Sivéry, "Le Hainaut et la Peste Noire," Mémoires et Publications de la Société des Sciences, des Arts et des Lettres du Hainaut, Vol. 79 (1965), 432 and 436; and John L. Fisher, "The Black Death in Essex," Essex Review, Vol. 52 (1943), 13-14.

[49]Ronald Hare, Pomp and Pestilence (New York, 1955), p. 28.

[50]F. Livesey, "Epidemics!" Manchester Medical Gazette, Vol. 50 (1971), 5.

[51]Erwin A. Ackerknecht, History and Geography of the Most Important Diseases (New York, 1965), p. 11.

[52]Shrewsbury, A History of Bubonic Plague, p. 5.

[53]Leszek Barg, "Epidemia Dzumy we Wroclawiu w Latach 1567-69," Archiwum Historii Medycyny, Vol. 33 (1970), 71.

[54]M. Marcel Fosseyeux, "Les Épidémies de Peste à Paris," Société Français d'Histoire de la Médicine, Vol. 12 (1913), 120.

[55]J. Hughes, "The Plague in Carlisle 1597/98," Cumberland and Westmoreland Antiquarian and Archeological Society, (1971), 62.

[56]E.A. Wrigley, Population and History (New York, 1969), p. 82.

[57]The Tractate of Pietro de Tossignano, 1398 in Dorothea W. Singer, "Some Plague Tractates (Fourteenth and Fifteenth Centuries)," Royal Society of Medicine Proceedings, Vol. 9 (1916), 187.

[58]The Treatise of Bengt Knutsson in Singer, "Some Plague Tractates," 183.

[59]Quoted in George Deux, The Black Death 1347 (London, 1969), p. 149.

[60]Quoted in R.S. Roberts, "The Place of Plague in English Society," Royal Society of Medicine Proceedings, Vol. 59 (1966), 103.

[61]Roberts, "The Place of Plague," 101.

[62]A. Neumayr, L. Mazakarini and O. Potuzhek, "Zur Geschichte der Pestepidemien in Wien," Wiener Zeitschrift für Innere Medizin und ihre Grenzgebiete, Vol. 45 (1964), 261-63; and Leopold Senfelder, "Die ältesten Pesttractate der Wiener Schule," Wiener Klinische Rundschau, Vol. 12 (1898), 7.

[63]Harold Avery, "Plague Churches, Monuments and Memorials," Royal Society of Medicine Proceedings, Vol. 59 (1966), 12.

[64]Henri Dubled, "Les Épidémies de Peste à Carpentras et dans le Comtat Venaissin," Provence Historique, Vol. 19 (1969), 20.

[65]Sylvette Guilbert, "A Chalons-sur-Marne au XVe Siècle: Un Conseil Municipal Face aux Épidémies," Annales: Économies, Sociétés, Civilisations, Vol. 23 (1968), 1286.

[66]Roland Goertchen, "Über die Geschichte der Pest in Mecklenburg," NTM: Schriftenreihe für Geschichte der Naturwissenschaften Technik und Medizin, Vol. 8 (1971), 75-76.

[67]Biraben, Les Hommes et La Peste, Vol. I, p. 193.

[68]Mullett, The Bubonic Plague, pp. 14-15, 86, 107, 195-96; Shrewsbury, A History of Plague, p. 487; John T. Alexander, "Catherine II, Bubonic Plague and the Problem of Industry in Moscow," American Historical Review, Vol. 79 (1974), 661; M. Hille and E. Ehler, "Zum medizinischen Wissen über die Pest in der ersten Hälfte des 17. Jahrhunderts im Norddeutschen Raum," Medizinische Klinik, Vol. 63 (1968), 1696; Roberts, "The Place of Plague," 104; and Jean-Noël Biraben, "Certain Demographic Characteristics of the Plague Epidemic in France, 1720-22," Daedalus, Vol. 97 (1968), 538.

[69]Thomas Jordanus, Pestis Phaenomena (Frankfurt, 1576), p. 5.

[70]Massa, Liber de Pestilentiali, pp. 21-22.

[71]Gilbert Skeyne, Ane Breve Descriptioun of the Pest (Edinburg, 1568), p. 14.

[72]Quoted in Frank G. Clemow, Notes of Some Past Epidemics of Plague in Russia (London, 1894), p. 225.

[73]John Swan (ed.), The Entire Works of Dr. Thomas Sydenham (London, 1742), 72.

[74]Thomas Lodge, A Treatise of the Plague (London, 1603), p. 5.

[75]Nicholas Culpepper, A Treatise of the Pestilence (Cornhill, 1655), pp. 9-10.

[76]Cartwright and Biddiss, Disease and History, p. 37; and Carlo M. Cipolla, Cristofano and the Plague (Berkeley, 1973), p. 15.

322

[77] John Graunt, <u>Natural and Political Observations Mentioned in a Following Index and Made upon the Bills of Mortality</u> (London, 1662), p. 7.

[78] Quoted in Cipolla, <u>Cristofano and the Plague</u>, pp. 15-16.

[79] Ernst Rodenwalt, "Die Entseuchungsverfahren des Venezianischen Gesundheitsdienstes im 16. Jahrhundert," <u>Sudhoff's Archiv für Geschichte der Medizin</u>, Vol. 38 (1954), 1.

[80] Antonio Brighetti, <u>Bologna e la Peste del 1630</u> (Bologna, 1968), pp. 199-200.

[81] Quoted in Luis G. Ballester and Jose M. Benitez, "Aproximacion a la Historia Social de la Peste de Orihuela de 1648," <u>Medicina Espanola</u>, Vol. 65 (1971), 321.

[82] Joshua O. Leibowitz, "Bubonic Plague in the Ghetto of Rome (1656): Descriptions by Zahalon and Gastaldi," <u>Koroth</u>, Vol. 4 (1967), xxvi-xxvii.

[83] Hille and Ehler, "Zum medizinischen Wissen," 1696.

[84] Quoted in G.R. Owen, "The Poore's Plague and Mr. Pepys," <u>Annals of Medical History</u>, Vol. 8 (1926), 250.

[85] Walter G. Bell, <u>The Great Plague in London in 1665</u> (New York, 1924), pp. 38ff; Jacques Revel, "Autour d'une Épidémie Ancienne: La Peste de 1666-1670," <u>Revue d'Histoire Moderne et Contemporaine</u>, Vol. 17 (1970), 954; and Egon Schmitz-Cliever, "Ein Beitrag zur Epidemiologie der Pestpandemie von 1664/67," <u>Archiv für Hygiene und Bakteriologie</u>, Vol. 138 (1954), 440-41.

[86] Vincent, <u>God's Terrible Voice</u>, p. 29.

[87] Theophilus Garencieres, <u>A Mite Cast into the Treasury of the Famous City of London</u> (London, 1665), p. 1.

[88] Garencieres, <u>A Mite Cast</u>, p. 1.

[89] Hodges, <u>Loimologia</u>, p. 3.

[90] <u>A Collection of the Yearly Bills of Mortality from 1657 to 1758 Inclusive</u> (London, 1759), <u>passim</u>.; Bell, <u>The Great Plague</u>, p. 92; and Leonard W. Crowie, <u>Plague and Fire, London 1665-66</u> (New York, 1970), p. 43.

[91] Vincent, <u>God's Terrible Voice</u>, p. 31.

323

[92]Quoted in Owen, "The Poore's Plague," 259.

[93]Quoted in K. Bryn Thomas, "Daniel Defoe and the Great Plague of London," Royal Society of Medicine Proceedings, Vol. 59 (1966), 6.

[94]Bell, The Great Plague, p. 91.

[95]Revel, "Autour d'une Épidémie," 980.

[96]Andrew P. Trout, "The Municipality of Paris Confronts the Plague of 1668," Medical History, Vol. 17 (1973), 418.

[97]Schmitz-Cliever, "Ein Beitrag zur Epidemiologie," 440-41.

[98]Quoted in Neumayr, et. al., "Zur Geschichte der Pestepidemien," 266.

[99]Hille and Ehler, "Zum medizinischen Wissen," 1696.

[100]Peter Diosi, "Aufzeichnungen eines Augenzeugen über die Pestepidemie der Jahre 1718-1720 in Siebenbürgen," Janus: Revue Internationale de l'Histoire des Sciences, Vol. 51 (1964), 221-22; and J.C. McDonald, "The History of Quarantine in Britain during the 19th Century," Bulletin of the History of Medicine, Vol. 25 (1951), 22.

[101]Biraben, "Certain Demographic Characteristics," 536-38.

[102]De Croissainte, A Brief Journal, p. 53 (1st Report).

[103]De Crossainte, A Brief Journal, p. 6 (3rd Report).

[104]John T. Alexander, "Plague in Russia and Danilo Samoilovich: An Historiographical Comment and Research Note," Canadian-American Slavic Studies, Vol. 8 (1974), 530.

[105]Alexander, "Catherine II," 637, 660.

[106]Alexander, "Plague in Russia," 526-27.

[107]W. Kemp, A Brief Treatise of the Nature, Causes, Signs, Preservation From, and Cure of the Pestilence (London, 1665), p. 46.

[108]Areto O. Kowal, "Danilo Samoilowitz: An Eighteenth-Century Ukranian Epidemiologist and His Role in the Moscow

Plague (1770-72)," Journal of the History of Medicine and Allied Sciences, Vol. 27 (1972), 440.

[109]John Howard, An Account of the Principal Lazarettos in Europe (London, 1789), p. 25.

[110]Howard, An Account, p. 25.

[111]Theophilus Lobb, Letters Relating to the Plague and Other Contagious Distempers (London, 1745), pp. 4-5.

[112]Biraben, Les Hommes et La Peste, Vol. I, pp. 195-96.

[113]Cartwright and Biddiss, Disease and History, p. 37.

[114]Author's conversation with A.A. Arata, World Health Organization, October 19, 1977.

[115]Fernand Braudel, Capitalism and Material Life 1400-1800, trans. by Miriam Kochan (New York, 1973), p. 43.

[116]Brighetti, Bologna e la Peste, pp. 173-74.

[117]Cowie, Plague and Fire, p. 43.

[118]Birben, "Certain Demographic Considerations," 536-39.

[119]Neumayr, et. al., "Zur Geschichte der Pestepidemien," 270.

[120]Livesey, "Epidemics!" 5.

[121]Hare, Pomp and Pestilence, p. 191.

Chapter 2: Syphilis

[1]Alfred W. Crosby, Jr., The Columbian Exchange: Biological and Cultural Consequences of 1492 (Westport, 1972), 122.

[2]Ulrich von Hütten, De Morbo Gallico: A Treastise of the French Disease, trans. by the Canon of Marten-Abbye (London, 1730), p. 12.

[3]Desiderius Erasmus, Colloquies (New York, 1964), p. 401.

325

[4]N.D. Falck, A Treatise on the Venereal Disease (London, 1772), p. 68.

[5]B. Scheube, "Über den Ursprung der Syphilis," Janus: Revue Internationale de l'Histoire des Sciences, de la Médicine, de la Pharmacie et de la Techique, Vol. 7 (1902), 39.

[6]Hütten, De Morbo Gallico, p. 5.

[7]For an opposing view, see Karl Sudhoff, "The Origin of Syphilis," Bulletin of the Medical Society of Chicago, Vol. 2 (1917), 16-17.

[8]Francisco Lopez de Villalobos, Sur les Contagieuses et Maudites Bubas: Historie et Médicine, trans. by E. Lanquetin (Paris, 1890), p. 39.

[9]Iwan Bloch, Der Ursprung der Syphilis, 2 vols. (Jena, 1901-1911), Vol. II, p. 141; and C.S. Butler and Vincent Hernandez, "Our Inheritance of Fallacy from Chapter XIV of Oviedo's Historia General y Natural," Southern Medical Journal, Vol. 22 (1929), 1099.

[10]Sudhoff, "The Origins of Syphilis," 17.

[11]Arthur W. Stillians, "The Introduction and Spread of Syphilis in Europe," International College of Surgeons Journal, Vol. 37 (1962), 595.

[12]A.N.R. Sanchez, Dissertation sur L'Origine de la Maladie Vérénienne (Paris, 1752), p. 96.

[13]William Clowes, A Briefe and Necessarie Treatise Touching the Cure of the Disease called Morbus Gallicus (London, 1585), p. 38.

[14]Charles C. Dennie, A History of Syphilis (Springfield, 1962), pp. 58-61.

[15]Quoted in D'Arcy Power, "The Venereal Diseases," in W.R. Bett (ed.), A Short History of Some Common Diseases (Oxford, 1934), pp. 37-38.

[16]Theodor Mildner, "Durch Jahrhunderte Hindurch Immer noch Mecurius," Medizinische Klinik, Vol. 70 (1975), 341.

[17]W.A. Pusey, "The Beginning of Syphilis," American Medical Association Journal, Vol. III (1915), 1962.

[18]Hieronymi Fracastorii, Syphilis, Sive Morbus Gallicus (Verona, 1530), Book I, lines 41-45.

[19]Pusey, "The Beginning of Syphilis," 1962.

[20]N. Sönnischen, "Fritz Richard Schaudinn zum 100. Geburtstag," Dermatologische Monatsschrift, Vol. 158 (172), 74.

[21]Karl Sudhoff, "The End of the Fable of the Great Syphilis Epidemic in Europe following the Discovery of the Antilles," Bulletin of the Society of Medical History of Chicago, Vol. 2 (1917), 24-25.

[22]Quoted in Ralph Flenley (ed.), Six Town Chronicles of England (Oxford, 1911), p. 188.

[23]C. Binz, "Die Einschleppung der Syphilis in Europa," Deutsche Medicinishe Wochenschrift, Vol. 19 (1893), 1058.

[24]J. Johnston Abraham, "The Early History of Syphilis," The British Journal of Surgery, Vol. XXXII (1944), 225.

[25]Sudhoff, "The End of the Fable," 24.

[26]Fracastorii, Syphilis, Book I, lines 123-24.

[27]John Vigo, Practica in Arte Chirurgica Copiosa (Lyons, 1516), p. 126.

[28]Hütten, De Morbo Gallico, p. 7. See also Edward Jeanselme, et. al., Histoire de la Syphilis (Paris, 1931), 81ff.

[29]M. Lazerme, Historia de Morbis Internis Capitis, Unpublished Manuscript No. 3201 - Wellcome Institute for the History of Medicine (Montpellier, 1750), p. 1.

[30]Quoted in J.D. Rolleston, "Venereal Disease in Literature," British Journal of Venereal Diseases, Vol. 10 (1934), 154.

[31]Ambroise Paré, "Traitant de la Grosse Verole," in J.-F. Malgaigne (ed.), Oeuvres Complètes d'Ambroise Paré, 3 vols. (Paris, 1840-1841), Vol. II, p. 527.

[32]Joannes Manardus, Epistolae Medicinales (Ferrara, 1521), Book Seven, letter two.

[33]Clowes, A Briefe and Necessairie Treatise, p. 4.

[34]R.C. Holcomb, "Christopher Columbus and the American Origin of Syphilis," U.S. Naval Medical Bulletin, Vol. 32 (1934), 405. See also Heinrich Haeser, Lehrbuch der Geschichte der Medicin und der Epidemischen Krankheiten, 3rd ed., 3 vols. (Jena, 1875-1882), Vol. III, p. 297.

[35]Thomas Jordanus, Luis Novae in Moravia Exportae Descriptio (Frankfurt, 1580), p. 1.

[36]Herman Goodman, Notable Contributions to the Knowledge of Syphilis (New York, 1943), p. 18.

[37]Ellis H. Hudson, "Villalobos and Columbus," American Journal of Medicine, Vol. 32 (1962), 578-83.

[38]R.S. Morton, "Another Look at the Morbus Gallicus," British Journal of Venereal Diseases, Vol. 44 (1968), 175.

[39]Iwan Bloch, "History of Syphilis," in D'Arcy Power and J. Keogh Murphy (eds.), A System of Syphilis, 6 vols. (London, 1908), Vol. I, p. 12.

[40]Pusey, "The Beginning of Syphilis," 1963.

[41]Quoted in Abraham, "The Early History of Syphilis," 228.

[42]Pusey, "The Beginning of Syphilis," 1964; and Holcomb, "Christopher Columbus," 407.

[43]Quoted in Alfred W. Crosby, Jr., "The Early History of Syphilis," American Anthropologist, Vol. 71 (1969), 222. See also Gonzalo Fernando di Oviedo y Valdez, Librio Secondo delle Indie Occidentali (Venice, 1534), p. 8.

[44]Quoted in Abraham, "The Early History of Syphilis," 228.

[45]Quoted in C.S. Butler and J.A. Biello, "The Influence of Ruy Diaz de Isla upon the Question of the American Origin of Syphilis," Southern Medical Journal, Vol. 26 (1933), 439. See also Bartolome de las Casas, Relation des Voyages et des Découvertes que les Espagnoles ont font dans les Indes Occidentales (Amsterdam, 1698), pp. 225-76.

[46]Quoted in Abraham, "The Early History of Syphilis," 229.

[47]Ellis H. Hudson, "Treponematosis and African Slavery," British Journal of Venereal Diseases, Vol. 40 (1964), 46.

[48]Ellis H. Hudson, "Historical Approach to the Terminology of Syphilis," Archives of Dermatology, Vol. 84 (1961), 65.

[49]Peter Wingate, The Penguin Medical Encyclopedia, 2nd ed. (Aylesburg, 1976), p. 430.

[50]Goodman, Notable Contributions, p. 18.

[51]Paré, "Traitant de la Grosse Verole," Vol. II, p. 27.

[52]Derek J. Cripps and Arthur C. Curtis, "Syphilis Maligna Praecox: Syphilis of the Great Epidemic? An Historical Review," Archives of Internal Medicine, Vol. 119 (1967), 412-14.

[53]Falck, A Treatise on the Venereal Disease, p. 247.

[54]Jordanus, Luis Novae in Moravia, p. 2. See also, E. Lancereux, Traité Historique et Pratique de la Syphilis (Paris, 1866), p. 26.

[55]Maurice Saint-Martin, "La Syphilis, Maladie d'Hier et Aujourd'hui," L'Union Médicale du Canada, Vol. 93 (1964) 1327-28.

[56]C. Kopp, "Ueber Syphilis Maligna," Münchener Medicinische Wochenschrift, Nr. 42 (1887), 813-14.

[57]H.C. French, "Malignant Syphilis," Royal Army Medical Corps Journal, Vol. 4 (1905), 477-79. See also A. Geigel, Geschichte, Pathologie und Therapie der Syphilis (Würzburg, 1867), pp. 4-7.

[58]Ellis H. Hudson, Non-Venereal Syphilis (Edinburg, 1958), p. 2; and Abner I. Weisman, "Syphilis: Was it Endemic in Pre-Columbian America or Was it Brought Here from Europe?" Bulletin of the New York Academy of Medicine, Vol. 42 (1966), 285.

[59]Quoted in Ralph H. Major, A History of Medicine, 2 vols. (Springfield, 1954), Vol. II, p. 934.

[60]John Hunter, A Treatise on Venereal Disease (London, 1787), p. 334.

[61]Max Isenberg, "Syphilis in the Eighteenth and Early Nineteenth Century," International Record of Medicine, Vol. 152 (1940), 460.

[62]Major, A History of Medicine, Vol. II, p. 931.

[63]Paul Ehrlich, "Über Laboratoriumsversuche und Klinische Erprobung von Heilstoffen," Chemiker-Zeitung, Vol. 36 (1912), 637-38.

[64]Weisman, "Syphilis," 285.

[65]R.S. Morton, "Some Aspects of the Early History of Syphilis in Scotland," British Journal of Venereal Diseases, Vol. 38 (1962), 176-77.

[66]Griffith Evans, Latent Syphilis and the Autonomic Nervous System, 2nd ed. (Bristol, 1937), p. 5.

[67]Paul Bru, Histoire de Bicêtre (Paris, 1890), p. 36.

[68]N.I. Gusakov, "Neopublikovannye Raboty Russikikh Virachei 18-19 Stoletii po Sifilidologii," Vestnik Dermatologii i Venerologii, Vol. 48 (1972), pp. 63-64.

[69]Lancereux, Traité Historique, p. 33.

[70]Olwen Hufton, The Poor of Eighteenth-Century France, 1750-1789 (Oxford, 1974), pp. 238, 308.

[71]Olwen Hufton, Bayeux in the Eighteenth Century (Oxford, 1967), pp. 70-71; and J. Rousset, "Les Épidémies à Lyon," Congrès des Sociétés Savants de Paris et des Départments - Actes, Vol. 89 (1964), 176-77.

[72]French, "Malignant Syphilis," 477.

[73]Aertzlicher Bericht des K.K. Allgemein Krankenhauses zu Wien vom Jahre 1886 (Vienna, 1888), p. 119.

[74]Richard Carmichael, An Essay on the Venereal Diseases (London, 1814), p. 92.

[75]Bulletin de la Société Médicale des Hospitaux de Paris (Paris, 1861), p. 338.

[76]Fifth Annual Report of the Board of Superintendence of Dublin Hospitals (Dublin, 1862), pp. 13-14.

[77]Bericht der K.K. Krankenanstalt Rudolph-Stiftung in Wien vom Jahre 1888 (Vienna, 1889), p. 40.

[78]Statistical Tables of the Patients under Treatment in the Wards of St. Bartholomew's Hosptial during 1895 (London, 1896), p. 72.

[79]Glasgow Royal Maternity and Women's Hospital, Medical Reports for the Year 1926 (Glasgow, 1927), pp. 9-10.

[80]Abstracts of Some of the Medical and Surgical Cases Treated at the General Hospital for Sick Children, Pendlebury, Manchester during the Year 1885 (Manchester, 1886), p. 37.

[81]Philippe Ricord, Traité Pratique des Maladies Vénériennes (Paris, 1838), pp. 279-377. See also Progrès de l'Enquête International sur le Traitement de la Syphilis, League of Nations Committee on Hygiene (Geneva, 1931), p. 3.

[82]The Liverpool and Manchester Medical and Surgical Reports (Manchester, 1875), p. 81.

[83]French, "Malignant Syphilis," 477.

[84]Sanitäts-Bericht über die Deutschen Heere im Kriege gegen Frankreich 1870/71 (Berlin, 1891), p. 105.

[85]A Statistical Return of the Health of the Royal Navy for the Year 1859 (London, 1862), p. 62.

[86]Statistical Report of the Health of the Navy for the Year 1906 (London, 1907), pp. 1 and 40.

[87]McNeil, Plagues and Peoples, p. 285.

[88]Annual Summary of Births, Deaths, and Causes of Death in London and Other Large Cities (London, 1871), p. XII.

[89]Evans, Latent Syphilis, p. 2.

[90]Bernhard Dattner, The Management of Neurosyphilis (London, 1944), p. 17.

[91]Georgii Baglivi, Opera Omnia: Medico-Practica et Anatomica (Lugundi, 1710), p. 95.

[92]Hunter, A Treatise, p. 23.

[93]Falck, A Treatise, p. 92.

[94] John Astruc, A Treatise of the Venereal Disease, 2 vols, trans. by William Barrowby (London, 1737), Vol. I, p. 49.

[95] Astruc, A Treatise, Vol. I, p. 282.

[96] Ricord, Traité Pratique, p. 171.

[97] St. George's Hospital Reports (London, 1868). p. 60.

[98] Dattner, The Management of Neurosyphilis, p. 17.

[99] P. Fildes and R.J.G. Parnell, "An Investigation into the Ultimate Results of the Treatment of Syphilis with Arsenical Compounds," in Medical Research Committee Reports (London, 1918), p. 14.

[100] J.B. van Helmont, Ortus Medicinae (Amsterdam, 1652), p. 848. See also R.R. Willcox, "Changing Patterns of Treponemal Disease," British Journal of Venereal Diseases, Vol. 50 (1974), 169-78.

[101] Zinsser, Rats, Lice and History, p. 60.

[102] Harold C. Cole, "Antiquity of Syphilis with Some Observations on Its Treatment Through the Ages," Archives of Dermatology, Vol. 64 (1951), 12-22; and Ellis H. Hudson, "Diagnosing a Case of Venereal Disease in Fifteenth Century Scotland," British Journal of Venereal Diseases, Vol. 48 (1972), 146-153.

[103] M.P. Morel, "La Syphilis Pré-Colombienne," Lyon Médical, Vol. 93 (1960), 1669.

[104] F.E. Rabello, "Les Origines de la Syphilis," La Nouvelle Presse Médicale, Vol. 2 (1973), 1379-1380.

[105] Crosby, "The Early History of Syphilis," 218-27.

[106] L.W. Harrison, "The Origin of Syphilis," British Journal of Venereal Diseases, Vol. 35 (1959), 1.

Chapter 3: Smallpox

[1]Genevieve Miller, The Adoption of Inoculation for Smallpox in England and France (Philadelphia, 1957), p. 29.

[2]Quoted in S. Monckton Copeman, Vaccination: Its Natural History and Pathology (London, 1899), p. 2.

[3]J.D. Rolleston, The History of the Acute Exanthemata (London, 1937), p. 6; and Miller, The Adoption, p. 27.

[4]Quoted in Rolleston, The History, p. 7.

[5]W. Kaiser and K. Werner, "Die Anfänge der Pockenschutzimpfung (Variolation) in Halle und Umgebung," Zeitschrift für die Gesamte Hygiene und ihre Grenzgebiete, Vol. 19 (1973), 807.

[6]M.P.M. Cooray, "Epidemics in the Course of History," Ceylon Medical Journal, Vol. 10 (1965), 88; and Livesey, "Epidemics!" 8.

[7]Émile Morat, Étude sur Les Idées et Les Faits Relatifs au Virus Variolique au XVIIIe Siècle (Paris, 1911), p. 18.

[8]C.W. Dixson, Smallpox (London, 1962), pp. 190-91; and John F.H. Broadbent, "Acute Infectious Disease," in Bett, A Short History, p. 5.

[9]Quoted in Dixson, Smallpox, p. 193.

[10]M.J.J. Paulet, Histoire de la Petite Vérole (Paris, 1768), p. 176.

[11]Braudel, Capitalism, p. 43.

[12]Quoted in Dixson, Smallpox, p. 193.

[13]J. Helvétius, An Essay on the Animal Oeconomy, trans. from the French (London, 1723), p. 114.

[14]Pierre de Baux, Parallèle de la Petite Vérole Naturelle avec L'Artificielle, ou Inoculée (Avignon, 1761), p. vi.

[15]Edward J. Edwardes, A Concise History of Small-Pox and Vaccination in Europe (London, 1902), p. 12.

[16]J. Rousset, "Essai de Pathologie Urbaine: Les Causes de Morbidité et de Mortalité à Lyon aux XVIIe et XVIIIe Siècles," Cahiers d'Histoire, Vol. 8 (1963), 91.

[17]Charles Singer and E. Ashworth Underwood, A Short History of Medicine, 2nd ed. (Oxford, 1962), p. 199.

[18]John Haygarth, A Sketch of a Plan to Exterminate the Casual Smallpox from Great Britain, 2 vols. (London, 1793), Vol. I, pp. 59-60.

[19]Edmund Massey, A Sermon Against the Dangerous and Sinful Practice of Innoculation, 2nd ed. (London, 1772), p. 15.

[20]Graunt, Natural and Political Observations, p. 9.

[21]A Collection (1759).

[22]William A. Guy, "Two Hundred and Fifty Years of Smallpox in London," Journal of the Royal Statistical Society, Vol. XLV (1882), 431-33.

[23]A.H. Gale, Epidemic Disease (London, 1959), p. 55.

[24]A Collection (1759); Laübstein, "Über einen frühen Geübten," 313; and E. Ashworth Underwood, "Edward Jenner: The Man and His Work," British Medical Journal, Vol. 1 (1949), 882.

[25]Paul Cassar, "Edward Jenner and the Introduction of Vaccination in Malta," Medical History, Vol. 13 (1969), 68.

[26]Norbert D. Zólyomi, "La Faculté de Médicine de Nazgszombat et Les Problèmes de L'Hygiène Publique Notamment La Variolisation," Orvostorteneti Kozlemenyek, Vols. 57-59 (1971), 249.

[27]August von Schlözer, Von der Unschädlichkeit der Pocken in Russland und von Russlands Bevölkerung (Göttingen, 1768), pp. 67-68.

[28]A.T. Kravchenko, "I Istorii Likvidatsii Ospy v SSR," Zhurnal Mikrobiologii, Epidemiologii i Immunobiologii, Vol. 47 (1970), 3.

[29]Timoteo O'Scanlan, Practica Moderna de La Inoculacion (Madrid, 1784), p. 12.

[30]E. LaGrange, "La Variole en Belgique," Le Scapel, Vol. 121 (1968), 293.

[31]M. Gatti, Nouvelles Réflexions sur La Pratique de L'Inoculation (Paris, 1767), p. 155.

[32]C. Brunel, "Un Projet D'Establissement D'Hôpital pour L'Inoculation de la Variole à Bruxelles," Cahiers Bruxellois, Vol. 35 (1968), 79.

[33]LaGrange, "La Variole," 293; and J. Cuvelier, "Avant Jenner," Revue de L'Instruction Publique en Belgique, Vol. 50 (1907), 364.

[34]William Rowley, Cowpox Inoculation No Security Against Smallpox (London, 1805), pp. 20-21.

[35]Benenson, Control, pp. 288-89.

[36]John Haygarth, An Inquiry How To Prevent The Smallpox (Chester, 1785), pp. 19-20.

[37]Haygarth, An Inquiry, pp. 55-56.

[38]Wingate, Medical Encyclopedia. p. 407.

[39]Thomas Dimsdale, The Present Method of Inoculating For The Smallpox (London, 1767), pp. 61-62.

[40]Wingate, Medical Encyclopedia, p.407.

[41]Theophilus Lobb, A Treatise of the Smallpox (London, 1731), p. 4.

[42]John Friend, Nine Commentaries Upon Fevers: And Two Epistles Concerning The Smallpox, trans. by Thomas Dace (London, 1730), pp. 32-33.

[43]A. Herrlich, Die Pocken (Stuttgart, 1967), pp. 155-56 and 205-6.

[44]Haygarth, A Sketch, Vol. I, p. 31.

[45]Arthur S. MacNalty, "The Prevention of Smallpox: From Edward Jenner to Monckton Copeman," Medical History, Vol. 12 (1968), 3.

[46]Quoted in Kenneth Dewhurst, Dr. Thomas Sydenham (1624-1689), His Life and Original Writings (London, 1966), p. 111.

[47]MacNalty, "The Prevention," 3.

[48]Charles G. Custom, "Historical Notes on Smallpox and Inoculation," Annals of Medical History, Vol. 6 (1924), 465-66.

[49]O'Scanlan, Practica Moderna, p. 12.

[50]Haygarth, A Sketch, Vol. I, p. 31.

[51]Rudolf Möller, "Die Pockenimpfung im Gebiet der Herzogtums Sachsen-Altenburg," Deutsche Medizinisches Journal, Vol. 16 (1965), p. 619.

[52]Marie-Louise Dufrenoy and Jean Dufrenoy, "Variolisation et Vaccination: Contribution à L'Histoire de La Pathologie Comparée," Revue de Pathologie Comparée, Vol. 64 (1965), 143; and Vincent J. Knapp, Europe in the Era of Social Transformation: 1700-Present (Englewood Cliffs, 1976), pp. 76-78.

[53]For a discussion of this point, see P. E. Razzell, "Population Change in Eighteenth-Century England: A Reinterpretation," The Economic History Review, 2nd Series, Vol. 18 (1965), pp. 312-32.

[54]Rousset, "Les Épidémies," 161.

[55]Cartwright and Biddiss, Disease and History, p. 121.

[56]Haygarth, An Inquiry, p. vii.

[57]Edwardes, A Concise History, p. 12.

[58]Emmanuel E. Duvillard, Analyse et Tableaux de L'Influence de La Petite Vérole sur La Mortalité Vérole (Paris, 1806), p. 169.

[59]Ackerknecht, History and Geography, p. 64.

[60]Ildikó Friedrich, "The Spreading of Jenner's Vaccination in Hungary," Orvostorteneti Kozlemenyck, Supplement 6 (1972), 140.

[61]Quoted in Friedrich, "The Spreading," 140.

[62]L. Griva, "Epidemia Vaiuolosa in Torino nel 1829," Minerva Medica, Vol. 61 (1970), 3127-28.

[63]Louis Chevalier, Laboring Classes and Dangerous Classes in Paris During the First Half of the Nineteenth Century, trans. by Frank Jellinek (New York, 1973), p. 332.

[64]George Rudé, Hanoverian London, 1714-1808 (London, 1971), p. 223.

[65]William A. Guy, "Two Hundred," 414-15.

[66]Weekly Returns of Births and Deaths in London in the Year 1857 (London, 1858), p. iii; and A General Bill of All the Christenings and Burials From December 15, 1807 to December 13, 1808 (London, 1809).

[67]Heinrich Bohn, Bedeutung und Werth der Schutzpockenimpfung (Berlin, 1867), p. 21.

[68]McNeill, Plagues and Peoples, p. 285.

[69]William B. Carpenter, "Smallpox and Vaccination in 1871-1881," The Nineteenth Century, Vol. II (1882), 529; and E. LaGrange, "La Variole," 293.

[70]Edwardes, A Concise History, pp. 112-14.

[71]John Moir, "Record of the Cases Treated in Hospital During the Smallpox Epidemic in West Ham in 1884 and 1885," Transactions of the Epidemiological Society, New Series, Vol. VI (1886-1887), 50.

[72]Moir, "Record," 50-51.

[73]"Smallpox Prevalence Throughout the World During and After the Second World War," World Health Organization, Epidemiological and Vital Statistics Report, (Geneva, 1950), 286.

[74]League of Nations, Minutes of the Health Committee Session, 1928 (Geneva, 1929), p. 71; and League of Nations, Epidemiological Report of the Health Section of the Secretariat (Geneva, 1929), p. 172.

[75]"Smallpox Prevalence," 286.

[76]B. Benjamin, "Statistics and Epidemiology," Scientific Basis of Medicine, Annual Review (Geneva, 1929), p. 172.

[77]Razzell, "Population Change," 319.

[78]Rousset, "Les Épidémies," 159-61.

[79]Guy, "Two Hundred," 427; and Edwardes, A Concise History, p. 12.

[80]Adna F. Weber, The Growth of Cities in the Nineteenth Century (New York, 1899), passim.

[81]Quoted in Edward Mellanby, "Jenner and His Impact on Medical Science," British Medical Journal, Vol. I (1949), 924.

[82]Edward Jenner, An Inquiry Into the Causes and Effects of Variolae Vaccinae (London, 1798), p. 45.

[83]Arnold Klebs, "The Historic Evolution of Variolation, Bulletin of the Johns Hopkins Hospital, Vol. 24 (1913), 70.

[84]James Jurin, An Account of the Success of Innoculating the Smallpox in Great Britain (London, 1724), p. iv.

[85]Derrrick Baxby, "Inoculation and Vaccination: Smallpox, Cowpox and Vaccinia," Medical History, Vol. 9 (1965), 384.

[86]Author's conversation with J.G. Breman, World Health Organization, October 19, 1977.

[87]W.R. LeFanu, "Edward Jenner," Royal Society of Medicine Proceedings, Vol. 66 (1973), 666.

[88]Baxby, "Inoculation," 384-85.

[89]Le Fanu, "Edward Jenner," 667.

[90]Baxby, "Inoculation, 384.

[91]Quoted in H.M. Koebling, "Edward Jenner (1749-1823): Vaccination versus Variolation," Agents and Actions: Swiss Journal of Pharmacology, Vol. 2, (1971), 41.

[92]C.L. Paul Trüb, Josef Posch and Karl-Heinz Richter, "Historische Studie über die Gesundheitsschüden nach Pockenschutzimpfungen," Medizinische Monatsschrift, Vol. 26 (1972), 167.

[93]Dale E. Ross, "Leicester and the Anti-Vaccination Movement," Leicestershire Archeological and Historical Society Transactions, Vol. 43 (1967), 39-40.

[94]Edwardes, A Concise History, p. 141.

[95]Knapp, Europe, pp. 59-64.

Chapter 4: Typhus and Cholera

[1]Henry E. Sigerist, Civilization and Disease (Ithaca, 1944), p. 118.

[2]Ackerknecht, History and Geography, pp. 33-34.

[3]Zinsser, Rats, Lice and History, p. 243.

[4]McNeill, Plagues and Peoples, p. 220.

[5]August Hirsch, Handbook of Geographical and Historical Pathology, trans. by Charles Creighton, 2 vols. (London, 1883-1885), Vol. I, pp. 83-84.

[6]McNeill, Plagues and Peoples, 220.

[7]Cartwright and Biddiss, Disease and History, p. 85.

[8]Schmitz-Cleaver, "Ein Beitrag," 440; and Cartwright and Biddiss, Disease and History, p. 85.

[9]Clara Lender, "A Dangerous Sickness Which Turned to a Spotted Fever," Studies in English Literature, Vol. 11 (1971), 97.

[10]Heinrich Haeser, Lehrbuch der Geschichte der Medicin und der Volkskrankheiten (Jena, 1845), pp. 475-76.

[11]Lieutenant-Colonel MacArthur, "Old-Time Typhus in Britain," Transactions of the Royal Society of Tropical Medicine and Hygiene, Vol. 20 (1927), 498.

[12]Lynn Thorndike, "Newness and Novelty in Seventeenth-Century Science and Medicine," in Philip P. Wiener and Aaron Noland (eds.), Roots of Scientific Thought (New York, 1957), p. 453.

[13]Edward Greaves, Morbus Epidemius Anni 1643, Or, The New Disease With the Signes, Causes, Remedies, Etc. (Oxford, 1643), p. 3.

[14]Quoted in Lander, "A Dangerous Sickness," 99.

[15]E. Ehler and M. Hille, "Über eine von M.J. Goniaeus im Jahre 1604 beschriebene Fleckfieberepidemie in Rostock und Umgebung," Medizinische Klinik, Vol. 64 (1969), 454-57; K. Schadelbauer, "Die Pest von 1611 in Innsbruck war Flecktyphus," Wiener Klinische Wochenschrift, Vol. 76 (1964), 550-52; and P. Diosi, "Epidemisches und sporadisches Fleckfieber in Schässburg," Zeitschrift für die Gesamte Hygiene und ihre Grenzgebiete, Vol. II (1965), 158.

[16]Thomas Bateman, A Succinct Account of the Contagious Fever of this Country, (London, 1818), p. vii.

[17]Hirsch, Handbook, Vol. I, p. 551.

[18]Singer and Underwood, A Short History, p.189; and MacArthur, "Old-Time Typhus," 490.

[19]Hufton, The Poor, p.64.

[20]G. Le Borgne, Recherches Historiques Sur Les Grandes Épidémies Qui Ont Régné à Nantes Depuis Le VIe Jusqua'au XIXe Siècle (Nantes, 1852), p. 97.

[21]William B. Adams, Ireland and Irish Emigration to the New World (New Haven, 1932), p. 111.

[22]H. F. Kramchaninov and F. V. Popova, "K Istorii Izucheniia Sypnogo Tifa v Rossi," Zhurnal Mikrobiologii, Epidemiologii i Immunobiologii, Vol. 43.

[23]Cartwright and Biddiss, Disease and History, p. 84.

[24]Folke Henschen, The History and Geography of Diseases, trans. by Joan Tate (New York, 1966), p. 64.

[25]F. Weyer, "Zur Entdeckungsgeschichte des Fleckfieberregers," Zeitschrift für Tropenmedizin und Parasitologie, Vol. 17 (1966), 478-80; and Cartwright and Biddiss, Disease and History, p. 86.

[26]H. da Rocha-Lima, "Zur Aetiologie des Fleckfiebers," Berliner Klinische Wochenschrift, Vol. 53 (1916), 567-68.

[27]François Blanc, "Charles Nicolle et Le typhus Exanthematique," Médicine Tropicale, Vol. 27 (1966), 465-66.

[28]H. Eyer, "Rudolf Weigl und die aetiologische Fleckfieberbekämpfung," Münchener Medizinische Wochenschrift, Vol. 109 (1967), 2185-87.

[29]League of Nations, Monthly Epidemiological Report of the Health Section of the Secretariat (Geneva, 1929), p. 172.

[30]William Cullen, First Lines of the Practice of Physic, 4 vols. (Edinburgh, 1786), Vol. I, p. 67.

[31]Bateman, A Succinct Account, p. 33.

[32]Bateman, A Succinct Account, pp. 53-54.

[33]Haeser, Lehrbuch, Vol. III, p. 599.

[34]J.R.L. de Kerchhove, Histoire Des Maladies Observées à La Grande Armée Française Pendant Les Campagnes De Russie en 1812 et D'Allemagne en 1813, 3rd ed. (Anvers, 1836), p. 410.

[35]Friedrich Prinzing, Epidemics Resulting From Wars (Oxford, 1916), p. 117.

[36]Ackerknecht, History and Geography, p. 36.

[37]Haeser, Lehrbuch, Vol. III, p. 611.

[38]Weekly Returns of Births and Deaths in London in the Year 1857 (London, 1858), p. 14; and The Sixty-Fourth Report of the London Fever Hospital (London, 1865), p. 5.

[39]Gale, Epidemic Disease, p. 74; and Rudé, Hanoverian London, p. 84.

[40]Annalen des Charité-Krankenhauses zu Berlin (Berlin, 1877), p. 708.

[41]Annalen der Städtischen Allgemeinen Krankenhauser zu München (Munich, 1878), p. 424a.

[42]A. Riffel, Mittheilungen über die Erblichkeit und Infektiosität der Schwindsucht (Braunschweig, 1892), p. 8 and passim.

[43]H. Vincent and L. Muratet, Dysentery, Asiatic Cholera and Exanthematic Typhus (London, 1917), pp. 177, 179.

[44]Bailey, The Mathematical Theory, p. 1.

[45]Report to the Health Committee of the League of Nations, Epidemiological Intelligence: Epidemics in Russia Since 1914 (Geneva, 1922), pp. 7, 35.

[46]H.C. Trizno, "Bor'ba Tifami y Nizov'iakh Volgi v Gody Grazhdanskoi Voiny," Zhurnal Mikrobiologii, Epidemiologii i Immunobiologii, Vol. 49 (1972), 147.

[47]Renseignements Epidémiologiques: Statistique des Maladies à Declaration Obligatoire (League of Nations, Geneva, 1923), pp. 17-18, 39-42.

[48]League of Nations, Epidemiological Report of the Health Section of the Secretariat (Geneva, 1929), p. 173.

[49]Wingate, Medical Encyclopedia, p. 460.

[50]Haeser, Lehrbuch, Vol. III, p. 599.

[51]Riffel, Mittheilungen, p. 8.

[52]Zinsser, Rats, Lice and History, p. 243.

[53]Nicholas Hahon (ed.), Selected Papers on Pathogenic Rickettsiae (Cambridge, Mass., 1968), p. 94.

[54]A.M. Geist-Hofman, J.V. Meininger and C.M. Verkoost, "Zinking, Zinkingskoorts en Zinkingsziekte," Nederlands Tijdschrift voor Geneeskunde, Vol. 116 (1972), 28-29; and Riffel, Mittheilungen, passim.

[55]William P. Alison, Observations on The Epidemic Fever of MDCCCXLII in Scotland and Its Consequences with The Destitute Condition of the Poor (Edinburgh, 1844), pp. 8-9.

[56]Greaves, Morbus Epidemius, p. 16.

[57]Vincent and Muratet, Dysentery, p. 192.

[58]Norman Longmate, King Cholera: The Biography of a Disease (London, 1966), pp. 1-2.

[59]Saul Jarcho, "Yellow Fever, Cholera and the Beginnings of Medical Cartography," Journal of the History of Medicine and Allied Sciences, Vol. 25 (1970), 133-34.

[60]For some of the statistics here, see Roderick E. McGrew, "The First Russian Cholera Epidemic: Themes and Opportunities," Bulletin of the History of Medicine, Vol. 36 (1962), 221.

[61]J.R. Lichtenstädt, Die asiatische Cholera in Russland in den Jahren 1829 und 1830 (Berlin, 1831), p. 19.

[62]Quoted in "Epidemic Cholera," Medico-Chirurgical Review, Vol. 16 (1832), 164.

[63]Quoted in Robert Pollitzer, "Cholera Studies," Bulletin of the World Health Organization, Vol. 10 (1954), 422.

[64]Pollitzer, "Cholera Studies," 421-28.

[65]Fraser Brockington, "Public Health at the Privy Council 1831-34," Journal of the History of Medicine and Allied Sciences, Vol. 16 (1961), 161.

[66]Roderick E. McGrew, Russia and the Cholera (Madison, 1965), p. 99.

[67]Karl C. Hille, Beobachtungen über die asiatische Cholera (Leipzig, 1831), pp. 24-25.

[68]Auguste Gerardin and Paul Gaimard, Du Choléra-Morbus en Russe, en Prusse et en Autriche (Paris, 1832), p. 12.

[69]Quoted in Longmate, King Cholera, p. 1.

[70]Quoted in "Epidemic Cholera," 194.

[71]Chevalier, Laboring Classes, pp. 344-47; and N.R. Barrett, "A Tribute to John Snow, M.D., London, 1813-1815," Bulletin of the History of Medicine, Vol. 19 (1946), 521-22.

[72]Jacques Poulet, "L'Épidémie de Choléra de 1832 à Paris," Semaine des Hôpitaux de Paris, Vol. 46, (1970), 3845.

[73]Quoted in "Epidemic Cholera," 194.

[74]Chevalier, Laboring Classes, p. 345; and Longmate, King Cholera, p. 228.

[75]Charles Gaselee, Practical Treatise on Cholera (London, 1832), p. 11.

[76]Onofrio Mitaritonna, "Misure Contro il Colera nel Ducato di Moderna nel 1836, Vers la Fine della Seconda Pandemia," Pagine di Storia della Medicina, Vol. 12 (1968), 60.

[77]McGrew, Russia, p. 5.

[78]E. Bozzi, "Un Frammento Storico del Colera che Dominò in Toscana nel 1854-1855," Minerva Medica, Vol. 62 (1971), 3250-54.

[79]A. Proust, La Défense de l'Europe contre Le Choléra (Paris, 1892), p. 116; W.R.W. Drew, "Cholera," Royal Army Medical Corps Journal, Vol. 107 (1961), 211; and Thomas Sheppard, London 1808-1870: The Infernal Wen (London, 1971), p. 273.

[80]Reiner Olzscha, "Die Epidemiologie und Epidemiographie der Cholera in Russland," Zeitschrift für Hygiene und Infektionskrankheiten, Vol. 21 (1938-39), 7.

[81]Stanislaw Koba, "Epidemie Cholery w Powiecie Kieleckim w Latach 1837-1867," Przeglad Lekarski, Vol. 27 (1971), 676.

[82]Olzscha, "Die Epidemiologie," 7; and Koba, "Epidemie," 676.

[83]E.A. Parkes, Researches into the Pathology and Treatment of the Asiatic or Algide Cholera (London, 1847), pp. 133, 137.

[84]Eugene J. Gangarosa, "The Epidemiology of Cholera: Past and Present," Bulletin of the New York Academy of Medicine, Vol. 47 (1971), 1141.

[85]Author's conversation with Branko Cvjetanovic, World Health Organization, October 19, 1977.

[86]Gangarosa, "The Epidemiology," 1142.

[87]Norman Howard-Jones, "Choleranomolies: The Unhistory of Medicine as Exemplified by Cholera," Perspectives in Biology and Medicine, Vol. 15 (1972), 422.

[88]Fausto Bonora, "Axel Munthe e la Epidemia di Colera in Napoli del 1886," Pagine de Storia della Medicina, Vol. 8 (1964), 25.

[89]Filippo Pacini, Sulla Causa Specifica del Colera Asiatico (Florence, 1865), p. 16.

[90]A. Briere-de-Boismont, Relation Historique et Médicale du Choléra-Morbus de Pologne (Paris, 1832), pp. 54-55.

344

[91]Ferdinand Foy, Histoire Médicale du Choléra Morbus de Pologne (Paris, 1832), p. 30.

[92]Foy, Histoire, p. 45.

[93]Quoted in Brockington, "Public Health," 167.

[94]Parkes, Researches, pp. 7-19.

[95]Giovanni B. Scarano, "Cenni Sull'Epidemia di Colera del 1835 in Venezia e Sugli Esperimenti Instituiti dal Dott. Giacinto Namais," Rivista di Storia della Medicina, Vol. 11 (1967), 82-83.

[96]William Baly and William W. Gull (eds.), Reports of the Cholera Committee of The Royal College of Physicians (London, 1854), p. 16.

[97]Barrett, "A Tribute," 523.

[98]James Keir, Practical Observations on the Prevailing Epidemic Called Cholera (Edinburgh, 1848), p. 3.

[99]Daniel E. Lipschutz, "The Water Question in London, 1827-1831," Bulletin of the History of Medicine, Vol. 42 (1968), 524-25.

[100]William Farr, Report on the Mortality of Cholera in England 1848-49 (London, 1852), p. lii.

[101]P.E. Brown, "John Snow," Anathesia and Analgesea: Current Researches, Vol. 43 (1964), 650.

[102]John Snow, On the Mode of Communication of Cholera, 2nd ed. (London, 1854), p. 23.

[103]H. Harold Scott, Some Notable Epidemics (London, 1934), pp. 3-6.

[104]Howard-Jones, "Choleranomolies," 423.

[105]McGrew, "The First Russian," 221.

[106]Henry M. Madden, "The Cholera in Pest, 1831," Bulletin of the History of Medicine, Vol. 13 (1943), 481.

[107]P. Frequr et. al., "L'Épidémie de Choléra à Bordeaux en 1832," Journal de Médicine de Bordeaux, No. 6 (1958), 548.

345

[108]Margaret C. Barnet, "The 1832 Cholera Epidemic in York," Medical History, Vol. 16 (1972), 28; and Thomas Shapter, The History of Cholera in Exeter in 1832 (London, 1849), p. 216.

[109]McGrew, Russia, p. 161; Sheppard, London, pp. 248-49, 273, 277; Chevalier, Laboring Classes, pp. 345-46; Shapter, The History, p. 216; Longmate, King Cholera, p, 288; Pollitzer, "Cholera Studies," 444, 449-50; B. Woelderink, "De Cholera-Epidemie van 1866 in Rotterdam," Rotterdam Jahrbuch, Vol. 4 (1966), 312; and U.A. Salchow, "Vor 75 Jahren: Cholera in Hamburg," Medizinische Klinik, Vol. 63 (1968), 149.

[110]Pollitzer, "Cholera Studies," 443-44.

[111]Woelderink, "De Cholera," 305.

[112]Ph. Hauser, Le Choléra en Europe (Paris, 1897). p. 334.

[113]Frank Clemow, The Cholera Epidemic of 1892 in the Russian Empire (London, 1893), p. 30.

[114]Salchow, "Vor 75 Jahren," 149.

[115]Olzscha, "Die Epidemiologie," 7.

[116]Wingate, Medical Encyclopedia, pp. 101-2.

[117]Norbert Hirschhorn and William B. Greenbough III, "Cholera," Scientific American, Vol. 225 (1971), 15-21.

[118]R.B. Hornick, et. al., "The Broad Street Pump Revisited: Response of Volunteers to Ingested Cholera Vibrios," Bulletin of the New York Academy of Medicine, Vol. 47 (1971), 1183-85; and Treatment and Prevention of Dehydration in Diarrhoel Diseases (World Health Organization, Geneva, 1976), pp. 10-15. For more information here, see two unpublished WHO documents, Strategy of Cholera Control and Epidemiological Model of Cholera, available at the World Health Organization, Geneva.

[119]Knapp, Europe, pp. 178-81.

Chapter 5: Tuberculosis

[1]Quoted in J. Arthur Myers, "Eighty Years after the First Glimpse of the Tubercle Bacillus," Diseases of the Chest, Vol. 51 (1967), 500.

[2]Ermar Junker, "Die Entwicklung der Tuberkulose in Mitteleruropa," Münchener Medizinische Wochenschrift, Vol. 112 (1970), 990.

[3]Sol Roy Rosenthal, "I Consume," Quarterly Bulletin of the Northwestern University Medical School, Vol. 35 (1961), 157.

[4]H.D. Chalke, "Some Historical Aspects of Tuberculosis," Public Health, Vol. 74 (1959), 84.

[5]P. James Bishop, "Some Recent Papers on the History of Tuberculosis," Tubercle, Vol. 46 (1965), 303.

[6]Henschen, The History, p. 97.

[7]Lewis J. Moorman, "Tuberculosis," in William R. Bett (ed.), The History and Conquest of Common Diseases (Norman, 1954), p. 100.

[8]John Fraser, "Tuberculosis," in Bett, A Short History, pp. 19-20.

[9]Lawrason Brown, The Story of Clinical Pulmonary Tuberculosis (Baltimore, 1934), pp. 32-33.

[10]Sylvius de le Boë, Opera Medica (Leyden, 1679), p. 74.

[11]R.R. Trail, "Richard Morton (1637-1698)," Medical History, Vol. 14 (1970), 169.

[12]Richard Morton, Phthisiologia, or, a Treatise of Consumptions, 2nd ed. (London, 1720), p. 14.

[13]Morton, Phthisiologia, p. 2.

[14]Trail, "Richard Morton," 169.

[15]Lawrence F. Flick, Development of our Knowledge of Tuberculosis (Philadelphia, 1925), pp. 256-57.

[16]Graunt, Natural and Political Observations, p. 9.

[17]A Collection (1759).

[18]Benjamin Marten, A New Theory of Consumptions, More Especially of Phthisis, 2nd ed. (London, 1722), pp. 6-7.

[19]John Haygarth, Observations on the Bills of Mortality in Chester for the Year 1772 and 1773 in James H. Cassedy (ed.), Mortality in Pre-Industrial Times: Contemporary Verdict (Westmead, 1973), pp. 88-89.

[20]Thomas Bateman, Reports on the Diseases of London, and The State of The Weather (London, 1819). p. 22.

[21]Robert W. Philip, Collected Papers on Tuberculosis (London, 1937), p. 67.

[22]Thomas Beddoes, Essay on the Causes, Early Signs and Prevention of Pulmonary Consumption (London, 1799), pp. 8-9.

[23]C.J. Wherrett, "Tuberculosis: A World Problem," Michigan Medicine, Vol. 64 (1965), 182.

[24]M. Michel Möring and M. Charles Quentin, Collection de Documents pour Servir a L'Histoire des Hôpitaux de Paris, 4 vols. (Paris, 1881-1887), Vol. I, p. 189.

[25]Gazette des Hôpitaux Civils et Militaries (Paris, 1839), p. 1.

[26]Hirsch, Handbook of Pathology, Vol. II, pp. 610-11.

[27]General Report of the Royal Hospitals of Bridewell and Bethlem (London, 1858), p. 58.

[28]Quoted in Flick, Development, p. 257.

[29]G.-L. Bayle, "Recherches sur La Phthisie Pulmonaire," in Encyclopédie des Sciences Médicales (Paris, 1838), p. 393.

[30]Theodor Mildner, "Mann Kann die Phthisis auch so heilen!" Praxis der Pneumologie, Vol. 18 (1964), 37-43.

[31]Quoted in Harley Williams, Requiem for a Great Killer: The Story of Tuberculosis (London, 1973), p. 20.

[32]Robert Koch, "Die Aetiologie der Tuberculose," Berliner Klinische Wochenschrift, Vol. 19 (1882), 221-24.

[33]F.V. Shebanov, "Evoliutsiia Ucheniia o Tuberkuleze i Razvitie Medtodov Lecheniia Ego v SSR za 50 Let," Problemy Tuberkuleza, Vol. 45 (1967), 3.

[34]Henry H. Southey, Observations on Pulmonary Consumption (London, 1814), p. 24.

[35]P.C.A. Louis, Recherches Anatomico-Pathologiques sur la Phthisie (Paris, 1825), p. 4.

[36]P.C.A. Louis, Pathological Researches on Phthisis, Anonymous trans. (London, 1835), p. 357.

[37]William Allison, Experimental and Practical Researches on Inflammation and on the Origin and Nature of Tubercles of the Lungs (London, 1843), p. 59.

[38]M. Pidoux, Études Générales et Pratiques sur la Phthisie (Paris, 1873), p. 291.

[39]Henry Ancill, A Treatise on Tuberculosis, The Constitutional Origin of Consumption and Scrofula (London, 1852), p. 39.

[40]John Hogg, Practical Observations on the Prevention of Consumption (London, 1860), p. 16.

[41]Rosenthal, "I Consume," 157.

[42]The Dublin Hospital Reports and Communications in Medicine (Dublin, 1827), p. 78.

[43]R.T.H. Laennec, A Treatise on the Diseases of the Chest in Which they are Described According to their Anatomical Characters and their Diagnosis, trans. by John Forbes (London, 1821), p. 23.

[44]Junker, "Die Entwicklung," 185.

[45]Williams, Requiem, pp. 11-12.

[46]Otto Hildebrand, Tuberculose und Scrophulose (Stuttgart, 1902), p. 2.

[47]Paul Dionne and Jacques Gougoux, "Notions Toujours Actuelles en Tuberculose," Union Médicale du Canada, Vol. 93 (1964), 1334.

[48]A Collection of the Yearly Bills of Mortality from December 14, 1813 to December 3, 1814 (London, 1815), passim.

[49]Weekly Returns of Births and Deaths in London in the Year 1857 (London, 1858), p. 111.

[50]Hogg, Practical Observations, pp. 90-91.

[51]J. Brownlee, "Investigations into the Epidemiology of Phthisis in Great Britain and Wales," in Medial Research Committee Reports (London, 1918), p. 39.

[52]Philip, Collected Papers, p. 361.

[53]Halliday G. Sutherland, et. al. (eds.), The Control and Eradication of Tuberculosis (Edinburgh, 1911), p. 6.

[54]Benjamin, "Statistics," 210.

[55]Godwin Timms, On Consumption: Its Nature and Successful Treatment (London, 1860), p. 134.

[56]Rosenthal, "I Consume," 157-58; and Timms, On Consumption, p. 134.

[57]Bericht 1889, pp. 30-31.

[58]F. Kreuser, "70 Jahre Deutsches Zentralkomitee zur Bekämpfung der Tuberkulose," Münchener Medizinische Wochenschrift, Vol. 108 (1966), 1172-73.

[59]H. Barbier and B. Boudin, "Recherches Statistiques sur la Fréquence de la Tuberculose Chez les Enfants Parisiens Hospitalises," Tuberculosis: Monthly Publication of the International Anti-Tuberculosis Association, Vol. VIII (1908), p. 237.

[60]R. Bandelier and R. Roepke, Lehrbuch der Spezifischen Diagnostik und Therapie der Tuberkulose (Würzburg, 1911), p. 79.

[61]Bateman, Reports, p. 23.

[62]Bericht über die V. Versammlung der Tuberkulose-Ärzte Berlin (Berlin, 1908), p. 47.

[63]Robert Koch, Ueber neue Tuberkulinpräparate," Deutsche Medicinische Wochenschrift, Vol. 23 (1897), 209-13.

[64]Wingate, Medical Encyclopedia, p. 456.

[65]Ermar Junker, "Tuberkulinreihenuntersuchungen in Wien seit 1907," Wiener Medizinische Wochenschrift, Vol. 122 (1972), 228-30.

[66]N.S. Altschuler, "Privlechenie Obschchestvennosti k Bor'be s Tuberkulezom," Problemy Tuberkuleza, Vol. 48 (1970), 88-91; K. Breu, "Die Geschichte der Tuberkulosefürsorge in Deutschland," Das Offentliche Gesundheitswesen, Vol. 33 (1971), 37; and A.T. Wallace, "Sir Robert Philip: A Pioneer in the Campaign against Tuberculosis," Medical History, Vol. 5 (1961), 56-59.

[67]Annual Epidemiological Report, Collected Statistics of Notifiable Deaths for the Year 1935 (League of Nations Health Organization, Geneva, 1937), p. 74.

[68]Die Tuberkulosestatistik (League of Nations Health Organisation, Geneva, 1925), pp. 4-5.

[69]Note on Tuberculosis in Greece (League of Nations Health Organisation, Geneva, 1923), p. 1; and La Tuberkulose dans Le Milieu Rural en Roumanie (League of Nations Committee on Hygiene, Geneva, 1937), p. 5.

[70]Junker, "Tuberkulinreiheuntersuchungen," 231.

[71]Rudoph Brauer (ed.), Der Tuberkulose-Fortbildungskurs des Allgemeinen Krankenhauses Hamburg-Eppendorf, 2 vols. (Würzburg, 1913), Vol. I, p. 7.

[72]The First Medical Report of the Hospital for Consumption and Diseases of the Chest-Brompton (London, 1849), p. 9.

[73]Reiner W. Müller, "Die Tuberkulose in ländlichem Milieu in Europa," Zeitschrift für Tuberkulose und Erkrankungen der Thoroxorgane, Vol. 122 (1964), 332.

[74]Junker, "Die Entwicklung," 986-87.

[75]Arthur Newsholme, "Relative Importance of the Constituent Factors Involved in the Control of Pulmonary Tuberculosis," Transactions of the Epidemiological Society of London, Vol. XXV (1906), 47.

[76]Williams, Requiem, p. 33.

[77]Chalke, "Some Historical Aspects," 90.

[78]J. Burns Amberson, "A Retrospect of Tuberculosis: 1865-1965," The American Review of Respiratory Diseases, Vol. 93 (1966), 343.

[79]Alain Rousseau, "Gaspard-Laurent Bayle," Clio Medica, Vol. 6 (1971), 207-8.

[80]P.J. Bishop, "Thomas Young and His 'A Practical and Historical Treatise on Consumptive Deseases,' 1815," Tubercle, Vol. 54 (1973), 163.

[81]The Middlesex Hospital -- Reports of the Medical, Surgical, Obstretic and Pathological Registrars for the Year 1902 (London, 1904), p. 123.

[82]J. A. Villemin, "De La Virulence et De La Spécificité de La Tuberculose," Gazette Hebdomadaire De Médicine et De Chirurgie, Vol. 5 (1868), 537.

[83]Koch, "Die Aetiologie," 221.

[84]Alfred Hillier, Tuberculosis Its Nature, Prevention and Treatment (London, 1900), p. 10.

[85]John Fraser, Tuberculosis of the Bones and Joints in Children (London, 1914), p. 7.

[86]Reports of the Society for the Study of Disease in Children, 1904-1905 (London, 1905), p. 11.

[87]The Middlesex Hospital -- Reports of the Medical, Surgical, Obstretic and Pathological Registrars for the Year 1900 (London, 1902), p. 9.

[88]Bulletin et Mémoires de la Société Médicale des Hôpitaux de Bucarest (Bucharest, 1928), p. 122.

[89]C. Gernez-Rieux and M. Gervois, "Le Role de la Lutte Antituberculeuse dans Le Developpement des Programmes Generaux de Santé," International Union Against Tuberculosis, Vol. 43 (1970), 186.

[90]Anthon Ghon, The Primary Lung Focus of Tuberculosis in Children, trans. by Barty King (London, 1916), p. 171.

[91]Franz Hamburger, Die Tuberkulose des Kindesalters (Leipzig, 1912), p. 1.

[92]Albert Calmette, L'Infection Bacillaire et la Tuberculose Chez L'Homme et Chez Les Animaux (Paris, 1920), p. 158.

[93]George E. Bushnell, A Study in the Epidemiology of Tuberculosis (New York, 1920), pp. 1-2.

[94]Mittheilungen aus der Chirurgischen Klinik zu Tübingen (Tübingen, 1884), pp. 249-50.

[95]Comrie, History, Vol. II, p. 683.

[96]A. Calmette, C. Guerin and B. Weill-Hallé, "Essais d'Immunisation contre L'Infection Tuberculeuse," La Presse Médicale, Vol. 32 (1924), 553-55.

[97]B. Weill-Hallé, R. Turpin and A. Maas, "Étude Clinique des Réactions à L'Infection Tuberculeuse des Nourrisons Vaccinés par Ingestion de BCG," La Presse Médicale, Vol. 40 (1932), 1605-7.

[98]Selman A. Waksman, The Conquest of Tuberculosis (London, 1964), p. 130.

[99]E. Kurz, "Die Tuberkulosesituation in Stadt und Land: Eine Vergleichende Untersuchung der Jahre 1958 bis 1962," Praxis der Pneumologie mit der Tuberkuloseartz Vereignt, Vol. 18 (1964), 461-64.

[100]Brauer, Die Tuberkulose-Fortbildungskurs, Vol. I, p. 1.

[101]F. Kreuser, "Bedeutung der Umgebungsuntersuchungen bei Tuberkulose," Oeffentliche Gesundheitsdienst, Vol. 26 (1964), 73-80.

[102]John Francis, "The Work of the British Royal Commission on Tuberculosis, 1901-1911," Tubercle, Vol. 40 (1959), 127.

[103]R.W. Philip, A Thousand Cases of Tuberculosis with Etiological and Therapeutic Considerations (Edinburgh, 1892), p. 10.

[104]Hermann Brehmer, Die Chronische Lungenschwindsucht und Tuberkulose der Lunge, 2nd ed. (Berlin, 1869), p. 33.

[105]Philip, A Thousand, p. 11.

[106]Philip, Collected Papers, pp. 356-66.

[107]Bushnell, A Study, p. 16.

[108]Knapp, Europe, pp. 178-81.

Chapter 6: Influenza

[1]Georg F. Most, Influenza Europaea oder die Grösseste Krankheits-Epidemie der neuern Zeit (Hamburg, 1820), p. 64; and R.S. Roberts, "A Consideration of the Nature of the English Sweating Sickness," Medical History, Vol. 9 (1965), 385-86.

[2]P.L. Mondani, "L'Influenza dal Punto di Vista Storico," Scientia Veterum, Vol. 129 (1968), 123.

[3]F.B. Alexandrov, "O Tsiklichnosti Épidemicheskogo Protsessa pri Grippe v Sviazi s Periodichnost' iu Solnechnoi Deiatel'nosti," Zhurnal Mikrobiologii, Epidemiologii i Immunobiologii, Vol. 43 (1966), 127.

[4]Otto Leichtenstern, Influenza und Dengue (Vienna, 1896), pp. 5-6.

[5]Quoted in Hans Zinsser, "The Etiology and Epidemiology of Influenza," Medicine, Vol. I (1922), 215-16.

[6]Quoted in Archibold W. Sloan "The Sweating Sickness in England," South African Medical Journal, Vol. 45 (1971), 473.

[7]John Caius, A Boke or Counseill against the Disease called the Sweate (London, 1552), folio 9.

[8]Caius, A Boke, folio 14; and J.F.C. Hecker, Der englische Schweiss (Berlin, 1834), p. 1.

[9]Arpad G. Gester, "What was the English Sweating Sickness or Sudor Anglicus of the Fifteenth and Sixteenth Centuries?" Johns Hopkins Hospital Bulletin, Vol. 27 (1916), 332-33.

[10]Quoted in E. Symes Thompson, Influenza or Epidemic Catarrhal Fever: An Historical Survey of Past Epidemics in Great Britain from 1510 to 1890 (London, 1890), p. 3.

[11]J. Brossollet, "Expansion Européenne de la Suette Anglaise," International Congress of the History of Medicine, Proceedings, Vol. 23, (1974), 595.

[12]Haeser, Lehrbuch der Geschichte, Vol. III, pp. 328-29.

[13]Adam Patrick, "A Consideration of the Nature of the English Sweating Sickness," Medical History, Vol. 9 (1965), 274.

[14]Roberts, "A Consideration," 386.

[15]Quoted in Hirsch, Handbook, Vol. I, pp. 83-84.

[16]Patrick, "A Consideration," 272.

[17]Quoted in Maurice B. Strauss, "A Hypothesis as to the Mechanism of Fulminant Course and Death in the Sweating Sickness," Journal of the History of Medicine, Vol. 28 (1973), 49.

[18]F.G. Crookshank, "The Trousse-galants of 1528-29 and 1545-45," Royal Society of Medicine Proceedings, Vol. 15 (1921-1922), 33.

[19]Quoted in Theophilus Thompson (ed.), Annals of Influenza or Epidemic Catarrh Fever in Great Britain from 1510 to 1837 (London, 1852), p. 9.

[20]Warren T. Vaughan, Influenza: An Epidemiological Study (Baltimore, 1921), p. 19.

[21]Zinsser, "The Etiology," 215.

[22]Stevenson, "New Diseases," 8.

[23]Thompson, Annals of Influenza, p. 23.

[24]Quoted in Charles Creighton, A History of Epidemics in Britain, 2 vols., 2nd ed. (London, 1965), Vol. II, p. 338.

[25]Creighton, A History, Vol. II, pp. 339-40.

[26]Marco C. Nannini, "L.A. Muratori Cronista della Febbre Influenzale a Capri Nell'Anno 1773," Pagine di Storia della Medicina, Vol. 14 (1970), 65.

[27]Rousset, "Les Épidémies," 164-65.

[28]Brossollet, "Expansion," 596.

355

[29]M. Saillant, Tableau Historique et Raisonné des Épidémies Catharrales Vulgairement dites La Grippe (Paris, 1780), pp. 70-71.

[30]Most, Influenza Europaea, p. 68.

[31]Brossollet, "Expansion," 597.

[32]Wilson Smith, C.H. Andrewes and P.O. Laidlow, "A Virus Obtained from Influenza Patients," Lancet, Vol. 225 (1933), 66-68.

[33]Thomas P. Magill, "A Virus from Cases of Influenza-like Upper-respiratory Infection," Society for Experimental Biology and Medicine, Vol. 45 (1940), 162-164. See also, Thomas Francis, "New Type of Virus from Epidemic Influenza," Science, Vol. 92 (1940), 405-9.

[34]Benenson, Control, p. 160.

[35]Cooray, "Epidemics," 93.

[36]Paul Brown, D. Carleton Gajdusek and J. Anthony Morris, "Virus of the 1918 Influenza Pandemic Era: New Evidence about Its Antigenic Character," Science, Vol. 166 (1969), 117-19.

[37]J.C. McDonald, "Asian Influenza in Great Britain 1957-58," Proceedings of the Royal Society of Medicine, Vol. 51 (1958), 36.

[38]J. Pesek and J. Vobecky, "Attempt to Apply the Results of Serological Surveys in Epidemiological Practice in Influenza," Journal of Hygiene, Epidemiology, Microbiology and Immunobiology, Vol. 8 (1964), 34-35.

[39]Charles H. Stuart-Harris, "Pandemic Influenza: An Unresolved Problem in Prevention," Journal of Infectious Diseases, Vol. 122 (1970), 108.

[40]L. Gaillard, La Grippe (Paris, 1898), pp. 5-6.

[41]Stuart-Harris, "Pandemic Influenza," 110.

[42]Ernst von Feuchtersleben, Mundirte Manuscripte, Unpublished Manuscript No. 2355 - Wellcome Institute for the History of Medicine (Vienna, 1845), pp. 1-3; and Franz Seitz, Catarrh und Influenza: Eine medizinische Studie (Munich, 1865), p. 103.

[43]Gaillard, La Grippe, pp. 5-6.

[44]Thomas B. Peacock, On the Influenza or Epidemic Catarrhal Fever of 1847-8 (London, 1848), 27.

[45]Gale, Epidemic Disease, pp. 47-48.

[46]Arthur Newsholme, "Discussion on Influenza," Royal Society of Medicine Proceedings, Vol. 12 (1918), 2-4.

[47]Local Government Report on the Epidemic of 1889-90 (London, 1891), p. 1.

[48]F.A. Dixey, Epidemic Influenza: A Study in Comparative Statistics (Oxford, 1892), pp. 5-10, 13.

[49]John W. Moore, The Influenza Epidemic of 1889-90 as Observed in Dublin (Dublin, 1890), p. 11.

[50]Julius Althaus, Influenza: Its Pathology, Symptoms, Complications and Sequels (London, 1892), p. 79.

[51]Local Government, Further Report and Papers on Epidemic Influenza, 1889-92 (London, 1893), p. 12.

[52]Thomson, "Change in Epidemiology," 835.

[53]Dixey, Epidemic Influenza, p. 24.

[54]Newsholme, "Discussion," 4.

[55]Edinburgh Hospital Reports (Edinburgh, 1893), p. 147.

[56]Edwin O. Jordan, Epidemic Influenza: A Survey (Chicago, 1927), p. 11.

[57]Livesey, "Epidemics!" 5.

[58]R. Pfeiffer and M. Beck, "Weitere Mittheilungen über den Erreger der Influenza," Deutsche Medicinische Wochenschrift, Vol. 18 (1892), 465-67.

[59]Adolphe Abrahams, "Influenza: Some Clinical and Therapeutic Considerations," in Francis G. Crookshank (ed.) Influenza (London, 1922), pp. 314-15.

[60]Alfred W. Crosby, Jr., Epidemic and Peace, 1918 (Westport, 1976), pp. 25-26, 159, 181-82.

[61]Jose W. Tobias, <u>La Epidemia de Grippe de 1918-19</u> (Buenos Aires, 1920), p. 6.

[62]<u>London Times</u>, October 14, 1918, p. 15.

[63]Crosby, <u>Epidemic</u>, p. 5.

[64]Quoted in Crosby, <u>Epidemic</u>, p. 27.

[65]Quoted in Richard Collier, <u>The Plague of the Spanish Lady: The Influenza Pandemic of 1918-19</u> (London, 1974), p. 111.

[66]Zinsser, "The Etiology," 223.

[67]Abrahams, "Influenza," 321-22.

[68]Adolph A. Hoehling, <u>The Great Epidemic</u> (Boston, 1961), p. 104.

[69]Crosby, <u>Epidemic</u>, p. 159.

[70]Marguerite Aitoff, "Quelques Observations sur L'Étiologie de la Maladie Espagnole," <u>Société de Biologie et des ses Filiales: Comptes Rendus Hebdomaires des Séances et Memoires</u>, Vol. 81 (1918), 974.

[71]J.J. Keegan, "The Prevailing Epidemic of Influenza," <u>American Medical Association Journal</u>, Vol. 71 (1918), 1051.

[72]Harlow Brooks and Curtenius Gillette, "The Argonne Influenza Epidemic," <u>International Record of Medicine</u>, Vol. 100 (1919), 925.

[73]Quoted in Gladys Morton, "The Pandemic Influenza of 1918," <u>Canadian Nurse</u>, Vol. 69 (1973), 25.

[74]E. Seligmann and G. Wolff, "Die Influenzapandemie in Berlin," <u>Zeitschrift für Hygiene</u>, Vol. 101 (1924), 163.

[75]M. Bettex, "La Grippe de 1918 à La Tour-de-Peilz," <u>Revue Médicale de la Suisse Romande</u>, Vol. 87 (1967), 836.

[76]Stuart-Harris, "Influenza," p. 77.

[77]<u>Weekly Return of Births and Deaths Registered: -London and Ninety-Five Other Great Towns</u> (London, 1918), 680; <u>Weekly Return of Births and Deaths Registered: -London and Ninety-Five Other Great Towns</u> (London, 1919), p. 105.

358

[78]Z. Deutschman, "Trend of Influenza Mortality During the Period 1920-51," World Health Organization Bulletin, Vol. 8 (1953), 638.

[79]Stuart-Harris, "Influenza," p. 76.

[80]Renseignements Épidémiologiques: Statistique des Maladies à Declaration Obligatoire (League of Nations, Geneva, 1923), pp. 39-42.

[81]Influenza Epidemic of 1926-27, and Action Taken by the Health Section in Connection Therewith (League of Nations, Geneva, 1927), pp. 4-5.

[82]Chester A. Darling, "The Epidemiology and Bacteriology of Influenza," American Journal of Public Health, Vol. 8 (1918), 751.

[83]Robert Donaldson, "The Bacteriology of Influenza: With Special Reference to Pfeiffer's Bacillus," in Crookshank, Influenza, pp. 143-154.

[84]Francis G. Crookshank, Epidemiological Essay (London, 1930), p. 48.

[85]F. Trémolières and M. Rafinesque, "Sur L'Épidémie de Grippe," La Presse Médicale, Vol. 27 (1919), 98-101.

[86]Epidemiological Report of the Health Section of the Secretariat (May-June, 1933), (League of Nations, Geneva, 1934), pp. 127-28.

[87]Francis G. Crookshank, "Some Historical Aspects of Influenza," in Crookshank, Influenza, pp. 31-63.

[88]Jane E. Brody, "Influenza Virus Continues to Keep Scientists Guessing," The New York Times, July 23, 1976, p. A22.

[89]Cockburn, The Evolution, p. 241.

[90]V.M. Zdanov and I.V. Antonova, "The Hong Kong Influenza Virus Epidemic in the USSR," Bulletin of the World Health Organization, Vol. 41 (1969), 381.

[91]W.K. Chang, "National Influenza Experience in Hong Kong, 1968," Bulletin of the World Health Organization, Vol. 41 (1969), 349.

[92]Stuart-Harris, "Influenza," pp. 80-82.

Part Two: The Consequences

[1]Ariès, Western Attitudes, pp. 103-4.

[2]G.A. Wehrli, "Das Wesen der Volksmedizin und die Notwendigkeit einer Geschichtlichen Betrachtungsweise Derselben," in Charles Singer and Henry E. Sigerist (eds.), Essays on the History of Medicine (London, 1924), pp. 369-81.

[3]John P. Dolan, "Jerome Fracastoro, Physician, Philosopher and Poet," South Carolina Medical Association Journal, Vol. 38 (1972), 455-57.

[4]G.L. Hendrickson, "The Syphilis of Girolamo Fracastoro," Bulletin of the Institute of the History of Medicine, Vol. II (1934), 516-17.

[5]Burnet and White, Natural History, p. 70.

Chapter 7: Popular Attitudes and Accepted Cures

[1]Langer, "The Black Death," 114.

[2]Mullett, The Bubonic Plague, p. 40.

[3]Ariès, Western Attitudes, pp. 103-4.

[4]Sheppard, London, p. 247.

[5]Hecker, The Black Death, pp. 104-5.

[6]Shrewsbury, A History of Bubonic Plague, p. 5.

[7]Kowal, "Danilo Samoilowitz," 437.

[8]McGrew, Russia, pp. 10-11; and Longmate, King Cholera, p. 4.

[9]Robert Hoeniger, Der Schwarze Tod in Deutschland (Berlin, 1882), p. 50.

[10]Raymond Crawford, Plague and Pestilence in Literature and Art (Oxford, 1914), p. 125.

[11]Peter Burke (ed.) Economy and Society in Early Modern Europe (New York, 1972), p. 2.

[12]N. Zaprjanov, "Smallpox and Variolisation in the Populations on Bulgarian Soil," Folia Medica, Vol. 9 (1967), 300.

[13]Gaselee, Practical Treatise, p. 6.

[14]Shapter, The History, p. 115.

[15]Henschen, The History, p. 54.

[16]Hodges, Loimologia, p. 21.

[17]Diosi, "Aufzeichnungen," 222.

[18]Charles E. Rosenberg, "Cholera in Nineteenth-Century Europe: A Tool for Social and Economic Analysis," Comparative Studies in History and Society, Vol. 8 (1965-66), 454-55.

[19]Ackerknecht, History and Geography, p. 17.

[20]Cowrie, Plague and Fire, pp. 28-29.

[21]Jordanus, Luis Novae, p. 3.

[22]Quoted in Thomas, "Daniel Defoe," 107.

[23]Hille and Ehler, "Zum medizinischen Wissen," 1697.

[24]Quoted in F.P. Wilson, The Plague in Shakespeare's London (Oxford, 1927), p. 45.

[25]G. Serison, La Tuberculose Considerée comme Maladie du Peuple (Paris, 1902), pp. 15-21.

[26]Geigel, Geschichte, p. 4.

361

[27]Hodges, Loimologia, p. 19; and Leon Bernard, The Emerging City: Paris in the Age of Louis XIV (Durham, 1970), p. 211.

[28]R.S. Morton, "St. Denis Patron Saint of Syphilitics," British Journal of Venereal Diseases, Vol. 37 (1961), 286.

[29]Poulet, "L'Épidémie," 3488.

[30]Dubled, "Les Épidémies," 22.

[31]Hemphill, "Society, Artists and Plague," 2.

[32]Fielding H. Garrison, "The New Epidemiology," in Singer and Sigerist, Essays, p. 256.

[33]Antero di San Bonaventura, Li Lazareti della Citta e Riviere di Genova (Genoa, 1658), p. 268.

[34]Logan Clending, "The Plague Saints," Bulletin of the Society of Medical History of Chicago, Vol. IV (1930), 134-35.

[35]McGrew, Russia, p. 97.

[36]Jeanselme, Histoire, p. 104; and Major, A History, Vol. I, p. 368.

[37]Hirst, The Conquest of Plague, p. 24.

[38]Quoted in Chevalier, Laboring Classes, p. 334.

[39]Trüb, Posch and Richter, "Historische Studie," 119-20.

[40]Preuner, "Epidemien im Wandel," 1.

[41]Rowley, Cowpox, p. 6.

[42]Friedrich Flückinger and Daniel Hanbury, Pharmacographie: A History of the Principal Drugs of Vegetable Origin (London, 1874), pp. 685-704.

[43]Wehrli, "Das Wesen der Volksmedizin," pp. 370-81.

[44]Fracastorii, Syphilis, Book II, lines 165, 167-69.

[45]Hendrick Halmael, Accounts for Medicine, Unpublished Manuscript No. 328 - Wellcome Institute for the History of Medicine (n.p., 1618), pp. 1-3.

⁴⁶McDonald, "The History of Quarantine," 29; and Hughes, "The Plague in Carlisle," 54.

⁴⁷Hughes, "The Plague in Carlisle," 56.

⁴⁸Thomas Vicary, The English Mans Treasure, or Treasor for Englishmen: With the True Anatomy for Mans Body (London, 1586), p. 7.

⁴⁹The Kings Medicines for the Plague, Prefcribed for the Yeare 1604, by the Whole College of Physiticians (London, 1636), p. 2A.

⁵⁰Quoted in E.A. Hammond and Claude E. Sturgill, "A French Plague Recipe of 1720," Bulletin of the History of Medicine, Vol. 46 (1972), 594.

⁵¹John Andree, Observations on the Theory and Cure of the Venereal Disease (London, 1799), p. 24.

⁵²Andree, Observations, p. 25.

⁵³Lazerme, Historia, p. 4.

⁵⁴Sudhoff, "The Origin of Syphilis," 20; and Power, "The Venereal Diseases," 42.

⁵⁵Crosby, The Columbian Exchange, pp. 153-54.

⁵⁶Abraham, "The Early History of Syphilis," 230.

⁵⁷Fracastorii, Syphilis, Book II, lines 270-71.

⁵⁸Power, "The Venereal Diseases," pp. 43-44.

⁵⁹Astruc, A Treatise, Vol. I, p. 282.

⁶⁰Mildner, "Durch Jahrhunderte," 342-43.

⁶¹Quoted in Robert S. Munger, "Guaiacum, the Holy Wood from the New World," Journal of the History of Medicine and Allied Sciences, Vol. 4 (1949), 200.

⁶²Hütten, De Morbo Gallico, p. 13.

⁶³Paré, Traitant, Vol. II, p. 535.

[64]Munger, "Guaiacum," 196-229.

[65]Arnold H. Rowbotham, "The Philosophes and the Propaganda for Inoculation of Smallpox in Eighteenth Century France," University of California Publications in Modern Philology, Vol. 18 (1935), 265, 279.

[66]Laubstein, "Über einen früher Geübten," 313.

[67]C. Canby Robinson, "The Therapeutic Use of Digitalis," Medicine, Vol. I (1922), pp. 4-17 and 42-50.

[68]Douglas Guthrie, Janus in the Doorway (London, 1963), p. 231.

[69]Quoted in Kenneth D. Keele, "The Sydenham-Boyle Theory of Morbific Particles," Medical History, Vol. 18 (1974), 243.

[70]Stevenson, "New Diseases," 12.

[71]Keele, "The Sydenham-Boyle Theory," 243.

[72]A. Dodin and J. Brossollet, "Thérapeutiques au Cours de Épidémie de Choléra de 1832," Bulletin de la Société de Pathologie Exotique, Vol. 64 (1971), 617-18; and Norman Howard-Jones, "Cholera Therapy in the Nineteenth Century," Journal of the History of Medicine and Allied Sciences, Vol. 27 (1972), 374-82.

[73]McGrew, "The First Russian Cholera," 229.

[74]Parkes, Researches, 208.

[75]Howard-Jones, "Cholera Theory," 380.

[76]Hervé Glorennec, "Le Choléra de 1832 à Quimper," Société Archeologique du Finistère Bulletin, Vol. 96 (1970), 244.

[77]McDonald, "The History of Quarantine," 29.

[78]McGrew, "The First Russian Cholera," 229-30.

[79]Howard-Jones, "Cholera Therapy," 383.

[80]Quoted in Howard-Jones, "Cholera Therapy," 381.

[81]George Gregory, Elements of the Practice of Medicine, 6th ed. (London, 1846), 460.

[82]Gregory, Elements, p. 460.

[83]Flick, Development, pp. 256, 285-86.

[84]B.J. Bishop, "Thomas Young," 161; and Louis Perret, "Retrospective Aspects of Pulmonary Tuberculosis in Finland," Scandinavian Journal of Respiratory Diseases, Supplement, Vol. 65 (1968), 84.

[85]Brown, The Story, pp. 54-55.

[86]The Year-Book of Treatment for 1899 (London, 1899), p. 57.

[87]Fraser, Tuberculosis, p. 7.

[88]Ehrlich, "Das Laboratoriumsversuche," 637-38.

[89]Fildes and Parnell, "An Investigation," pp. 32-36, 68.

[90]A.W. Hewlett and W.M. Alberty, "Influenza at Navy Base Hospital in France," American Medical Association Journal, Vol. 71 (1918), 1057-58.

[91]Brooks and Gillette, "The Argonne Influenza," 929.

[92]Devonshire Hospital and Buxton Bath Charity Annual Report for the Year 1878 (Buxton, 1879), p. 1.

[93]Cartwright and Biddiss, Disease and History, pp. 56-57.

[94]Hornick, "The Broad Street Pump," 1184-1185.

[95]E.I. Grin and T. Guthe, "Evaluation of a Previous Mass Campaign against Endemic Syphilis in Bosnia and Herzegovina," British Journal of Venereal Diseases, Vol. 49 (1973), 1.

[96]Dionne and Gougoux, "Notions Toujours," 1334-35; and Wherrett, "Tuberculosis," 185-86.

[97]Knapp, Europe, pp. 178-81.

[98]Rowley, Cowpox, p. 6.

[99]Wherrett, "Tuberculosis," 183.

[100]Wherrett, "Tuberculosis," 183-84.

Chapter 8: Medical Opinion

[1]Esmond R. Long, A History of Pathology, Revised ed. (New York, 1965), pp. 31-72.

[2]Oswei Temkin, "An Historical Analysis of the Concept of Infection," in Johns Hopkins University History of Ideas Club: Studies in Intellectual History (New York, 1968), pp. 126-27.

[3]Quoted in Major, A History of Medicine, Vol. I, p. 368.

[4]Richard Kephale, Medela Pestilentiae: Theological Queries Concerning the Plague (London, 1665), p. 3.

[5]Edmund Massey, A Sermon Against the Dangerous and Sinful Practice of Innoculation, 2nd ed. (London, 1772), p. 15.

[6]Thomson, "Change in Epidemiology," 831.

[7]L. Fabian Hirst, The Conquest of Plague (Oxford, 1953), p. 25.

[8]Hudson, "Villalobos," 582.

[9]Quoted in Hirst, The Conquest, p. 26.

[10]Temkin, "An Historical Analysis," 127.

[11]Sloan, "Medical and Social Aspects," 270.

[12]Fracastorii, Syphilis, Book I, lines 123-24.

[13]Skeyne, Ane Breve Descriptioun, p. 4.

[14]Haygarth, An Inquiry, pp. 19-20.

[15]Keir, Practical Observations, p. 3.

[16]Clowes, A Briefe and Necessarie Treatise, p. 4.

[17]Dieter Wagner, "Zeitgenössische Darstellungen zur Ätiologie-Auffassung von Infektionskrankheiten im 18. Jahrhundert," Beiträge zur Geschichte der Universität Erfurt, Vol. 14 (1968-69), 83-89.

[18]Caius, A Boke or Counseill, folio 15.

[19]Astruc, Dissertation, p. 98.

[20]R.S. Roberts, "Epidemics and Social History," Medical History, Vol. 12 (1968), 307.

[21]De Villalobos, Sur les Contagieuses, p. 47.

[22]Lobb, Letters, pp. 4-5.

[23]Quoted in Wilson, The Plague, p. 5.

[24]Kemp, A Brief Treatise, p. 46.

[25]August Hirsch, Ueber die Verhütung und Bekämpfung der Volkskrankheiten mit specieller Beziehung auf die Cholera (Berlin, 1875), p. 5.

[26]Greaves, Morbus Epidemius, p. 16.

[27]Quoted in Keele, "The Sydenham-Boyle Theory," 241.

[28]Swan, The Entire Works, p. 109.

[29]Edna H. Lemay, "Thomas Hérier, A Country Surgeon Outside Angoulême at the End of the XVIIIth Century: A Contribution to Social History," Journal of Social History, Vol. 10 (1977), 528.

[30]Howard-Jones, "Cholera Therapy," 373.

[31]On this point, see Alexander, "Plague in Russia," 526-27.

[32]Quoted in William Bullock, The History of Bacteriology (Oxford, 1960), p. 11.

[33]Erwin A. Ackerknecht, A Short History of Medicine (New York, 1955), p. 162.

[34]Quoted in Charles-Edward Winslow, The Conquest of Epidemic Disease: A Chapter in the History of Ideas (Princeton, 1943), p. 147.

[35]Winslow, The Conquest, p. 157.

[36]Scott, Some Notable Epidemics, p. 3.

[37] Morton, Phthisiologia, p. 2.

[38] Henry Gaulter, The Origin and Progress of the Malignant Cholera in Manchester (London, 1833), p. 127.

[39] Quoted in Richard C. Holcomb, Who Gave the World Syphilis? (New York, 1937), p. 105.

[40] See, for example, Clowes, A Briefe and Necessarie Treatise, p. 4; and Alexander, "Plague in Russia," 526-27.

[41] Douglas Guthrie, A History of Medicine (Philadelphia, 1946), p. 204.

[42] Long, A History, p. 51.

[43] Baglivi, Opera Omnia, p. 51.

[44] R. S. Morton, Venereal Diseases (London, 1966), p. 21.

[45] Bloch, "History of Syphilis," pp. 32-33.

[46] Custom, "Historical Notes," 465-69.

[47] Philip H. Clendenning, "Dr. Thomas Dimsdale and Smallpox Inoculation in Russia," Journal of the History of Medicine and Allied Sciences, Vol. 28 (1973), 109-10.

[48] H. J. Parish, Victory With Vaccines (Edinburgh, 1968), p. 9.

[49] W. R. Le Fanu, A Bio-Bibliography of Edward Jenner (London, 1951), p. 58; and Erna Lesky, Die Wiener Medizinische Schule im 19. Jahrhundert (Graz, 1965), pp. 28-29.

[50] Maurice Bariéty and Charles Coury, Histoire de la Médicine (Paris, 1963), p. 653.

[51] Wingate, Medical Encyclopedia, pp. 345-46.

[52] Ackerknecht, A Short History, pp. 162-63.

[53] Winslow, The Conquest, p. 182.

[54] Erwin A. Ackerknecht, "Anticontagionism Between 1821 and 1867," Bulletin of the History of Medicine, Vol. 22 (1948), 562-63.

[55]Villemin, "De La Virulence," 1012-15.

[56]Ackerknecht, A Short History, pp. 164-66.

[57]Arturo Castiglioni, A History of Medicine (New York, 1958), pp. 735-36.

[58]Rosenberg, "Cholera," 455.

[59]Brown, "John Snow," 650.

[60]Quoted in Hirshhorn and Greenough, "Cholera," 15.

[61]Bruce S. Shoenberg, "Snow on the Water of London," Mayo Clinic Proceedings, Vol. 49 (1974), 681.

[62]Hornick, "The Broad Street Pump," 1181.

[63]Max von Pettenkofer, "Boden und Grundwasser in ihren Beziehungen zu Cholera und Typhus," Zeitschrift für Biologie, Vol. 5 (1869), 171.

[64]McGrew, "The First Russian Cholera," 228.

[65]Howard-Jones, "Choleranomalies," 422; and Rosenberg, "Cholera," 455.

[66]Baly and Gull, Reports, p. 16.

[67]Fifteenth Annual Report of The Local Government Board 1885-86; Supplement Containing Reports and Papers on Cholera Submitted by the Board's Medical Officer (London, 1886), p. xvi.

[68]Briggs, "Cholera and Society," 78.

[69]Bayle, Recherches, p. 393.

[70]C.J.B. Williams and Charles T. Williams, Pulmonary Consumption: Its Nature, Varaties, and Treatment (London, 1871), pp. 110-11.

[71]Quoted in Bushnell, A Study, p. 1.

[72]Dubos, The White Plague, pp. 69-70.

[73]Jean-Antoine Villemin, De la Virulence et de la Specificité de la Tuberculose (Paris, 1868), pp. 3-32.

[74]Villemin, "De la Virulence," 537-38.

[75]Koch, "Die Aetiologie," 221.

[76]P.J. Bishop, "The Brompton Hospital and Its First Medical Report," Tubercle, Vol. 48 (1967), 353.

[77]Paul Röthlisberger, "Der Zürcher Arzt Conrad Meyer-Ahrens (1813-1872) -- Medizinhistoriker, Epidemiologie und Balneograph," Gesnerus, Vol. 30 (1973), 131-32.

[78]Huldrych M. Koebling, "Alexander Spengler als Tuberkulose-Arzt und Klimatotherapeut." Gesnerus, Vol. 23 (1966) 79-82.

[79]Koch, "Ueber neue Tuberkulinpräparate," 209-13.

[80]Robert Koch, "Weitere Mittheilungen über ein Heilmittel gegen Tuberculose," Deutsche Medicinische Wochenschrift, Vol. 16 (1890), 1029; and Richard Bochalli, Robert Koch: Der Schöpfer der Modernen Bakteriologie (Stuttgart, 1954), pp. 84-85.

[81]Junker, "Tuberkulinreiheuntersuchungen," 228-29.

[82]J. Edward Squire, The Hygienic Prevention of Consumption (London, 1893), p. 21, 93-94; Noel D. Bardswell and John C. Chapman, Diets in Tuberculosis: Principles and Economics (London, 1908), 58-59; and W. Löffler, "Tuberkulose und Tuberkulosebekämpfung im Wandel der Zeiten," Schweizerische Medizinische Wochenschrift, Vol. 100 (1970), 1790.

[83]Squire, The Hygienic Prevention, p. 21.

[84]K. Lydtin, "In Memoriam Bruno Lange--1885 bis 1942," Praxis der Pneumologie, Vol. 21 (1967), 723-27.

[85]Hillier, Tuberculosis, p. 10.

[86]Carl Spengler, Tuberculose-und Syphlisarbeiten (Davos, 1911), p. ix.

[87]A. Calmette and C. Guérin, "Origine Intestinale de La Tuberculose Pulmonaire et Mécanisme de L'Infection Tuberculeuse," Annals de L'Institut Pasteur, Vol. 20 (1906), 613.

[88]Williams, Requiem, pp. 55-56.

[89]Quoted in Weill-Hallé, "Étude Clinique," 1607.

[90]Ehrlich, "Über Laboratoriumsversuche," 637; and Paul Ehrlich, Beiträge zur Experimentellen Pathologie und Chemotherapie (Leipzig, 1909), p. 47.

[91]Waksman, The Conquest, p. 121.

[92]Smith, "A Virus," 65-66; and Magill, "A Virus," 162-64.

[93]Francis, "The Type of Virus," 405-9.

Chapter 9: Public Health Measures

[1]W.M. Frazer, A History of English Public Health, 1834-1939 (London, 1950), pp. 1-2; and Kreuser, "70 Jahre," 1172-73.

[2]Ackerknecht, History and Georgaphy, p. 171.

[3]Quoted in Hille and Ehler, "Zum medizinischen Wissen," 1697.

[4]Garrison, "The New Epidemiology," 257.

[5]Quoted in S. Simpson, "Notices of the Appearance of Syphilis in Scotland in the Last Years of the Fifteenth Century," Lancet, November 24, 1860, 513.

[6]Sudhoff, "The End of the Fable," 24.

[7]Dieter Jetter, "Erwägungen beim Bau französischer Pesthäuser," Archives Internationales d'Histoire de Sciences, Vol. 19 (1966), 247.

[8]Hemphill, "Society, Artists and the Plague," 2.

[9]Quoted in Cipolla, Cristofano and the Plague, p. 27.

[10]Sudhoff, "The Origin of Syphilis," 19.

[11]Munger, "Guaiacum," 209.

[12]Comrie, Scottish History of Medicine, Vol. 1, p. 200.

[13]Mullett, The Bubonic Plague, p. 90.

[14]Ziegler, The Black Death, p. 53.

[15]Quoted in Wilson, The Plague, p. 45.

[16]Dieter Jetter, "Das Isolierungsprinzip in der Pestkämpfung des 17. Jahrhunderts," Medizinhistorisches Journal, Vol. 5 (1970), 115-16.

[17]Cipolla, Cristofano and the Plague, p. 27.

[18]Howard, An Account, p. 4.

[19]Ballester and Benitz, "Aproximacion a la Historia," 320.

[20]Jarcho, "Yello Fever, Cholera," 131-32.

[21]Gunther E. Rothenberg, "The Austrian Sanitary Cordon and the Control of the Bubonic Plague: 1710-1871," Journal of the History of Medicine, Vol. 28 (1973), 15-20; and Erna Lesky, "Die österreichische Pestfront an der k.k. Militärgrenze," Saeculum, Vol. 8 (1957), 89 and 93-94.

[22]Longmate, King Cholera, pp. 3-4.

[23]Alex Berman, "The Scientific Tradition in French Hospital Pharmacy," American Journal of Hospital Pharmacy, Vol. 18 (1961), 110; and Guillaume Valette, "Évolution du Rôle de L'Internat en Pharmacie dans les Hôpitaux de Paris depius un Siècle," Revue de l'Assistance Publique à Paris (1954), 395-96.

[24]Imhof, "The Hospital," 451; and Marcel Fosseyeux, "Histoire de l'Hospitalisation des Maladies en France," in Maxine Laignel-Lavastine, Histoire Générale de la Médicine, de la Pharmacie, de l'Art Dentaire et de l'Art Vétérinaire (Paris, 1949), 681-82.

[25]Dora A. Weiner, "The French Revolution, Napoleon, and the Nursing Profession," Bulletin of the History of Medicine, Vol. 46 (1972), 274-305.

[26]Marcel Candille, "Évolution des Principes d'Assistance Hospitalière," Revue de l'Assistance Publique à Paris, Vol. 9 (1958), 43-51.

[27]George Rosen, "Society and Medical Care: An Historical Analysis," McGill Medical Journal, Vol. 17 (1948), 414.

[28]McNeill, Plagues and Peoples, p. 253.

[29]Dimsdale, The Present Method, pp. 61-62.

[30]Klebs, "The Historic Evolution," 76.

[31]Quoted in Koebling, "Edward Jenner," 40.

[32]Rousset, "Les Épidémies," 160; and Möller, "Die Pockenimpfung," 619-20.

[33]Razzell, "Population Change," 313.

[34]F. Dawtrey Drewitt, The Life of Edward Jenner, 2nd ed. (London, 1933), p. 69; and Heinrich A. Gins, Krankheit wider den Tod: Schicksal der Pockenschutzimpfung (Stuttgart, 1963), p. 10.

[35]Dorothy Fisk, Dr. Jenner of Berkeley (London, 1959), pp. 156-61.

[36]Razzell, "Population Change," 317-21.

[37]Quoted in Chevalier, Laboring Classes, p. 334.

[38]Quoted in Chevalier, Laboring Classes, p. 334.

[39]Leonello Manzi and Pietro Ascanelli, "Vaiolo e Vaccinazione a Bologna dal 1815 al 1860," Bulletino delle Scienze Mediche, Vol. 140 (1968), 234-35, 258.

[40]Ross, "Leicester," 39.

[41]W. Fröbelius, "Eine geschichtliche Notiz über die Vaccination im St. Petersburger Findelhause," St. Petersburger Medicinische Zeitschrift, Vol. 16 (1869), 2.

[42]Guy, "Two Hundred," 419.

[43]Rose, "Leicester," 39.

[44]Quoted in Gale, Epidemic Disease, p. 61.

[45]R.M. MacLeod, "Law, Medicine and Public Opinion: The Resistance to Compulsory Health Legislation 1870-1907," Public Law (1967), 110.

[46]Archives of the Public Health Laboratory of the University of Manchester (Manchester, 1906), p. 125.

[47]MacNalty, "The Prevention," 12.

[48]Lawton and Surgalla, "Immunization," 39-42; Y. Biraud, État Actuel de La Vaccination Contre Le Typhus Exanthematique Epidemique à Poux (League of Nations Committee on Hygiene, Geneva, 1939), pp. 1-2; and Albert Calmette, Tubercle Bacillus Infection and Tuberculosis in Man and Animals, trans. by William S. Soper (Baltimore, 1923), p. 172.

[49]L. Lugosi, "La Vaccination par Le BCG à 50 Ans," Annals de Pédiatrie, Vol. 109 (1972), 9693-97.

[50]Waksman, The Conquest, p. 208.

[51]Le Borgne, Recherches Historiques, p. 97.

[52]Henry E. Sigerist, Grosse Ärzte: Eine Geschichte der Heilkunde in Lebensbildern (Munich, 1931), p. 251.

[53]Singer and Underwood, A Short History, pp. 213-16.

[54]Quoted in Carlo M. Cipolla, Public Health and the Medical Profession in the Renaissance (Cambridge, 1976), p. 17.

[55]Cipolla, Public Health, p. 18.

[56]Fosseyeux, "Les Épidémies," 117.

[57]Werner Piechocki, "Die Anfänge des Halleschen Stadtphysikats," Acta Historica Leopoldina, Vol. 2 (1965), 8-11.

[58]George Rosen, "Cameralism and the Concept of Medical Police," Bulletin of the History of Medicine, Vol. 27 (1953), 30-31.

[59]Caroline C. Hannaway, "The Société Royale de Médicine and Epidemics in the Ancien Régime," Bulletin of the History of Medicine, Vol. 46 (1972), 257-58.

[60]Rosen, "Cameralism," 39; and Zólyomi, "La Faculté de Medicine," 249-50.

[61]McGrew, "The First Russian Cholera," 234.

[62]Woelderink, "De Cholera," 307-8; and Salchow, "Vor 75 Jahren," 151-52.

[63]Glorrenec, "Le Choléra," 243-44.

[64]Quoted in Shapter, The History, p. 117.

[65]Quoted in Shapter, The History, p. 120.

[66]Pollitzer, "Cholera Studies," 427.

[67]C. Fraser Brockington, Public Health in the Nineteenth Century (Edinburgh, 1965), pp. 136-39.

[68]Kreuser, "70 Jahre," 1172-73.

[69]Altschuler, "Privlechenie Obschschestvennosti," 88-89.

[70]Quoted in Norman Howard-Jones, The Scientific Background to the International Sanitary Conference, 1851-1938 (Geneva, 1975), p. 14.

[71]Quoted in Howard-Jones, The Scientific Background, p. 12.

[72]Howard-Jones, The Scientific Background, pp. 17-87.

[73]Howard-Jones, The Scientific Background, p 93.

[74]Gottfried Frey, Les Services d'Hygiene Publique en Allemagne (League of Nations Committee on Hygiene, Geneva, 1923), pp. 5-6.

[75]M.D. Mackenzie, Rapport Preliminaire sur la Syphilis dans le District de Bourgas, Bulgarie (League of Nations Committee on Hygiene, Geneva, 1930), Appendix 3, pp. 1-2.

[76]N.M. Josephus Jitta, Organisation of the Public Health Services in the Kingdom of the Netherlands (League of Nations Committee on Hygiene, Geneva, 1924), p. 13.

[77]M. Kacprzak, L'Hygiene en Pologne (League of Nations Committee on Hygiene, Geneva, 1933), p. 3; and Alexander de Dobrovits, Public Health Services in Hungary (League of Nations Committee on Hygiene, Geneva, 1925), pp. 38-40.

[78]L'Hygiene Publique en Italie (League of Nations Committee on Hygiene, Geneva, 1928), p. 27.

[79]Biraud, État Actuel, pp. 1-2.

[80]Denis I. Duveen and Herbert S. Klickstein, "Antoine Laurent Lavosier's Contributions to Medical and Public Health," Bulletin of the History of Medicine, Vol. 29 (1955), 164-69.

[81]Olivier Faure, "Physicians in Lyon during the Nineteenth Century: An Extraordinary Social Success," Journal of Social History, Vol. 10 (1977), 511.

[82]Gernez-Rieux and Gervois, "Le Role," 185; and Bishop, "The Brompton Hospital," 344.

[83]Gernez-Rieux and Gervois, "Le Role," 186.

[84]Breu, "Die Geschichte," 37.

[85]C. Langer, "50 Jahre Lungenheilstätte Baumgartner Höhe (1923-1973)," Wiener Medizinische Wochenschrift, Vol. 123 (1973), 758-59.

[86]Quoted in Wallace, "Sir Robert Philip," 61.

[87]Albert Robin, Traitement de la Tuberculose (Paris, 1912), p. 69.

[88]Philip, Collected Papers, p. 69.

[89]Squire, The Hygienic Prevention, p. 101.

[90]Squire, The Hygienic Prevention, p. 101.

[91]Bardswell and Chapman, Diets in Tuberculosis, pp. 58-59; and Squire, The Hygienic Prevention, p. 101.

[92]Revel, "Autour d'une Épidémie," 968.

[93]Knapp, Europe, pp. 47-48.

[94]Jean-Pierre Goubert, "The Extent of Medical Practice in France around 1780," Journal of Social History, Vol. 10 (1977), 410-414.

[95]Rosen, "Society," 414.

[96]Rosen, "Society," 414.

[97]McGrew, Russia, pp. 13-14.

Chapter 10: Demographic and Sociological Consequences

[1]Knapp, Europe, pp. 78-81.

[2]Peter Laslett, The World We Have Lost (New York, 1965), p. 93.

[3]Dufrenoy and Dufrenoy, "Variolisation et Vaccination," 143.

[4]Pierre Goubert, "Recent Theories and Research in French Population between 1500 and 1700," in D.V. Glass and D.E.C. Eversley (eds.), Population in History: Essays in Historical Demography (Chicago, 1965), p. 408; and Braudel, Capitalism, p. 52.

[5]Thomas McKeown and R.G. Brown, "Medical Evidence Related to English Population Changes in the Eighteenth Century," in Glass and Eversley, Population, p. 293.

[6]Knapp, Europe, pp. 179-80.

[7]Goubert, "Recent Theories," 465.

[8]Knapp, Europe, pp. 78-79.

[9]On this point, see Thomas McKeown and R.G. Record, "Reasons for the Decline of Mortality in England and Wales during the Nineteenth Century," Population Studies, Vol. 16 (1962), 94-122.

[10]Burnet and White, Natural History, p. 1; and M.W. Flinn, "The Stabilisation of Mortality in Pre-Industrial Western Europe," The Journal of European Economic History, Vol. 3 (1974), 285-86.

[11]Langer, "The Black Death," 114.

[12]Bowsky, "The Impact, 1-34.

[13]Sivéry, "Le Hainaut," 432-36.

[14]Prat, "Albi et La Peste Noire," 17-18.

[15]Henri Dubled, "Conséquences Économiques et Sociales des Mortalités du XIVe Siècle, Essentiellement en Alsace," Revue d'Histoire Économique et Sociale, Vol. 37 (1959), 284-86.

[16]Ziegler, The Black Death, pp. 235-37.

[17]Bean, "Plague, Population," 432.

[18]Quoted in Ffrangcon Roberts, "The Effects of Epidemics on Population and Social Life," Royal Society of Medicine Proceedings, Vol. 48 (1955), 786.

[19]Carpentier, "Famines et Épidémies," 1065.

[20]Ballester and Benitz, "Aproximacion a la Historia," 325.

[21]Roberts, "The Effects," 786,

[22]Revel, "Autour d'une Épidémie," 979.

[23]Wrigley, Population and History, p. 115.

[24]W.G. Hoskins, "Epidemics in English History," The Listener, December 31, 1964, 1045; and J. Meuvert, "Demographic Crisis in France from the Sixteenth to the Eighteenth Century," in Glass and Eversley, Population, p. 515.

[25]Hoskins, "Epidemics," 1045.

[26]Major Greenwood, Epidemics and Crowd-Diseases (New York, 1935), p. 177.

[27]Riffel, Mittheilungen, pp. 1-164.

[28]Abraham, "The Early History of Syphilis," 228.

[29]Brossollet, "Expansion," 597.

[30]Knapp, Europe, p. 77.

[31]Flinn, "The Stabilisation," 285-318.

[32]John Brownlee, "The History of the Birth and Death Rates in England and Wales Taken as a Whole, from 1570 to the Present Time," Public Heath, Vol. 19 (1916), 211-12.

[33]McKeown and Record, "Reasons," 94-95.

[34]Dixson, Smallpox, pp. 195-96.

[35]Trüb, Posch and Richter, "Historische Studie," 119.

378

[36]Guy, "Two Hundred," 407.

[37]Cartwright and Biddiss, Disease and History, pp. 120-21.

[38]Duvillard, Analyse et Tableaux, p. 169.

[39]Goubert, "Recent Theories," 459.

[40]Jean Meyer, "Une Enquête de l'Academie de Médicine sur les Épidémies," Annales: Économies, Sociétés, Civilisations, Vol. 21 (1966), 286.

[41]J.A. Johnston, "The Impact of the Epidemics of 1727-1730 in South West Worcestershire," Medical History, Vol. 15 (1971), 742.

[42]Rosenthal, "I Consume," 157; and Trail, "Richard Morton," 169.

[43]Batemen, Reports, p. 22.

[44]Rosenthal, "I Consume," 157-58.

[45]Hamburger, Die Tuberkulose, p. 1.

[46]Filip Sylvan, Consumption and Its Cure by Physical Exercise (New York, 1915), p. 41.

[47]Bishop, "The Brompton Hospital," 9.

[48]Calmette, Tubercle Bacillus, pp. 584-85.

[49]Drew, "Cholera," 211; Ackerknecht, History and Geography, p. 26; McGrew, Russia, p. 4; and McGrew, "The First Russian Cholera," 221.

[50]Gerardin and Gaimard, Du Choléra-Morbus, p. 32A; and McGrew, Russia, p. 161.

[51]Olzscha, "Die Epidemiologie," 10.

[52]Augustin Fabre and Fortuné Charlan, Histoire du Choléra-Morbus Asiatique (Marseilles, 1835), p. 353.

[53]Jordan, The Influenza Epidemic, pp. 11 and 19; and Stuart-Harris, "Pandemic Influenza," 110.

[54]Moore, The Influenza Epidemic, p. 11.

[55]Crosby, Epidemic, p. 27.

[56]Riffel, Mittheilungen, pp. 1-164.

[57]Ricord, Traité Pratique, p. 30.

[58]Carlo M. Cipolla, Before the Industrial Revolution: European Society and Economy, 1000-1700 (New York, 1976), pp. 14-18.

[59]F.J. Fisher, "Influenza and Inflation in Tudor England," The Economic History Review, Second Series, Vol. XVIII (1965), 121.

[60]Razzell, "Population Change," 312-32.

[61]Quoted in George Rosen, "What is Social Medicine? A Genetic Analysis of the Concept," Bulletin of the History of Medicine, Vol. 21 (1947), 684.

[62]Bailey, The Mathematical Theory, p. 1.

[63]Sprössig, "Die Erfurter," 171.

[64]Crawford, Plague and Pestilence, p. 134.

[65]Cartwright and Biddiss, Diease and History, p. 53.

[66]G.C. Coulton, The Black Death (London, 1930), p. 37.

[67]Richard W. Emery, "The Black Death of 1348 in Perpignan," Speculum, Vol. 42 (1967), 614.

[68]Mullett, The Bubonic Plague, p. 135.

[69]Carpentier, "Famines et Épidémies," 1069.

[70]Meuvert, "Demographic Crisis," 509.

[71]Fosseyeux, "Les Épidémies," 118; and Bell, The Great Plague, p. 91.

[72]René Baehrel, "La Haine de Classe en Temps d'Épidémie," Annales: Économies, Sociétés, Civilisations, Vol. 7 (1952), 345.

[73]Hugues Neveux, "La Mortalité des Pauvres à Cambrai," Annales Démographie Historique (1968), 73-91.

[74]Comrie, Scottish History of Medicine, Vol. I, p. 203.

[75]Quoted in Braudel, Capitalism, p. 49.

[76]Quoted in Roberts, "The Place of Plague," 103.

[77]Quoted in Kirchner, "The Black Death," 432.

[78]D. Herlihy, "Population, Plague and Social Change in Rural Pistoia, 1201-1430," The Economic History Review, Second Series, Vol. XVIII (1965), 232.

[79]Stefan Winkle, "Die Verseuchung der Mittelalterlichen Städte," Muenchener Medizinische Wochenschrift, Vol. 116 (1974), 2081.

[80]Neumeyer, Mazarkini and Potuzek, "Zur Geschichte," 273; and Alexander, "Catherine II," 659-661.

[81]Abraham, "The Early History of Syphilis," 225.

[82]Quoted in Major, A History of Medicine," Vol. I, p. 225.

[83]Jeanselme et. al., Histoire, p. 106.

[84]Hudson, "Villalobos," 582.

[85]Roberts, "Epidemics," 312.

[86]Quoted in Patrick, "A Consideration," 273.

[87]Quoted in Gerster, "What was," 334.

[88]Quoted in Razzell, "Population Change," 323.

[89]Dixson, Smallpox, pp. 199-200.

[90]Guy, "Two Hundred," p. 415.

[91]Quoted in Chevalier, Laboring Classes, p. 338.

[92]Longmate, King Cholera, p. 4.

[93]Shapter, The History, p. 121.

[94]McGrew, Russia and the Cholera, p. 7.

[95]Farr, Report, p. lxvii.

381

96Snow, <u>On the Mode</u>, p. 123.

97Chevalier, <u>Laboring Classes</u>, pp. 320-49.

98George Rosen, "An Eighteenth Century Plan for a National Health Service," <u>Bulletin of the History of Medicine</u>, Vol. XVI (1944), 431.

99Sprössig, "Die Erfurter," 171.

100<u>The First Medical Report</u>, p. 14.

101Bateman, <u>Reports</u>, p. 23.

102Kreuser, "Bedeutung," 73-80.

103<u>Congrès International de la Tuberculose Tenu à Paris 1905</u>, 3 vols. (Paris, 1905), Vol. 2, pp. 474-75.

104Philip, <u>Collected Papers</u>, pp. 66-67.

105Junker, "Tuberulinreihenuntersuchungen," 229.

106Cockburn, <u>The Evolution</u>, p. 84.

107Calmette, <u>Tubercle Bacillus</u>, p. 584.

108Quoted in Harry Bloch, "Rudolf Virchow, M.D. (1821-1902)," <u>New York State Journal of Medicine</u>, Vol. 74 (1974), p. 1472.

INDEX

STUDIES IN HEALTH AND HUMAN SERVICES